GET INTO MEDICAL SCHOOL

1300 UCAT PRACTICE QUESTIONS

Includes Full Mock Exam

Comprehensive tips, techniques & explanations

Olivier Picard, Laetitia Tighlit, Sami Tighlit, David Phillips

Published by ISC Medical
97 Judd Street, London WC1H 9JG
Tel: 0203 507 0001 – www.iscmedical.co.uk

Fourth Edition: September 2021.
ISBN: 978-1-905812-27-1 "1300 UCAT Practice Questions"

Third Edition: May 2017.
ISBN: 978-1-905812-26-4 "1250 UKCAT Practice Questions"

Second Edition: May 2016.
ISBN: 978-1-905812-18-9 "1000 UKCAT Practice Questions"

First Edition: June 2009.
ISBN 978-1-905812-09-7 "600 UKCAT Practice Questions"

A catalogue record for this book is available from the British Library.

© Interview Skills Consulting Limited 2009-2021. All rights reserved.

The moral right of Olivier Picard, Laetitia Tighlit, Sami Tighlit and David Phillips to be identified as the authors of this work has been asserted in accordance with Sections 77 and 78 of the Copyright, Designs and Patents Act 1988.

No part of this publication may be reproduced, stored in a retrieval system, or transmitted in any form or by any means, electronic, mechanical, photo-copying, recording or otherwise, without prior permission of the publishers.

The information within this text is intended as a revision aid for the purpose of the UCAT only. Any information contained within the texts used in the verbal reasoning section should not be regarded as views held by the authors of this book, but simply as text used in a question-setting context with the view of preparing students for a competitive test.

Note: The information contained within this book is accurate as of August 2021. Any changes made after that to the exam may not be reflected in this edition.

Printed in the United Kingdom by:
Optichrome Ltd, 98-100 Maybury Road, Woking GU21 5HX

INTRODUCTION

The UCAT (University Clinical Aptitude Test) is designed to assess a spectrum of skills in candidates to medical and dental schools, ranging from their ability to manipulate data and numbers, to their ability to draw meaningful conclusions from somewhat incomplete or confusing data.

The difficulty in such tests does not rest so much in the actual difficulty of each question independently (ultimately, if given proper time to do the test, everyone would get a fairly high score) but in the fact that candidates only have a few seconds to get it right. It is that added pressure which makes many candidates stress on the day.

As a result, although there is no need to revise any specific material to answer any of the questions, those who have had a maximum amount of practice will fare much better than the others. Not only will they know what to expect from each type of question and will therefore spend less time on the day of the test to get used to the format of the test, they will also have familiarised themselves with all the potential traps that can be laid by the examiners. In addition, by practising intensely, candidates will have learnt valuable techniques that will save them a considerable amount of time on the day.

With over 1300 questions spanning over 800 pages, this book contains an overwhelming range of exercises that will enable all UCAT candidates to refine and optimise their technique to answer questions under strict time constraints.

This book replicates the breadth and depth of the different types of questions that can be asked in the live UCAT. The spectrum of difficulties that it covers (from normal to stretching) makes it an ideal preparation tool for all those who want to achieve a high score and maximise their chances of getting into the medical school of their choice.

Good luck with your preparation!

Olivier, Laetitia, Sami and David

CONTENTS TABLE

Section	Description	Page
INTRODUCTION TO THE UCAT		**5**
1	Background	6
2	How the UCAT is marked	9
QUANTITATIVE REASONING		**11**
3	Format, Purpose & Key Techniques	12
4	Practice Questions	19
5	Answers to Practice Questions	79
ABSTRACT REASONING		**119**
6	Format, Purpose & Key Techniques	120
7	Practice Questions	135
8	Answers to Practice Questions	210
VERBAL REASONING		**267**
9	Format, Purpose & Key Techniques	268
10	Practice Questions	275
11	Answers to Practice Questions	344
DECISION MAKING		**401**
12	Format, Purpose & Key Techniques	402
13	Practice Questions	407
14	Answers to Practice Questions	461
SITUATIONAL JUDGEMENT		**513**
15	Format, Purpose & Key Techniques	514
16	Practice Questions	521
17	Answers to Practice Questions	576
MOCK EXAM		**625**
	Mock Exam Instructions	626
	Quantitative Reasoning	627
	Abstract Reasoning	643
	Verbal Reasoning	657
	Decision Making	681
	Situational Judgement	701
	Mock Exam Answers	725
	Mock Exam Marking Schedules	791

INTRODUCTION TO THE UCAT

1 Background

INTRODUCTION

The UCAT was set up by a group of medical schools with the view of assisting in the selection of candidates for entry into medical and dental school by testing a range of abilities relevant in the context of their degrees and their subsequent professional life.

The testing is computerised and takes place under controlled conditions in each of the 150 testing centres every year, typically between early July and early October. Full details on how the exam is run and the universities to which the test applies can be found each year on the official UCAT website at www.ucat.ac.uk.

THE TEST

The test comprises five distinct sections, which are taken one after the other at the exam, and are timed separately. The five sections are as follows:

1 – Quantitative reasoning
This section tests the candidates' ability to manipulate data and interpret charts, tables and other numerical information in order to resolve problems. This quantitative reasoning section contains 36 numerical questions, which must be answered in a total of 24 minutes (plus one minute to read the instructions). For explanations, techniques and quantitative reasoning practice exercises, go to page 11.

2 – Abstract reasoning
The abstract reasoning section of the test assesses the candidates' ability to analyse information in an environment where there are distracting features, to derive and test hypotheses, and to query their judgement when needed. This is achieved by asking candidates to identify relationships between various abstract shapes. This section contains 55 questions, which much be answered in 13 minutes (plus one minute to read the instructions). For explanations, techniques and abstract reasoning practice exercises, go to page 119.

3 – Verbal reasoning

This section tests the candidates' ability to analyse an important amount of text in order to determine whether specific conclusions can be drawn from the information presented. The test includes 11 pieces of text, each of approximately 200 to 300 words. Each piece of text attracts 4 questions. All 44 resulting questions must be answered in 21 minutes (plus one minute to read the instructions). For explanations, techniques and verbal reasoning practice exercises, go to page 267.

4 – Decision making

This section tests the candidates' ability to solve problems, manage risk and deal with uncertainty. It consists of 29 questions (some of which contain several sub-questions) associated with texts, charts, tables, graphs and diagrams, which must be answered in 31 minutes (plus one minute to read the instructions). For explanations, techniques and decision making exercises, go to page 401.

5 – Situational judgement

This section assesses the candidates' ability to understand real world situations and to identify critical factors and appropriate behaviour in dealing with them. It consists of 69 questions relating to 22 different scenarios, which must be answered in 26 minutes (plus one minute to read the instructions). For explanations, techniques and situational judgement exercises, go to page 513.

USE OF CALCULATOR AND WHITEBOARD

Calculators are given on the day of the exam. You cannot use your own. The calculators given are simple calculators i.e. they contain no scientific functions and are available on screen only.

You are not allowed any paper to write calculations or information down; however you will normally be given a whiteboard and marker pens. Before the exam starts, check that all the marker pens you were given are in good working order. Check also whether the whiteboard can be erased. In some centres, you are deliberately given whiteboards which can't be erased and you are required to ask for a new one whenever one has been filled. If that is the case, ensure you know the local procedure to obtain a new whiteboard whenever you need one.

LEVEL OF DIFFICULTY OF UCAT QUESTIONS

Questions are drawn at random from a large database of questions and every candidate is therefore likely to be asked different questions (this reduces the possibility of cheating if the test is to be taken over a period of 3 months). Although the examiners are trying to ensure that the questions are carefully calibrated so that, on balance, the test remains fair, we know from experience that the level of difficulty of the questions asked can vary from candidate to candidate, particularly in the quantitative reasoning section. In the quantitative reasoning section, some past candidates were given a majority of relatively quick questions whereas others were given a majority of questions which required more thinking time and more calculations. The average candidate will be given a fair mix of both, but you should expect some variations.

SUMMARY TABLE

Test	Number of questions	Time for questions	Time for instructions	Total time
Quantitative Reasoning	36	24 min	1 min	25 min
Abstract Reasoning	55	13 min	1 min	14 min
Verbal Reasoning	44	21 min	1 min	22 min
Decision Making	29	31 min	1 min	32 min
Situational Judgement	69	26 min	1 min	27 min
TOTAL		1h 55 min	5 min	2h 00min

2 How the UCAT is marked

MARKING OF THE UCAT

Each subtest of the UCAT except the Situational Judgement section, is allocated a score between 300 and 900. The score is not a simple allocation of points for each correct answer; instead, your number of correct answers for each section is compared to how well candidates have done in previous years and scores are then allocated in relation to the performance of those candidates using complex statistical tools.

It means that in order to get the maximum score of 900, you do not necessarily need to answer every single question correctly. You simply need to do as well as some of the best candidate in previous years.

The Situational Judgement is marked using a complex matrix-based system (see the situational judgement marking schedule at the back of the mock exam section for more detailed explanations). The score is then converted into a band (Band 1 being the top, Band 4 being the bottom).

Once every section of the test has been marked, the scores are communicated to each university with the full breakdown for each subtest. Each university then uses the results that it receives about each candidate in a way that it sees fit.

Here are some examples of the ways in which universities have used the UCAT results in the past:

- The test results are averaged across all sections to give an overall score out of 900. Only applicants with a score above a given cut-off mark are considered. A score of 600 out of 900 has often been used, though some universities have been known to use lower cut off marks, and few universities have been known to use higher cut off marks, as high as 700. Universities may use a different cut-off point each year depending on the number of applicants which they are prepared to call for interview.

- The results of the four sections are considered separately; candidates are expected to achieve a given cut-off mark in <u>each</u> of the sections.

- Candidates are ranked according to their average UCAT test results and only those in the top x % (typically top 20%, 25% or 50% depending on the university and the year) are invited to interview.

WHAT THIS MEANS FOR YOU

The issue of a likely cut-off point being adopted by many universities means two things:

- You must identify your weaker areas and practise questions for the tests which cause you the most trouble so that you maintain a high average score as well as a high individual score for each section.

- You must consider the issue of the mark that you are targeting in relation to the time that you know it takes you to do an exercise within each type of test. For example, if you know that you keep getting your sums wrong when you calculate too quickly, you might want to attempt only 80% of the exercises in the quantitative reasoning test, with the view of getting 90% of the answers to those questions right, instead of rushing through all the questions and ending up getting only 20% of the questions right.

PRACTISE, PRACTISE, PRACTISE

Ultimately, your goal should be to achieve the highest possible score. Worrying unnecessarily about any cut-off point which may or may not exist in such and such a university is a secondary matter when it comes to the actual day of the test. To help you achieve this, the practice questions and the mock exam contained in this book will help you understand the requirements for each of the four main tests and will help you build a range of skills and techniques which will ensure you save a considerable amount of time.

QUANTITATIVE REASONING

TIPS & TECHNIQUES

+

204
PRACTICE QUESTIONS & ANSWERS

3 Quantitative Reasoning
Format, Purpose & Key Techniques

FORMAT

The quantitative reasoning section of the UCAT consists of nine scenarios, each consisting of:

- Numerical data, usually provided in the form of graphs or tables, but sometimes as part of a piece of text, and

- Four questions requiring calculations and interpretations to be carried out. For each question, you are provided with five possible answers, from which you must choose the correct one.

To answer all 36 questions, you are allocated 25 minutes. This includes one minute for reading the generic instructions provided and 24 minutes to answer the 36 questions. It represents 40 seconds per question.

The level of familiarity with numbers is that of a good GCSE pass. A basic calculator is provided on-screen on the day of the exam.

PURPOSE

The quantitative reasoning section of the UCAT tests your numerical problem-solving abilities and your ability to extract and manipulate information in doing so. As with any other scientific discipline, medicine requires a large degree of data analysis. This is sometimes based on readily available information and at other times based on more tenuous information. Whether you are attempting to calculate the dose of a drug that needs to be administered to a patient in relation to their weight, age and other key factors; whether you are designing a new rota for your team to make sure that it is fully compliant with regulations; or whether you are trying to make sense of statistics quoted in a research paper that you are reading, medicine requires an ability to use information in order to solve problems and therefore requires a degree of mental agility too.

LEVEL OF DIFFICULTY

At the exam, the difficulty level of questions varies, with some questions requiring a simple calculation that will take you 3 seconds and others requiring either longer calculations (e.g. adding and multiplying several numbers in a row) or involving two or three different calculations to get to the answer. Some questions also present a timing challenge because they contain a lot of text. At the exam, you will get a bit of everything and, overall, it should all average out, but you must make sure that you do the shorter questions in less than 40 seconds so that you have more time to handle the questions involving longer texts or longer steps.

This book offers a wide range of difficulty of questions so that you can gain the maximum practice. We did not want to fill page after page with really easy questions that would take 3 seconds to answer and would give you a false sense of security (there would be no real value in that!). As such, although we have obviously included some easy questions, we also wanted to provide you with a real opportunity to improve your technique and your timing. So, on average, this section will contain fewer easy questions than the exam might. The mock exam (p.625), however, is in line with what you can expect on the day.

KEY TECHNIQUES

Find a strategy that works for you

The main difficulty of this section is that you only have on average 40 seconds to find the answer to each question. Given that some questions and scenarios can be lengthy to read through, in reality you will probably find that you only have 20 seconds left for each question once you have finished reading everything. Different candidates will handle this matter in different ways and, before making decisions on your own strategy, you may wish to consider the following points (looking at the individual questions rather than the scenarios):

- Although you obviously need to aim for the highest possible score, it would be foolish to try to answer every single question if it means getting most of them wrong simply because you wanted to go quickly. It may be better to attempt 80% of the questions properly and get them all right rather than mess up on 100% of the questions provided because you rushed your calculations.

- The test is not negatively marked (i.e. you don't get penalised explicitly for getting an answer wrong). So, never leave a question unanswered. If you have not managed to come to a sensible answer for a specific question, or if you have run out of time, make sure that you give an answer, even if you have to guess it. Even if you answered randomly you would expect to get it right by chance 20% of the time since you have to pick one option out of five. If you make an educated guess rather than a random guess, the probability of getting it right is even higher. So, if you had to make a guess on, say, 25% of the questions because you did not have time to answer them, you would gain on average an additional score of 5% (20% of 25%). This could well tip you over the threshold of 600–625 marks that many medical schools seem to regard as a good score.

- You will find that some questions are much easier than others and that these easier questions are littered throughout the test. One strategy is to go through the questions systematically but picking out the easier ones to ensure that they get done quickly. Once you have done the easier questions then go back to the more difficult questions and address them until you run out of time. This strategy ensures that you do not get held up for prolonged periods of time by some of the more difficult questions and you score as many of the easy points as possible. It does, however, have three drawbacks:

    i. It requires some practice to identify at a glance whether a question is likely to be an easy, quick question or whether it will take some time to answer. However, with practice, this should be easily resolved. The questions in this book will help you with this.
    ii. When you go back to a previous difficult question, you have to remind yourself of the context of the question once again.
    iii. Going back and forth on the computer system may waste time by itself.

- Another strategy is to go through the questions in order and to force yourself to move on to another question once you have overstepped the 40-second target allocated to each question: unless you can see that you are about to get to a result quickly thereafter, in which case you can allow yourself a few more seconds. This has the advantage of not allowing you to get bogged down with the questions that are taking a long time and will also enable you to have a go at most of the questions. However, it presents a serious risk of making you rush for the sake of going through all the questions and of placing quantity over quality.

- A better strategy is to monitor your time carefully and to give yourself some time markers that you can use to determine whether you are on track or not. For example, you should have done the first 5 scenarios in the first 10 minutes. If you are lagging, then you need to speed up a little. Try not to time each question individually. Not only will you become so obsessed with time that you will lose valuable seconds looking at the clock, but you would be ignoring the fact that some scenarios are easier than others and therefore that it is the average of 2.5 minutes per scenario which counts rather than the timing on each individual scenario.

- If you are getting bogged down with one question and feel that you are not likely to find the answer easily despite your efforts, cut your losses and move on. You may have wasted valuable time, but you don't want to waste more through stubbornness if it means losing marks because you did not have time to do other questions. Simply take a guess and move on. You can always go back to it later.

- The strategy you should ultimately adopt will depend on your way of working, your attitude to risk and whether you get stressed or remain composed when facing pressure. Many candidates adopt a halfway strategy whereby they go systematically through every question, give it a shot for, say, 20 seconds and then decide whether it is worth investing more time in it or just taking a guess and moving on. If they have time at the end, they then go back to the answers they guessed and refine their answers as necessary.

Don't study the data in-depth immediately. Scan it intelligently
In some scenarios, the amount of data given could be such that it would take you 2 minutes just to read it all and understand it. In such cases, it will therefore be difficult to assimilate everything and answer the questions in 2 minutes. Rather than read and assimilate the full amount of data given, you may wish to scan through it quickly to understand the "type" of information that you are given. Then, when you read the question, you will be able to determine quickly what sort of data you need to answer it; having glanced at the data before, you will know exactly where to find it when you need it.

Use order of magnitudes whenever possible
Some questions give the choice between answers in a wide range. In some cases, you can derive the answer simply by looking at the data and the orders of magnitude of the different answers. For example, consider the following table:

Data set	143	176	129	172

If you were being asked the question "What is the average of the above numbers", with possible answers being 70, 100, 135, 155 and 170, you could answer quickly that the answer has to be 155 since 70 and 100 are lower than the smallest number in the list, 135 is very close to 129 and has to be too low, and 170 is almost equal to the highest number in the list.

This question could therefore be answered simply by glancing at the data and exercising judgement, without the need for any calculation. In many questions you will obviously be required to carry out some calculations but very often you can simplify your task drastically and save yourself a lot of time by identifying suitable shortcuts and narrowing down the scope of the calculations that you need to perform.

This technique will not work when the options are too close together so you will need to learn to recognise when such an approach is possible. Some of the exercises in this book will give you an opportunity to do this and we have provided full explanations in the answers.

When appropriate, start from the options given
In some questions, you may need to write an equation, which, although it looks simple, may take a few seconds too many to resolve. Rather than trying to find the answer by resolving the equation from a pure mathematical perspective, which could take some time, simply try the options given and see which one fits. If you have managed to rule out some of the options through pure logical deduction, then hopefully you will only have to try a few of the options on display.

Save valuable time by converting as few numbers as you can
Some questions provide numbers in one unit and ask for the result in another unit. For example, you may be given the lengths of two sides of a rectangle in metres and be asked to calculate the surface area in square

Quantitative Reasoning – Practice

feet. Rather than converting both lengths into square feet and then multiplying one by the other, it is quicker to calculate the area in square metres and then to convert that number into square feet.

Make full use of the whiteboard, if provided
Some questions may require a simple equation to be set and resolved. Although it will always be a simple one, solving it in your head will often result in a plus or minus sign being misplaced or inverted. In previous years, candidates have had access to a computerised whiteboard in the exam. For the more complex calculations, use it to keep track of your reasoning on the board so that you can easily spot any error you may have made.

Convert numbers the right way round
Candidates in a hurry often get their conversion rates the wrong way round. If the text states that the conversion rate is £1.5 = $2.1 then $100 will be equivalent to 100 / 2.1 x 1.5 = £71.43. This result will obviously appear in the list of options, but so will £140 (which is calculated as 100 x 2.1 / 1.5). It is therefore imperative that you check the units in which the data is expressed, that you check the unit in which the result is required and that you apply conversion rates the right way round.

Round numbers as specified or implied by the question
Some questions will ask you to calculate numbers that one would expect to be integers but which, in a calculation, may come out as decimal.

For example, if you are given a recipe that requires 1.5 kg of meat and you are told that the meat can only be purchased in packs of 600 g, you would need to buy 3 packs to make the dish, and not 1.5 / 0.6 = 2.5. It may well be that 2.5 and 3 are both options offered to you.

Read the text carefully to determine which one would fit best (e.g. if it asks for the average number of packs required to make the recipe, the answer would be 2.5. If it asks how many packs one particular customer should buy, it would be 3).

Follow the question through
It may sound obvious but reading a question too quickly may cause you to miss valuable terms, which will then lead you to calculate the wrong answer.

For example, you may have a scenario about two friends who are travelling using different routes. A question may ask "How many more days than Paul will Peter take to complete the journey?" This will mean computing the two different travelling times and then the difference between the two. In many cases, a rushed candidate may calculate both and forget to subtract one from the other. The two individual journey times are likely to feature in the options; the candidate will find an answer that matches his findings but which does not actually answer the full question posed.

Make sure you read the question carefully since, in most cases, the options will have anticipated your mistake.

Get the percentage increase/decrease the right way round
In some questions, you may be asked for the percentage increase or decrease from one year to the next. Remember that the percentage is calculated in relation to the starting point. For example, if sales in 2007 were £800 and sales in 2008 were £1,000 then the percentage increase between 2007 and 2008 was 25% (i.e. 200/800) and not 20% (i.e. 200/1000). Again, you can be sure that both 20% and 25% will feature in the options provided. In a rush, such a mistake is easy to make.

Practise, practise, practise
Although the level of mathematics that you require to solve each question is relatively simple, the main difficulty lies in the timing. Many of the questions are of a similar nature and, although you don't need to acquire or revise any specific knowledge for the quantitative reasoning test, it is important that you familiarise yourself with the various formats in which the information can be presented, and the various difficulties that you can encounter in your reasoning.

4 Quantitative Reasoning Practice Questions

In this section you will find 204 practice questions (36 scenarios, each containing between 4 and 10 practice questions). This is equivalent to nearly six full exams.

The questions have been carefully chosen to represent the different numerical reasoning approaches and levels of difficulty that you may encounter in the live exam. We have deliberately provided more questions per scenario than you would have at the exam to enhance your learning experience. At the end of the section we have also set out detailed explanations on how the answers can be derived. When relevant, we have provided several possible ways of getting to the answer.

Depending on your way of learning and working, you may decide to answer the questions in real time (in which case you would need to allocate an average of 36 seconds per question, i.e. a scenario with 7 questions should be done in just over 4 minutes) or to approach the questions at your own pace in order to build your awareness of the difficulties that you may encounter. The answers to all questions can be found from page 79 onwards.

Once you have practised answering all 204 questions, you should be ready to confront the mock exam at the back of the book and replicate the actual exam's format. You may want to wait until you have practised all sections in this book before going ahead with the mock exam.

QR 1 Practice — White Goods

An online store offers the following products for sale. Each product comes with various options, as follows:

Product	Price	Delivery	Installation
Washing machine	£349	£30	Not known
Washer dryer	£452	£25	£15
Dishwasher	£353	£35	£23
Fridge	£412	£23	Free
Freezer	£383	£25	Free
Fridge-freezer	£586	£38	Free

Prices for delivery are for weekday delivery only. Deliveries on a Saturday incur a surcharge of £15 for each item purchased.

Customers who order two items will need to pay the delivery charge for each item as if the items had been ordered separately.

PRACTICE QUESTIONS

Q1.1 What would be the cost of getting a dishwasher delivered and installed on a Monday?

a. £353   b. £376   c. £388   d. £411   e. £426

Q1.2 What would be the cost of getting a fridge delivered and installed on a Saturday?

a. £412   b. £435   c. £450   d. £475   e. £495

Q1.3 Tessa wants to buy a fridge-freezer instead of a fridge and a separate freezer. She can only take deliveries on Saturdays. How much would she save by buying a combined fridge-freezer compared to buying two separate appliances?

a. £209   b. £219   c. £224   d. £234   e. £249

Quantitative Reasoning – Practice

Q1.4 The installation price for the washing machine is missing from the website. However, a client would pay a total of £416 for delivery and installation of a washing machine on a Saturday. What is the installation cost?

a. Free   b. £15   c. £22   d. £23   e. £37

Q1.5 Julia has a voucher that gives her a 30% discount. The discount applies only to the price of the item, not on the delivery or installation charge, which she must pay in full. How much would she pay if she wanted the dishwasher, delivered and installed on a Tuesday?

a. £123.30   b. £163.60   c. £178.60   d. £305.10   e. £320.10

Q1.6 John has a voucher that gives him a 20% discount on any appliance sold on that online store. The discount applies only to the price of the item, not on the delivery or installation charge, which he must pay in full. He selects a product and opts for delivery and installation on a Thursday. The total invoice after discount is £401.60. Which product did he buy?

a. Washer dryer   b. Dishwasher   c. Fridge
d. Freezer   e. Fridge-freezer

Q1.7 The owners of the online shop are thinking of changing their policy for the delivery charge such that the delivery charge will be a flat fee for all products. They would like that the delivery charge does not exceed 10% of the purchase price of the item. What is the maximum delivery charge they can impose for all items?

a. £34.90   b. £35.30   c. £41.20   d. £45.20   e. £58.60

Q1.8 The owners are thinking of selling extended-warranty products for each appliance. The cost of such a warranty is £4 per month, for a maximum of 5 years. No warranty is offered after 5 years. If a customer decided to take out the 5-year warranty on a fridge, how much more expensive would this work out over the full 5-year period, assuming the fridge was delivered on a Tuesday and did not develop any fault over that period?

a. 11.1%   b. 11.7%   c. 33.2%   d. 55.2%   e. 58.2%

1300 UCAT Practice Questions

QR 2 Practice — Field Areas

Consider the following rectangular field (dimensions in metres (m)):

```
Length: 1,000 m
Width: 500 m
```

PRACTICE QUESTIONS

Q2.1 An architect has found a map on which the field is being shown with a width of 25 cm on paper. What scale was used?

a. 1:2000   b. 1:4000   c. 1:5000   d. 1:10000   e. 1:50000

Q2.2 If we extend the length of the field by 150 m and the width remains the same, by what percentage does the field's perimeter increase?

a. 2%   b. 10%   c. 15%   d. 30%   e. 45%

Q2.3 If we wanted a field with the same perimeter but in a square shape, how would the surface area of the square compare to that of the rectangle?

a. Greater   b. Equal   c. Lower   d. Requires further info

Q2.4 A lawnmower is used to mow the grass on the field. The lawnmower can mow strips that are 50 cm wide. What is the minimum distance the lawnmower will need to travel in order to cover the area of the whole field, assuming there is no overlap?

a. 1 km   b. 10 km   c. 100 km   d. 500 km   e. 1,000 km

Q2.5 If we wanted to draw the field on paper using a scale of 1:10000, what would the surface area of the drawn rectangle be?

a. 0.5 cm²   b. 5 cm²   c. 50 cm²   d. 500 cm²   e. 5000 cm²

QR 3 Practice: Actual v. Reading Age

The following scatter chart shows the actual age and reading age of 26 pupils in a school. Each dot represents a specific child.

PRACTICE QUESTIONS

Q3.1 What proportion of the children have a reading age equal to or greater than their actual age?

a. 5.5%   b. 11.5%   c. 21.5%   d. 41.5%   e. 61.5%

Q3.2 How many years behind is the worst performing pupil?

a. 1.5   b. 2.0   c. 2.75   d. 3.0   e. 3.5

Q3.3 What is the average age of the pupils with a reading age of 6?

a. 5   b. 5.375   c. 5.583   d. 5.75   e. 6

Q3.4 The four children currently showing an actual age of 6 increase their reading age by 0.75 years in the following year. How many of those four children are underperforming at age 7?

a. 0   b. 1   c. 2   d. 3   e. 4

QR 4 Practice — Stamp Duty

In England, Stamp Duty (tax) is payable to the government by the buyer of a flat or house. A different rate applies to different parts of the purchase price, as follows:

Value	Tax rate
Up to £125,000	0%
The next £125,000 (the portion from £125,000 to £250,000)	2%
The next £675,000 (the portion from £250,000 to £925,000)	5%
The next £575,000 (the portion from £925,000 to £1.5 million)	10%
The remaining amount (the portion above £1.5 million)	12%

For example, the buyer of a £200,000 house will pay stamp duty calculated as: 0 + 2% x (200,000 − 125,000) = £1,500. A similar calculation applied to a purchase price of £1.5m would give a stamp duty of £93,750.

PRACTICE QUESTIONS

Q4.1 How much stamp duty would someone purchasing a property for £1 million have to pay?

a. £2,500   b. £7,500   c. £33,750   d. £43,750   e. £100,000

Q4.2 John bought a house worth over £1.5m. In total he paid £100,000 of stamp duty. How much did he pay approximately for the house?

a. £1.500m   b. £1.512m   c. £1.525m   d. £1.552m   e. £1.600m

Q4.3 The government would like to introduce a 15% tax rate for the portion of the price over £2 million. How much more stamp duty would be payable on a £3 million mansion as a result?

a. £10,000   b. £30,000   c. £50,000   d. £70,000   e. £90,000

Q4.4 Denise has saved up a total of £250,000 and refuses to borrow any money to buy a property. She will therefore need to pay the purchase price of the property and the stamp duty out of that budget. What maximum price can she afford for the property?

a. £242,135   b. £245,000   c. £245,098   d. £247,500   e. £247,549

QR 5 Practice — Restaurant Pricing

A restaurant owner calculates the amounts he should charge his customers for each dish or bottle (the "menu price") with the following formulae:

Menu Price for food
= 3 x cost of the ingredients for the dish excluding VAT x (1+ VAT rate)

Menu Price for a bottle of wine
= 4 x purchase price of the bottle excluding VAT x (1 + VAT rate)

where VAT is calculated at a rate of 20%.

In addition, a 12% service charge is payable on the whole bill for groups of 6 or above only. Groups of 5 or fewer pay no service charge.

PRACTICE QUESTIONS

Q5.1 A couple visit the restaurant and decide to drink tap water only, which comes for free. The meal costs them a total of £158. How much did the ingredients cost for that meal (excluding VAT)?

a. £41.16   b. £42.13   c. £43.89   d. £44.37   e. £52.67

Q5.2 The restaurant has bought ingredients for a price excluding VAT of £50. If they used all the ingredients, what price would a party of 6 people pay for the meal in total, excluding any drinks?

a. £150   b. £165   c. £168   d. £180   e. £201.60

Q5.3 A couple incurs a total bill of £172, which includes £48 for a bottle of wine. How much is the average cost of ingredients per person (excluding VAT)?

a. £16.53   b. £17.22   c. £20.64   d. £34.44   e. £41.28

Q5.4 A lone customer has a total bill in which the drinks represent 60% of the total price. The restaurant spent £32 excluding VAT on ingredients. What was the total bill?

a. £115.20   b. £160   c. £192   d. £240   e. £288

QR 6 Practice — Distances & Journey Times

Here is a table showing distances in kilometres (km) between some European cities.

	Amsterdam	Barcelona	Brussels	Geneva	Madrid	Paris	Rome
Amsterdam		1530	200	990	1770	-------	1740
Barcelona	1530		1340	810	620	1030	1470
Brussels	200	1340		680	1570	300	1530
Geneva	990	810	680		1360	500	930
Madrid	1770	620	1570	1360		1260	2020
Paris	-------	1030	300	500	1260		1430
Rome	1740	1470	1530	930	2020	1430	

PRACTICE QUESTIONS

Q6.1 Tom needs to drive from Paris to Madrid. He expects to drive at an average speed of 90 km/hour. How long will his journey take?

   a. 8h40min   b. 10h30min   c. 12h10min   d. 13h00min   e. 14h00min

Q6.2 Paul wants to go from Geneva to Amsterdam. He drives at an average speed of 110 km/hour. Every time he has driven two hours, he takes a break of 20 minutes. How long will his journey last?

   a. 9h00min   b. 9h20min   c. 9h40min   d. 10h20min   e. 10h40min

Q6.3 Tracy wants to go from Rome to Brussels. How much further would it be to travel via Geneva compared to travelling direct?

   a. 4.97%   b. 5.07%   c. 5.23%   d. 6.07%   e. 7.23%

Q6.4 Suzie travelled from Geneva to Brussels. Her car uses 9 litres (L) of petrol per 100 km. If petrol costs £1.30/L and the toll fees amount to £30 for the journey, what was the cost of the journey?

   a. £41.70   b. £61.20   c. £79.56   d. £91.20   e. £109.56

Q6.5 Peter travelled from Paris to Amsterdam. He drove at an average speed of 100 km/h for the first 2h36min and then at an average speed of 90 km/h for the remaining 2h40min. What is the distance between Paris and Amsterdam?

   a. 452 km   b. 500 km   c. 512 km   d. 552 km   e. 570 km

Q6.6 David travels from Madrid to Barcelona. He drives the first 430 km in 2h40min. The rest of the distance takes him 5 hours because of roadworks. What was his average speed over the whole journey?

   a. 38 km/h   b. 57 km/h   c. 81 km/h   d. 90 km/h   e. 92 km/h

Q6.7 Rob travels from Barcelona to Brussels via another town "X". The total length of his journey is 1490 km. What town is "X"?

   a. Amsterdam   b. Geneva   c. Madrid   d. Paris   e. Rome

Q6.8 John travelled from Paris to Brussels. He drove the first half of the journey in 1h30min, stopped for a break and then drove the second half of the journey at a speed of 50 km/h. In total his journey lasted 5 hours. How long did he stop for?

   a. 15 min   b. 20 min   c. 30 min   d. 45 min   e. 50 min

Q6.9 Julia drives at an average speed of 60 miles/hour between Rome and Madrid. How long will it take her to cover the distance (to the nearest 10 minutes)? (Use 1 mile = 1.6 km.)

   a. 21h00min b. 21h10min c. 27h20min d. 27h40min e. 33h40min

Q6.10 An Englishman mistakenly thinks that the distances shown in the table are expressed in miles instead of kilometres. He thinks that the journey from Brussels to Geneva should take him 10 hours. How much shorter or longer will his actual journey be? Assume 1 mile = 1.6 km.

   a. 3h45 min shorter
   b. 1h20 min shorter
   c. 0h45 min shorter
   d. 1h20 min longer
   e. 3h45 min longer

QR 7 Practice: Sightseeing

The optician "For Your Eyes Only" offers the following prices:

Type of glasses	Classic frame	Lenses (Cost per lens)	Anti-reflection treatment (Cost per lens)
Single vision	£26	£15	£20
Bifocal	£34	£30	£25
Varifocal	£36	£38	£30

PRACTICE QUESTIONS

Q7.1 A client requires bifocal glasses with anti-reflection treatment. He chooses a designer frame, which is 20% more expensive than a classic frame. How much will his glasses cost?

 a. £95.80   b. £106.80   c. £125.80   d. £150.80   e. £172.80

Q7.2 The shop offers a 25% discount on the whole order to clients over the age of 60. How much would a 65-year-old client pay for varifocal glasses with a classic frame but no anti-reflection treatment?

 a. £55.50   b. £74.00   c. £84.00   d. £89.60   e. £112.00

Q7.3 A client is considering buying a classic frame with lenses and anti-reflection treatment. What is the ratio of the total cost of single vision glasses over the total cost of bifocal glasses?

 a. 1:3   b. 1:2   c. 61:89   d. 49:72   e. 2:3

Q7.4 Another optician "The Apple Of My Eye" sells classic frames with varifocal lenses and anti-reflection treatment for £159.96. What discount would the optician "For Your Eyes Only" need to apply in order to match that price?

 a. 7%   b. 7.53%   c. 8%   d. 8.6%   e. 9%

QR 8 Practice — Amateur Science

An amateur scientist buys a basic science kit, which contains a tank with the following dimensions: Length: 40 cm, Width: 20 cm, Height: 30 cm.

You are given: 1 litre (L) = 1 dm^3, where 1 dm = 10 cm.

PRACTICE QUESTIONS

Q8.1 What is the volume of the tank?

    a. 8 L   **b.** 24 L   **c.** 80 L   **d.** 120 L   **e.** 240 L

Q8.2 The amateur scientist makes 12,000 cm^3 of a salt solution of concentration 9 g/L. How much salt has he added?

    a. 90 g   **b.** 100 g   **c.** 108 g   **d.** 200 g   **e.** 208 g

Q8.3 The amateur scientist pours 4 L of water in the tank and places the tank in the freezer. The following morning, the ice within the tank has a height of 5.4 cm. By what percentage has the volume of water increased during the freezing process?

    a. 4%   **b.** 5.8%   **c.** 7.2%   **d.** 8%   **e.** 10%

Q8.4 The amateur scientist pours salted water in the tank so that the height of the water level is 15 cm. He then lets the water evaporate in order to recover the salt contained within it. If 1 L of water is expected to produce 30 g of salt, how much salt can he expect to recover?

    a. 300 g   **b.** 360 g   **c.** 400 g   **d.** 600 g   **e.** 625 g

Q8.5 In his tank, the amateur scientist pours 4,800 cm^3 of pure water, which has a concentration in oxygen of 89%. He also adds 3 fish. What is the average quantity of oxygen per fish?

    a. 0.1424 L   **b.** 1.424 L   **c.** 14.24 L   **d.** 142.4 L   **e.** 1,424 L

QR 9 Practice: Eye In The Sky

A number of Ferris wheels were built or considered around the world, consisting of capsules arranged in a circular pattern and rotating at slow speed to enable the passengers of each capsule to have aerial views of the city. The number of capsules varies from one wheel to another depending on its circumference. All capsules are spread evenly along the outside circle.

City	Height
Beijing	208.0 m
Singapore	165.0 m
London	135.0 m
Osaka	112.5 m
Paris	60.0 m

You are given the following:
Circumference: $= 2 \times \pi \times R$
$= \pi \times D$

where D is the diameter of the wheel and R is the radius of the wheel.
Use $\pi = 3.14$

PRACTICE QUESTIONS

Q9.1 What is the average circumference of the five wheels, to the nearest metre?

a. 136 m   b. 254 m   c. 272 m   d. 427 m   e. 855 m

Q9.2 A country plans to build a new wheel that is 12% taller than the Beijing Great Wheel. What will be the radius of the new wheel?

a. 24.96 m   b. 116.48 m   c. 184.72 m   d. 232.96 m   e. 249.60 m

Q9.3 The London Eye has 32 capsules. What is the distance between the centres of two consecutive capsules along the circumference?

a. 13.25 m   b. 24.36 m   c. 26.30 m   d. 30.54 m   e. 48.72 m

Q9.4 The Singapore Flyer makes one full rotation in 30 minutes. What is the average speed of one of the capsules along its path (in cm/s)?

a. 17 cm/s   b. 23 cm/s   c. 29 cm/s   d. 32 cm/s   e. 41 cm/s

Q9.5 The London Eye has 32 capsules and executes a full rotation in 30 minutes. It is open 24 hours a day for 350 days of the year, during which time it takes on 5 million tourists. How many tourists will a capsule contain on average per rotation?

a. 4.7   b. 5.3   c. 7.3   d. 9.3   e. 18.6

Q9.6 In the end, the Beijing wheel was never built. Had it been built, it would have had one capsule every 13.607 metres along its circumference. How many capsules would it have had?

a. 24   b. 30   c. 36   d. 42   e. 48

Q9.7 Berlin would like to build a wheel twice as tall as the Singapore Flyer, keeping the same distance between each pod. Which of the following sentences is definitely true?

a. The Berlin wheel will have 1.5 more pods than the Singapore Flyer.

b. If the two wheels rotate at the same speed, they will do a full rotation in the same amount of time.

c. The Berlin wheel will have twice as many capsules as the Singapore Flyer.

d. The perimeter of the Berlin wheel will be 6 times the diameter of the Singapore Flyer.

e. For the two wheels to execute a full rotation in the same amount of time, the speed of the Berlin wheel will need to be half the speed of the Singapore Flyer.

QR 10 Practice: Going Swimmingly

A medical school society organises a sponsored swim. Five students decide to take part and it is agreed that the money raised will be given to two charities: the Red Triangle and the Blue Moon in the ratio 2:1.

The following table summarises the number of lengths each student has swum and the amount of money they have raised.

Student	Number of lengths	Amount of money raised (£)
A	10	19.00
B	8	20.10
C	9	23.80
D	10	26.00
E	9	22.10

PRACTICE QUESTIONS

Q10.1 How much money has been given to the Red Triangle Charity?

a. £18.50   b. £37.00   c. £55.50   d. £74.00   e. £111.00

Q10.2 Which student has raised the most money per length?

a. A   b. B   c. C   d. D   e. E

Q10.3 A new student, F, only has enough stamina to swim 6 lengths. How much money will he need to raise in order to earn as much per length as Student D?

a. £2.60   b. £12.20   c. £15.60   d. £21.30   e. £26.00

Q10.4 The Blue Moon would like that the proceeds of the charity swim be distributed equally between each charity. If that were the case, how much extra cash would it receive?

a. £10.00   b. £18.50   c. £20.00   d. £25.50   e. £37.00

Quantitative Reasoning – Practice

QR 11 Practice — Insurance Claims

An insurance company has recorded the number of claims it experienced in five consecutive years as follows:

Year	Total number of claims	Change from previous year	Number of approved claims	Number of rejected claims
2010	1920	20% up	1217	703
2011	2039	6.2% up	1435	?
2012	1733	15% down	1211	?
2013	1633	5.8% down	915	?
2014	1933	18.4% up	1532	?
2015	2012	4.1% up	1263	749

A claim can only have one of two statuses: Approved or Rejected.

PRACTICE QUESTIONS

Q11.1 How many more claims did the company receive in 2015 compared to the year 2009?

    a. 82   b. 92   c. 232   d. 412   e. 476

Q11.2 By what percentage did the number of rejected claims increase between 2012 and 2013?

    a. 5.8%   b. 12.4%   c. 22.3%   d. 28.5%   e. 37.5%

Q11.3 Which year saw the lowest percentage of rejected claims?

    a. 2011   b. 2012   c. 2013   d. 2014   e. 2015

Q11.4 The insurance company estimates that the total number of claims it will receive in 2030 will be double the total number of claims it received in 2015. In 2030, it aims to approve the same percentage of claims as it approved in 2013. How many claims does it expect to reject in 2030?

    a. 885   b. 1127   c. 1524   d. 1769   e. 2255

QR 12 Practice: New Employees

A charity recruited 300 new employees in 2015. The following graphs record their education profile as well as the type of responsibility they were allocated.

Education profile
Stage at which candidate left education

- BSc 33%
- GCSE 30%
- A Level 37%

Responsibilities allocated

- Admin 4%
- Engineering 19%
- Sanitation 27%
- Education 17%
- Construction 33%

PRACTICE QUESTIONS

Q12.1 How many employees were recruited into sanitation in 2015?

    a. 11   b. 27   c. 31   d. 81   e. 90

Q12.2 How many more employees were allocated to sanitation than to engineering?

    a. 12   b. 24   c. 36   d. 57   e. 81

Q12.3 Two-thirds of those allocated to construction left education with a BSc. How many of them left school either at GCSE or A Level?

    a. 11   b. 22   c. 33   d. 44   e. 66

Q12.4 In 2016, the charity recruited exactly the same number of employees into each area as in 2015, except in admin where the number allocated in 2016 was 3 times higher than in 2015. What proportion of the total number of recruits was allocated to education in 2016?

    a. 15.2%   b. 15.7%   c. 16.2%   d. 16.7%   e. 17.0%

Q12.5 Following a review, the charity decided to recruit another 20 employees in 2015, to all be allocated to admin responsibilities. By what percentage has the number of admin recruits been increased for that year?

    a. 0.67%   b. 6.7%   c. 67%   d. 167%   e. 267%

Q12.6 What proportion of the sanitation recruits have a BSc?

    a. 11%   b. 22%   c. 33%   d. 100%   e. Can't tell

Q12.7 What is the minimum number of recruits who work in construction and have either A Levels or a BSc?

    a. 9   b. 10   c. 20   d. 30   e. Can't tell

Q12.8 It turns out that all recruits allocated to engineering have a BSc. What proportion of the non-engineering recruits have a BSc?

    a. 9%   b. 12.7%   c. 17.3%   d. 26.7%   e. 33%

QR 13 Practice — Riding Lessons

A horse-riding school charges an annual fee per person, on top of which tickets can be purchased to ride. Tickets are sold by the unit, by packs of 5 and packs of 10. One ticket gives the right to one ride. You should assume that users of the school will always choose the purchase method that is the cheapest for them and that they use all the tickets they purchase in the same year as they are purchased.

Horse type	Age of the rider	Annual fees	1 ticket	5 tickets	10 tickets
Shetland	3–6	£64	£15	£65	£120
Pony	7–17	£86	£25	£78	£150
Horse	Adult 18+	£110	£32	£90	£170

Q13.1 Kathy, 10 years old, bought 45 tickets this year. How much did she spend in total at the school for the year?

a. £86.00   b. £723.00   c. £764.00   d. £788.00   e. £1,211.00

Q13.2 Anna's total cost for one year was £710. She is 30 years old. How many lessons did she take?

a. 31   b. 32   c. 33   d. 34   e. 35

Q13.3 What discount is the riding school giving on Shetland lessons for those who purchase a block of 5 tickets instead of 5 individual tickets?

a. 13.3%   b. 15.4%   c. 18.3%   d. 19.6%   e. 37.6%

Q13.4 The parents of two children aged 9 and 5 respectively have a budget of £960. They wish to offer the two children the same number of lessons each, opting to purchase 10-ticket packs only. How many lessons will they purchase for each child?

a. 3   b. 10   c. 20   d. 30   e. 60

QR 14 Practice — Gravity

The weight P of a body is defined in Newton (N) by the formula P = m × g, where m is the mass (in kg) and g is the gravitational acceleration (in m/s^2).

The gravitational acceleration g differs depending on which planet the object is. It is given as follows:

On Pluto	On Jupiter	On the Moon	On Mars	On Earth
0.62	1.4	1.6	3.7	9.8

Q14.1 What is the weight of an object with a mass of 70 kg on Earth?

    a. 112 N   b. 259 N   c. 686 N   d. 712 N   e. 734 N

Q14.2 Given that the mass is constant, by what percentage does the weight of an object increase if transported from the Moon to Mars?

    a. 31%   b. 43%   c. 143%   d. 131%   e. 231%

Q14.3 An object has a weight of 95 N on Pluto. What weight would it have on Jupiter (to the nearest N)?

    a. 42 N   b. 95 N   c. 135 N   d. 215 N   e. 265 N

Q14.4 On 6 August 2012, NASA's rover Curiosity landed on Mars, having covered a distance of 563 million km in 255 days. What was its average speed, to the nearest km/s?

    a. 24   b. 25   c. 26   d. 613   e. 1533

Q14.5 The first data sent to NASA by the rover Curiosity left at 7:48 am on 6 August 2012, travelling at a speed of 300,000 km/s. On that day, Mars was at a distance of 248 million km from the Earth. At what time did the first item of data reach NASA?

    a. 8:02 am   b. 8:19 am   c. 12:47 pm   d. 9:34 pm   e. 9:48 pm

QR 15 Practice: Exchange Rate

A bank customer who lives in the UK and travels to the US can pay his way with a range of payment methods whilst abroad.

- When in the UK, he can go to a Bureau de Change and exchange Pounds Sterling (£) against US Dollars (US$ or $) in cash.

- Whilst in the US, he may wish to pay for purchases directly with his credit card, saving him the hassle of handling cash. If he does need cash during his trip, he can withdraw it from a cash machine (ATM) in the US.

		In the USA Cash withdrawal (ATM)	In the USA Credit card purchases	In the UK Buying US$
Bank A	Commission	3.00%	3.50%	1.50%
Bank A	Fee	£2	0	£6
Bank B	Commission	2.50%	3%	2.00%
Bank B	Fee	£3	£1	£5
Bank C	Commission	2.00%	3.20%	2.50%
Bank C	Fee	£4	£1	£4
Bank D	Commission	2.00%	3.30%	2.70%
Bank D	Fee	£4	£1.5	£4.50

- Exchange rate £1 = US$1.70.

- A fee is charged for each transaction.

- When a UK bank is given Pounds Sterling to change to US Dollars, it first deducts the fee from the amount tendered and then charges commission on the remaining amount. The remainder is converted into Dollars and given to the client.

- When a customer spends or withdraws money in the US, his UK bank calculates the commission on the amount of US Dollars withdrawn or paid, adds the commission to the amount, converts the total to Pounds and charges the amount to the customer's account, together with the fee.

PRACTICE QUESTIONS

Q15.1 A customer travels from the UK to the US and, before his departure, exchanges Pounds Sterling in cash at Bank A to obtain a sum of US$850. How much does he give the bank in Pounds Sterling to achieve this?

    a. £507.50   b. £507.61   c. £509.61   d. £513.50   e. £513.61

Q15.2 A customer banking with Bank A spends $3,570 on his credit card. How much should he expect to appear on his bank statement for this transaction?

    a. £2068.97 b. £2173.50 c. £5979.31 d. £6180.03 e. £6183.03

Q15.3 A customer of Bank B exchanged £380 against US Dollars in cash before his departure. In the US, he withdrew $780 in cash from an ATM in three separate transactions. How much has he spent in total, expressed in Pounds Sterling?

    a. £850.29   b. £853.29   c. £856.29   d. £859.29   e. £862.29

Q15.4 A customer has decided to shop around and wants to find the cheapest bank, given that he wishes to spend $3,400 on his credit card on one single transaction when he gets to the US. Which bank should he choose?

    a. Bank A   b. Bank B   c. Bank C   d. Bank D   e. Any bank

Q15.5 In the US, a Bank C customer wants to buy a US$2,000 present for his wife. How much cheaper in Pounds will it be to pay for it by withdrawing cash in the US, compared to paying by credit card?

    a. £10.12   b. £11.12   c. £14.12   d. £17.12   e. £18.12

Q15.6 Bank C has now decided that, for ATM cash withdrawals only, it will reduce its transaction fee to zero and will increase its commission rate instead. Based on a withdrawal of $2,000, what commission should the bank charge in order for the change to be neutral?

    a. 0.20%   b. 0.34%   c. 1.66%   d. 2.34%   e. 3.40%

QR 16 Practice — Amusement Park

This table represents the number of tickets sold by a UK amusement park and the ticket prices for the years 2004 to 2007.

	Ticket sales					
	Individual Children		Individual Adults		Groups	
Years	Low season	High season	Low season	High season	Low season Children	Low season Adults
2004	51,000	27,000	38,000	20,000	15,000	17,000
2005	47,000	24,000	34,000	17,000	12,500	13,500
2006	44,000	24,000	32,000	17,000	12,000	14,300
2007	46,000	21,000	34,000	15,500	11,500	13,400
	Ticket prices					
2004/2005	£3.05	£3.55	£5.10	£6.10	£2.05	£4.05
2006/2007	£3.35	£4.00	£5.35	£6.65	£2.00	£4.00

Notes:
- Group tickets are not available in high season.
- A group is defined as 15 or more adults and children aged over 3.

PRACTICE QUESTIONS

Q16.1 By what percentage did the total income from high season sales increase (or decrease) between 2004 and 2005?

 a. −15.33%   b. −13.29%   c. +7.24%   d. +13.29%   e. +15.33%

Q16.2 In 2006, what proportion of total income did group ticket sales represent?

 a. 10.34%   b. 13.34%   c. 15.67%   d. 17.57%   e. 18.35%

Q16.3 Between 2004 and 2005, all categories suffered a drop in the number of tickets sold. One of the six categories experienced a smaller loss than all others when measured as a percentage of the level of 2004 ticket sales. What is that percentage?

a. 7.84%   b. 11.53%   c. 22.50%   d. 23.23%   e. 23.33%

Q16.4 Managers of the amusement park are expecting to sell 17,504 Adult High Season tickets in 2008. By how much should the managers increase the ticket price in 2008 (from 2007 prices) in order to obtain the same income as in 2004 in that category?

a. 4.81%   b. 12.90%   c. 14.26%   d. 15.65%   e. 16.54%

Q16.5 Managers of the amusement park are thinking of charging the same price for all individual children, regardless of whether they come in low or high season. What price should the park have been charging for individual children throughout 2007 in order to earn the same income as it did in that year?

a. £3.35   b. £3.45   c. £3.55   d. £3.65   e. £4.00

Q16.6 The same group of 15 adults goes to the amusement park every year between 2004 and 2007 (both years included) in low season. What is the total saving made by the group over the four years by buying a group ticket instead of individual tickets?

a. £4.20   b. £4.80   c. £36.00   d. £72.00   e. £81.00

Q16.7 In 2007, a large company hired the entire amusement park for a day for its employees and their families. This represented 750 adults and 900 children, on the following terms:

- Each child was charged 70% of the group low season tariff for children.
- Each adult was charged 50% of the group low season tariff for adults.

What was the total cost for the company for the day?

a. £1,200   b. £2,760   c. £2,810   d. £2,990   e. £3,430

QR 17 Practice: The Hunters and the Hunted

A field bordering a forest is being regularly used by hunters to shoot game. Its characteristics are as follows:

```
A ─────────────────► C
        240 yards        F
                         O
                         R
   150 yards             E
                         S
                         T
B ─────────────────► D
```

Conversion: 1 metre(m) = 1.0936 yards(yd)

PRACTICE QUESTIONS

Q17.1 What is the area of the field?

a. 30,101m² b. 32,919m² c. 36,000m² d. 39,370m² e. 43,055m²

Q17.2 The field's owner is nearing retirement and wants to share the field between his four sons. He wishes to allocate:

- 1/6 of the field to his first son
- 2/7 of the field to his second son
- 1/5 of the field to his third son
- The remainder to his fourth son.

What is the area of the portion of the field allocated to the fourth son?

a. 12,514yd²   b. 15,895yd²   c. 17,657yd²
d. 18,343yd²   e. 23,486yd²

Q17.3 Two hunters have killed 14 animals in total (pheasants & rabbits). We are told that:

- Hunter A killed twice as many rabbits as Hunter B
- Hunter A killed three times fewer pheasants than Hunter B
- Hunter A killed 2 pheasants.

How many rabbits did Hunter B kill?

a. 2   b. 3   c. 4   d. 6   e. 8

Q17.4 The field's owner wants to use the field to plant potatoes in rows parallel to the AC edge of the field. The first row will be on line AC and the last row will be on line BD. In-between, he will plant one row every 6 inches. Given that there are 36 inches in a yard, how many rows of potatoes will he be able to plant?

a. 900   b. 901   c. 1440   d. 1441   e. 5400

Q17.5 The field owner runs along the edge of his field every morning in order to exercise. How long does it take him to run along the full perimeter of the field once, assuming that he runs at a speed of 5 km/h?

a. 5min 35s b. 8min 34s c. 8min 56s d. 9 min 22s e. 10min 14s

Q17.6 The field's owner is trying to keep hunters out of the field by installing an electric fence. However, for legal reasons, he can only install the fence one metre inside the field along the entire perimeter. What will be the perimeter of the fence (to the nearest metre)?

a. 705 m   b. 706 m   c. 709 m   d. 713 m   e. 714 m

Q17.7 Two hunters walk along the edge of the field, towards the forest. Hunter A walks clockwise from point A. He walks at 60 yd/min. Hunter B walks anticlockwise from point B at a non-specified speed. They meet along the edge of the forest after exactly 5 minutes. At what speed was Hunter B walking?

a. 50 yd/min b. 55 yd/min c. 56 yd/min d. 65 yd/min e. 66 yd/min

QR 18 Practice — Diamonds are Forever

Key facts about diamonds:
1. The weight of a diamond is measured in carats. A carat is equivalent to 0.2 grams.
2. The price of rough diamonds is proportionate to the square of the number of carats and is therefore calculated according to the following formula: **Price = (Price of 1 carat) x (Number of carats)^2**
3. The price of a 1-carat diamond varies according to market forces. Currently, a 1-carat rough diamond sells for $125. Hence a 2-carat rough diamond sells for 125 x 2^2 = $500, etc.
4. Diamonds are exported and imported by countries in rough or polished forms.

Diamond import/export figures for Country X for 2008

	Oct – Dec 2008 US$ millions	% change from 2007	Jan – Sep 2008 US$ millions	% change from 2007
Polished Exports	428	−62.1%	5,812	−2.2%
Polished Imports	594	−42.8%	3,787	7.6%
Rough Exports	141	−73.0%	3,173	11.0%
Rough Imports	315	−68.1%	4,165	1.7%

PRACTICE QUESTIONS

Q18.1 What is the cost of a rough diamond that weighs 2.6 g?

a. $2,275   b. $4,225   c. $12,653   d. $18,845   e. $21,125

Q18.2 How much money would a diamond cutter save by buying a 4-carat diamond and a 7-carat diamond, instead of an 11-carat diamond?

a. $7,000   b. $9,000   c. $8,125   d. $9,175   e. $12,125

Quantitative Reasoning – Practice

Q18.3 A diamond cutter has purchased a 5-carat rough diamond and must remove half of it in the process of shaping and polishing the rough diamond. He then sells the polished diamond at 20 times the price of a rough diamond of the same weight. How much profit will he make?

a. $12,125   b. $12,500   c. $13,225   d. $14,175   e. $15,625

Q18.4 A diamond cutter has heard rumours that the price of rough diamonds may change soon. He is told that a 4-carat rough diamond might now cost $640. If the new price were to be implemented, what would be the weight of a rough diamond costing $1,960?

a. 4 carats   b. 5 carats   c. 6 carats   d. 7 carats   e. 8 carats

Q18.5 What was the total value of exports in Oct–Dec 2007, to the nearest US$ million?

a. $340m   b. $421m   c. $920m   d. $1,652m   e. $2,117m

Q18.6 By what percentage has the value of polished imports increased or decreased between 2007 and 2008?

a. −35.2%   b. −4.04%   c. −3.88%   d. +3.88%   e. +4.04

Q18.7 The diamond industry for Country X expects that, for the first quarter of 2009, the net export figure (i.e. the difference between total exports and total imports) will be 20% higher than the average quarterly net export figure over the period Jan–Sep 2008. What is the expected net export figure for the period Jan–Mar 2009 (to the nearest $ million)?

a. $70m   b. $413m   c. $810m   d. $1,033   e. $1,240m

Q18.8 What is the average quarterly income from polished exports in 2008?

a. $428m   b. $1,453m   c. $1,560m   d. $1,937m   e. $3,120m

45

QR 19 Practice — Printing

Printing costs

Digital printing (normal quality):
- Initial set-up cost: none
- 6p per page up to total 300,000 pages
- 5p per page between 300,001 pages and 600,000 pages
- 4p per page above 600,001 pages
- The total quantity printed determines the price per page. The same price is charged for all pages, e.g. for 500,000 pages, all pages will be charged at 5p.

Litho printing (higher quality):
- Initial set up cost: £1000
- 6p per page up to total 200,000 pages
- 4.5p per page between 200,001 and 550,000 pages
- 3.5p per page above 550,001 pages
- The total quantity printed determines the price per page. The same price is charged for all pages, e.g. for 300,000 pages, all pages will be charged at 4.5p.

Cover printing

- One colour only:
  - £1.50 per book if ordering 1599 books or less
  - £1.40 per book if ordering between 1600 and 1999 books
  - £1.00 per book if ordering 2000 or more books
- More than one colour: Add 20% to the cost of "one colour only" printing regardless of the number of colours.

Lamination of the cover
- Matt laminate: 20p per book
- Gloss laminate: 12p per book

Retail data
- Bookshops purchase books directly from the publisher at 75% of the Recommended Retail Price (RRP)

PRACTICE QUESTIONS

Q19.1 Mr Scribbler wants to print 1600 copies of his 126-page book. He wants the book printed using the litho technique, with a cover printed with one colour only and laminated in gloss. How much will it cost?

    a. £10,547   **b.** £11,664   **c.** £12,504   **d.** £12,654   **e.** £14,678

Q19.2 A customer needs 3,000 covers, and hesitates between 2 options:
- Option A: 1 colour, matt laminate
- Option B: 2 colours, gloss laminate

How much cheaper is Option A compared to Option B?

    a. £ 0   **b.** £ 80   **c.** £360   **d.** £960   **e.** £1,034

Q19.3 A publisher had one of his titles printed at a cost of £34,500. He sold all copies of the book to a bookshop and made a profit of £9,672. The Recommended Retail Price for the book is £16. How many copies of this book did he sell to the bookshop?

    a. 2156   **b.** 2761   **c.** 3681   **d.** 4256   **e.** 6783

Q19.4 On 1 January, the publisher asked the printer for a quote based on 2000 copies of a book of 300 pages to be printed using digital technology with a one-colour gloss-laminated cover. On 10 January, he realised the book had, in fact, 400 pages. What is the difference between the actual price paid for the printing of the 400-page books, and the price originally quoted for 300 pages?

    a. £1,690   **b.** £2,000   **c.** £4,690   **d.** £8,000   **e.** £10,000

Q19.5 A customer wants 50 copies of a 30-page book printed but cannot afford to pay the full price. The book is to be printed using digital technology and has a three-colour cover which is to be laminated gloss. As a gesture of goodwill, the printer charges him a lower printing cost per page and hands out a total invoice for £156. What price did the printer charge per page?

    a. 2p   **b.** 3p   **c.** 4p   **d.** 5p   **e.** 5.5p

QR 20 Practice — Fishy Business

A fish enthusiast buys a fish tank with the following characteristics:

Dimensions
Rectangular base (Length: 2 m, Width: 1.50 m), Volume: 2,250 litres.

Filling the tank with water
In order to avoid excessive pressure on the glass panels of the tank, the fish tank should be filled so that the water level does not go over 80% of its height.

Water treatment
If using tap water, new water added to the tank should be treated with a special solution. Dosage: 1 drop of the solution per litre of water added. The solution is available in bottles of 250 ml. Each drop has a volume of 0.05 ml.

Fish population
In order to avoid illnesses and stress to the fish population, fish enthusiasts should avoid populating the tank with too many fish. On average there should be no more than 2.5 cm of fish per 4.5 litres of water, e.g. a 9-litre tank could take 1 fish of 5 cm, 2 fish of 2.5 cm each, etc.

PRACTICE QUESTIONS

Q20.1 The fish enthusiast decides to clean the tank before using it by filling it completely with water up to the very top, ignoring the 80% rule. He places the tank under a tap which has a flow rate of 6 litres per minute. How long will it take to fill the tank?

  a. 2h 50min **b.** 4h 10min **c.** 4h 15min **d.** 6h 15min **e.** 6h 25min

Q20.2 The fish enthusiast decides to fill the tank with just water, i.e. no ornaments, gravel or plants, filling it to the maximum level recommended. What volume of water treatment solution will he need to add to the water?

  a. 9 ml **b.** 90 ml **c.** 112.5 ml **d.** 900 ml **e.** 1125 ml

Q20.3 The fish enthusiast decides to introduce 60 fish into the tank and notices that, once he has done so, the level of the water has risen by 0.5 cm. What is the average volume of a fish?

a. 190 cm³   b. 210 cm³   c. 250 cm³   d. 320 cm³   e. 450 cm³

Q20.4 The fish enthusiast decides to place gravel on the floor of his tank. The gravel occupies 15% of the total volume of the tank. The enthusiast then fills up the tank to the maximum recommended limit. What is the maximum recommended number of fish of 10 cm each which the enthusiast will be able to place in the tank?

a. 81   b. 82   c. 83   d. 84   e. 85

Q20.5 The fish enthusiast prefers to tile the bottom of the tank with decorative tiles which are square-shaped and measure 12.5 cm on each side. How many tiles will he require?

a. 72   b. 96   c. 192   d. 194   e. 204

Q20.6 The fish enthusiast wants to supplement the tank with a special lighting unit which fits on top of the tank and would add 18% to its height. What is the total height of the combined tank and lighting unit?

a. 50.75cm   b. 75cm   c. 88.5cm   d. 94.7cm   e. 98.6cm

Q20.7 Gravel for the tank can be bought in bags of 5 kg. The label on the bag states that the contents of the bag are enough to cover a surface of 1 m² with a thickness of 7 cm of gravel. The fish enthusiast lays down 3 cm of gravel at the bottom of the tank, covering the entire surface evenly. What is the weight of the gravel that he has placed into the tank?

a. 2.1 kg   b. 3.9 kg   c. 5.0 kg   d. 6.4 kg   e. 11.7 kg

Q20.8 A tank's price is proportionate to its volume. A cubic tank with edges of 30 cm costs £47. How much would the fish enthusiast's tank cost?

a. £2,350   b. £3,133   c. £3,917   d. £4,549   e. £4,551

QR 21 Practice — World News

Number of newspapers sold over Years 1 to 5

	Newspaper A	Newspaper B	Newspaper C
Year 1	130,000	110,000	98,700
Year 2	230,000	140,000	100,000
Year 3	135,000	110,000	190,000
Year 4	136,000	156,000	167,000
Year 5	133,000	176,000	156,000

Newspaper A:

- Sold in New Zealand, Australia and West Africa.
- Price is 70p in all years.

Newspaper B:

- Sold only in Europe.
- Years 1, 2 and 3: Price is 65p.
- Years 4 and 5: Price is 60p.

Newspaper C:

- 37% of copies sold in Europe. 63% of copies sold in Asia.
- Years 1, 2 and 3: Price is 55p in all regions.
- Years 4 and 5: Price is 50p in Europe and 60p in Asia.

Quantitative Reasoning – Practice

PRACTICE QUESTIONS

Q21.1 In Year 1, what proportion of the total number of newspapers sold that year did Newspapers A and C represent?

    a. 59%   b. 63%   c. 68%   d. 76%   e. 79%

Q21.2 What was the income for Newspaper C in Year 5?

    a. £86,166   b. £86,245   c. £87,135   d. £87,576   e. £87,828

Q21.3 What was the total income for Europe in Year 4?

    a. £91,585   b. £110,165   c. £111,350   d. £124,495   e. 134,460

Q21.4 Between Year 5 & Year 6, the <u>number</u> of newspapers sold changed as follows:
- Newspaper A: sales dropped by 50%
- Newspaper B: sales increased by 133%
- Newspaper C: sales increased by 5/9ths.

How many newspapers were sold in Year 6 (nearest thousand)?

    a. 231,000   b. 384,000   c. 543,000   d. 719,000   e. 923,000

Q21.5 In Year 3, the cost of printing Newspaper B was 30p per copy. The cost of printing increases by 10% every year. In what year will the cost of printing become greater than the income generated by the sales of Newspaper B, assuming that the retail price of Newspaper B remains at Year 5 level?

    a. Year 8   b. Year 9   c. Year 10   d. Year 11   e. Year 12

Q21.6 What proportion of all newspaper copies were sold in Europe in Year 3?

    a. 16.2%   b. 25.3%   c. 35.3%   d. 41.4%   e. 47.4%

Q21.7 What was the average yearly income for Newspaper C over the five years (to the nearest pound)?

    a. £ 66,842   b. £ 79,127   c. £ 142,340   d. £ 253,256   e. £ 376,199

QR 22 Practice — D.I.Y.

An architect has drawn up plans for an apartment using a scale of 1:200.

```
      3.20 m      1.20 m  1.80 m      3.30 m
   |<--------->|<------>|<------>|<------------>|
                       Bathroom
                          ▼
   ┌─────────────────┬──────┬──────────────────┐  ▲
   │                 │      │                  │  │
   │    Bedroom      │      │                  │  │
   │                 ├──────┤   Dining room    │ 3.60 m
   │                 │Kitchen                  │  │
   │                 │      │                  │  │
1.20 m▲├─────────────┴──────┴──────────────────┤  ▼
     ▼│         Hall                           │
      └──────────────────┬──────────────────┐──┘  ▲
                         │                  │    │
                         │                  │    │
                         │     Lounge       │   3.10 m
                         │                  │    │
                         │                  │    │
                         └──────────────────┘    ▼
                          |<----3.50 m---->|
```

Although the plans only show the surface area at floor level, we know that, in the dining room, there is:

- One French window (1.50 m wide and 2 m high) on the side opposite to the lounge
- One door (60 cm x 2 m) between the hall and the dining room
- One door (90 cm x 2 m) between the lounge and the dining room

The walls are 2.65 m high.

Metre to feet conversion rate: 1 m = 3.27 ft

PRACTICE QUESTIONS

Q22.1 What is the surface area of the apartment?

    a. 69.68 ft²   **b.** 181.99 ft²   **c.** 208.14 ft²   **d.** 481.72 ft²   **e.** 680.61 ft²

Q22.2 What is the surface area occupied by the hall on the architect's plans on paper?

    a. 1.86 cm²   **b.** 2.84 cm²   **c.** 3.60 cm²   **d.** 3.72 cm²   **e.** 7.44 cm²

Q22.3 The bedroom has a surface area of 8.76 m². What is the length of the longer portion of wall separating the bedroom and the bathroom?

    a. 1.20 m   **b.** 1.25 m   **c.** 1.30 m   **d.** 1.45 m   **e.** 1.50 m

Q22.4 The landlord wishes to paper over the walls of the dining room. What is the surface covered by the wallpaper?

    a. 13.80 m²   **b.** 24.80 m²   **c.** 25.48 m²   **d.** 30.57 m²   **e.** 36.57 m²

Q22.5 What is the total length of the outside walls of the apartment?

    a. 26.2 m   **b.** 29.3 m   **c.** 32.4 m   **d.** 35.4 m   **e.** 35.7 m

Q22.6 The landlord is contemplating laying down a wooden floor in the lounge. Wooden floors come in planks of 1 m length and 10 cm width. The planks are laid one after the other in a row; the last plank of a row can be cut easily to fit the dimensions of the room. The part which was cut out can then be used to start the next row. There are no gaps between planks. Planks are sold in packs of 25, with one pack costing £27.53. How much will the owner need to spend to buy the required number of packs?

    a. £119.48   **b.** £137.65   **c.** £143.46   **d.** £164.78   **e.** £166.34

1300 UCAT Practice Questions

QR 23 Practice — Going for a Ride

The following graph shows distances between 8 towns named A to H. Travel between towns is always done using the shortest route.

```
A •
     \ 7 km                    B •
      \                         \ 6.5 km    9 km
       \                         \         /      • C
        D •                       E •     F •
       /  \—————— 47 km ——————————>•<————•       | 8 km
6 km  /                              3 km  7.5 km |
    G •                                           • H
```

PRACTICE QUESTIONS

Q23.1 It takes 20 minutes for a car to travel from Town E to Town C using the shortest route. How long will the car take to travel from town E to town H using the most direct route, assuming that it goes at the same average speed?

    a. 17min 30s   b. 17min 40s   c. 17min 50s
    d. 18min 10s   e. 18min 20s

Q23.2 A cyclist can ride along the following route: D-E-F-C-H-F-E-B in 10 hours and 30 minutes. What is his average speed?

    a. 7.1 km/h   b. 7.6 km/h   c. 8.0 km/h   d. 8.2 km/h   e. 8.4km/h

Q23.3 Mr Smith works in Town G. He has 2 hours and 25 minutes free. He decides to go for a ride in his car. He calculates that he has just enough time to go to a certain town, stay there for 49 minutes and get back to work. Which town does he intend to visit, assuming that he drives at an average speed of 70 km/h?

    a. Town B   b. Town C   c. Town E   d. Town F   e. Town H

Q23.4 A cyclist starts riding from Town C at an average speed of 18 km/h and arrives at his destination 40 minutes later. What is his destination?

    a. Town B   **b.** Town D   **c.** Town E   **d.** Town F   **e.** Town H

Q23.5 A cyclist rides from Town D to Town H along the road D-E-F-H. He calculates that if he could ride at a certain average speed, he would arrive into Town H 15 minutes earlier than if he was travelling at 18.4 km/h. What is that speed?

    a. 5 km/h   **b.** 10 km/h   **c.** 15 km/h   **d.** 20 km/h   **e.** 25 km/h

Q23.6 As well as a road network, the towns are linked by a tube network which runs exactly underneath the roads. The tube stations are where the dots are shown on the map.

Two passengers leave Town C at the same time to go to Town G, using the route C-F-E-D-G. One passenger travels by tube (no changes necessary) and the other one by car. Between stations, the tube drives at 30 km/h, stopping at each intermediary station for exactly 1 minute. On the road, the car driver drives at 94 km/h between D and E, and at 72 km/h on all other roads. How much later than the car driver will the tube passenger arrive in Town G?

    a. 45 min   **b.** 59 min   **c.** 1h 28min   **d.** 1h 47min   **e.** 2h 13min

Q23.7 The local authorities have organised a bus service as follows:

- Line FCH: the bus goes in a loop from Town F to Town C to Town H to Town F and so on at 49 km/h (including stops).

- The bus starts at 5am from Point F and stops running at 11pm.

During a one-day shift, how many times will the bus have driven through Town C?

    a. 12 times   **b.** 18 times   **c.** 36 times   **d.** 48 times   **e.** 54 times

QR 24 Practice: Hot Chocolate

A chocolate lover purchases a 360 g box of powdered drinking chocolate. The label states the following:

NUTRITIONAL INFORMATION			INSTRUCTIONS
	Per 100 g (dry powder)	Per 18 g serving (with 200 ml whole milk)	Put 3 heaped teaspoons (18 g) into a mug. Add 200 ml of hot milk and stir well. Sit back and relax! For a diet drink, you can use semi-skimmed or skimmed milk. Semi-skimmed milk contains 1.7 g of fat per 100 ml. Skimmed milk contains 0.3 g of fat per 100 ml.
Energy (kJ)	1555	845	
kCal	372	200	
Protein (g)	8.9	8.0	
Carbohydrate (g)	65.2	20.4	
Fat (g)	8.4	9.6	

PRACTICE QUESTIONS

Q24.1 How much fat is contained in 200 ml of whole milk (to the nearest 0.1 g)?

a. 1.2 g   b. 3.4 g   c. 6.8 g   d. 8.1 g   e. 9.6 g

Q24.2 The customer finds whole milk a bit rich and decides to use a mix of semi-skimmed milk and water instead. He then adds 200 ml of the mixed liquid to 18 g of powdered chocolate. The total fat content of the resulting drink is 2.464 g. Given that water does not contain any fat, what volume of semi-skimmed milk did he use?

a. 56.0 ml   b. 81.5 ml   c. 144.9 ml   d. 118.5 ml   e. 170.4 ml

Q24.3 The customer uses up the whole box of powdered chocolate, making hot drinks according to the instructions. How many pints of milk will he have used (1 pint = 570 ml)?

a. 0.35   b. 4.4   c. 7.0   d. 14.1   e. 20.0

Q24.4 The customer is on a diet and, in an effort to reduce his weight, he decides to limit the total daily calories that he gets from the chocolate drink to a strict maximum of 800 kCal. To achieve his objective, he decides to make three chocolate drinks per day using water only (water does not contain any calories) and to make any other chocolate drink using his usual whole milk.

What is the maximum number of whole-milk-based chocolate drinks that he can have in addition to his three daily water-based drinks in order not to breach his resolution?

a. 0 drink   b. 1 drink   c. 2 drinks   d. 3 drinks   e. 4 drinks

Q24.5 The customer buys semi-skimmed milk with a label that states that its protein content is 3.3 g per 100 ml. What is the total amount of protein that he will have drunk once he has made drinks with the entire box of chocolate using standard proportions and semi-skimmed milk instead of whole milk (to the nearest gram)?

a. 66 g   b. 160 g   c. 164 g   d. 244 g   e. 272 g

Q24.6 The calorific value of food is measured in kCal and is calculated by adding the calorific values of protein, carbohydrate and fat. The calorific value of 1 g of protein is 4 kCal and the calorific value of 1 g of carbohydrate is 4 kCal.

What is the calorific value of 1 g of fat, to the nearest gram?

a. 4 kCal   b. 6 kCal   c. 9 kCal   d. 21 kCal   e. 44 kCal

1300 UCAT Practice Questions

QR 25 Practice — Time Traveller

A traveller is looking at a variety of options to travel. All possible connections are shown on the diagram below and can be made by plane.

```
                                            ● London
                         ● New York (NY)

  Los Angeles
  (LA)       ●                              ● Paris
```

The timetables for the various flights are as follows (all times expressed in local times):

	London to Paris	London to NY	Paris to NY	Paris to LA	NY to LA	London to LA
Departs:	7:50	7:25	6:15	11:15	11:30	10:15
Arrives:	10:15	10:25	8:15	13:25	14:50	13:20
Departs:	9:25	9:10	8:55	13:00	15:50	12:00
Arrives:	11:50	12:10	10:55	15:10	19:10	15:05
Departs:	10:30	11:45	13:20	16:10	17:20	15:10
Arrives:	12:55	14:45	15:20	18:20	20:40	18:15
Departs:	12:25	13:55	15:40	19:45	20:10	18:15
Arrives:	14:50	16:55	17:40	21:55	23:30	21:20

In addition, the traveller is aware that when it is 12 noon in London, the time in:
- Paris is 1pm
- New York is 7am
- Los Angeles 4am

Quantitative Reasoning – Practice

PRACTICE QUESTIONS

Q25.1 What is the duration of a flight from NY to LA?

a. 20min   b. 2h 20min   c. 3h 30min   d. 5h 20min   e. 6h 20min

Q25.2 A client wants to travel along the route London → Paris → Los Angeles. He takes the first plane of the day from London and then transfers to the next plane available whenever he reaches a new destination. How much time will have elapsed between his departure from London and his arrival in Los Angeles?

a. 5h35min   b. 12h35min   c. 13h35min   d. 14h35min   e. 15h35min

Q25.3 The plane from Paris to New York flies at an average speed of 730 km/h. What is the distance between the two airports?

a. 1,460km   b. 2,920km   c. 4,380km   d. 5,840km   e. 7,300km

Q25.4 Jack and John want to travel from London to Los Angeles. Jack decides to fly via Paris, whilst John decides to fly via New York. It is 9am and they decide to take the first plane available to them. On arrival at their intermediate destination (Paris or New York), they jump on the first available plane to Los Angeles. When they meet up in Los Angeles, they compare the time it took them to travel from the moment their first plane left to the time their second plane arrived. What is the difference between their respective times?

a. 1h 55min   b. 2h 35min   c. 2h 45min   d. 3h 35min   e. 4h 15min

Q25.5 The airline wants to introduce a new flight from Paris to New York such that the flight should arrive in New York 30 minutes before the last flight from New York to Los Angeles departs. At what time should this new flight leave Paris (expressed in local Paris time)?

a. 11:40   b. 13:40   c. 15:40   d. 17:40   e. 19:40

Q25.6 A plane travels on average at 730 km/h and consumes on average 2.1 litres of fuel per kilometre flown. How much fuel does the airline use in 1 day for the Paris to Los Angeles flights?

a. 3,321   b. 13,286   c. 17,119   d. 68,474   e. 75,486

QR 26 Practice — Conferencing & Banqueting

A company specialising in organising conferences has a choice between two different types of contracts at one venue.

- A **Daily Delegate Rate (DDR)** contract, whereby they pay a fixed price per delegate which entitles them to a comprehensive range of services (e.g. use of the room, flipchart, water, tea and coffee, lunch, etc.).

- A **Room-Basis (RB)** contract, whereby each service used is charged individually.

The company has collected a brochure from a potential conference venue, which provides the following tariff information:

The Red Rag Conference Centre	
DDR contract	**RB contract**
£45 per participant (weekend) £50 per participant (weekdays) Includes: • Use of conference room • Projector • Flipchart • 3 tea/coffee breaks • Sit-down lunch • Orange juice at lunch time (1 jug for 5 people) • 1 bottle of water per person NOTE Minimum of 8 participants applies. If the number of participants is less than 8, the fee will be charged for 8 people.	Room hire: • £250 (weekend) • £350 (weekdays) Facilities (per room): • Projector: £189 • Flipchart: £15 Refreshments / Food: • Coffee break: £2.50 per break per person • Orange juice: £10 per jug (serves 5 people) • Sit-down lunch: £20 per person • Buffet lunch: £17 per person • Water: £5 per bottle No minimum requirement on the number of participants applies.

All prices quoted above include VAT on all items.

Quantitative Reasoning – Practice

PRACTICE QUESTIONS

Q26.1 What is the cost for 7 participants on a DDR contract on a Monday?

   a. £315   b. £350   c. £360   d. £400   e. £450

Q26.2 How much would it cost on the RB contract to replicate the package of services provided under the DDR package for 10 participants on a Sunday?

   a. £450   b. £500   c. £650   d. £799   e. £817

Q26.3 The company needs the following for a Saturday conference:
- Room
- Flipchart
- 3 servings of tea and coffee
- Sit-down lunch

They are hesitating between the RB rate and the DDR rate (they don't mind getting more than they require if the price is cheaper). For which number of participants would the total DDR cost be greater than the RB cost?

   a. 10   b. 13   c. 14   d. 15   e. 16

Q26.4 All costs quoted include VAT at 17.5%. The government decides to reduce the VAT rate to 15% for the foreseeable future and the hotel wishes to alter its rates accordingly. What is the new week-end DDR rate after allowance has been made for the new 15% VAT rate?

   a. £38.30   b. £39.13   c. £44.04   d. £45.98   e. £46.74

Q26.5 The company organises a conference for 50 participants on a Monday, hiring a room by itself and using their own caterer, which charges £30 per person. To authorise the customer to use their own caterer, the hotel adds a surcharge of 12% on the room hire cost. What is the average cost per person?

   a. £30.00   b. £32.67   c. £35.00   d. £37.84   e. £40.00

QR 27 Practice: Milking It

A farmer owns 15 cows. Each cow produces an average of 8.75 litres of milk per day. He sells his milk to a local cooperative at 33p per kilo. Once milk has been obtained from a cow, 15% of its weight can be extracted to obtain cream. 25% of the weight of the extracted cream represents butter.

1 litre of milk weighs 1.034 kg. 1 litre of water weighs 1 kg.

PRACTICE QUESTIONS

Q27.1 What weight of butter can the farmer extract on average every day?

　a.4.921 kg　**b.**4.967 kg　**c.**5.021 kg　**d.**5.089 kg　**e.**5.124 kg

Q27.2 In April, the farmer sold his entire milk production to the same cooperative. How much did he earn?

　a.£1,299.37　**b.**£1,342.68　**c.**£1,343.55　**d.**£1,364.56　**e.**£1,388.34

Q27.3 With a view to inflate his profit, the farmer engages in the dishonest activity of adding water to his milk. The volume of water added is 25% of the volume of raw milk. How much does 1 litre of the new mixture weigh?

　a. 1.000 kg　**b.** 1.025 kg　**c.** 1.027 kg　**d.** 1.200 kg　**e.** 1.250 kg

Q27.4 During the 160 days that the winter season lasts, the farmer requires 19,800 kg of hay to feed his 15 cows. He has purchased all the hay required before winter started. After 42 days of winter, the farmer decides to purchase 3 new cows. What additional quantity of hay will he require to feed all the cows for the remainder of the winter period if he wishes each cow to be fed on average the same as each was consuming before the purchase?

　a.1,039.5kg　**b.**2,135.0kg　**c.**2,920.5kg　**d.**3,052.0kg　**e.**3,960.0kg

QR 28 Practice — A Colourful Life

A paint shop allows its customers to produce any paint colour they like from the three primary colours: red, blue and yellow. Its most popular colours are made by mixing as follows:

Colour	% of Red	% of Blue	% of Yellow
Chocolate	33%	33%	34%
Amazon	10%	80%	10%
Rosebud	50%	45%	5%
Violet	40%	40%	20%
Crimson	70%	20%	10%

PRACTICE QUESTIONS

Q28.1 What volume of yellow paint do 2 litres of Amazon paint contain?

   a. 100ml   b. 200ml   c. 300ml   d. 500ml   e. 800ml

Q28.2 The shop owner mixes 100 ml of Crimson with 400 ml of Amazon. What proportion of red paint does the resulting colour contain?

   a. 10%   b. 12%   c. 22%   d. 40%   e. 70%

Q28.3 The shop owner has a 1-litre pot of Violet. He wants to add yellow to it in order to obtain Chocolate. Once the yellow paint has been added, what will be the total quantity of Chocolate paint obtained (in litres)?

   a. 0.212   b. 0.412   c. 0.812   d. 1.2   e. 1.212

Q28.4 An eccentric customer wants to invent a new paint colour obtained by mixing all five mixed colours (i.e. Chocolate, Amazon, Rosebud, Violet and Crimson) in equal quantities. What proportion of blue paint would the resulting colour contain?

   a. 15%   b. 21.8%   c. 43.6%   d. 60.3%   e. 70.8%

1300 UCAT Practice Questions

QR 29 Practice — Advertising Rates

A magazine offers businesses an opportunity to purchase advertising space in its pages. The cost of adverts is linked to the number of columns which they span, and their height measured in centimetres. The data and rates available are as follows:

Page sizes
- Width: 4 columns
- Height: 28 cm

Advertising rates
- Single column: £50 per cm
- Double column: £75 per cm
- Spanning four columns: £150 per cm
- Advert sizes must be measured in exact number of columns by a whole number of centimetres, i.e. one cannot have an advert measuring 1.5 columns by 3.5 cm
- Minimum height of advert charged for: 3 cm (all adverts of less than 3 cm will be charged as if they had a height of 3 cm)

Add-on for colour
- Black and white: No additional cost
- Full colour: Add 20%

Packages available
- Quarter-page: £1,000 black and white, +20% for colour
- Half-page (vertical or horizontal): £2,000 black and white, +20% for colour
- Full-page: £3,800 black and white, +20% for colour

PRACTICE QUESTIONS

Q29.1 A customer wants to place a full colour advert across two columns, which is 8 cm tall. What will the cost be?

a. £400   b. £480   c. £600   d. £720   e. £800

64

Q29.2 A customer wants to place a black and white advert across four columns which is 7 cm tall. How much is the cheapest possible option?

a. £900   b. £950   c. £1,000   d. £1,050   e. £1,400

Q29.3 Consider the following two scenarios:

Scenario 1
The magazine sells one page of advertising to a lot of small customers who all take out black and white single column adverts. All adverts are more than 3 cm long and are laid out one after the other and side by side without any space between them. The page is completely full, i.e. there is no space left.

Scenario 2:
The magazine sells one page of advertising to a single customer who takes out a full-page black and white advert.

What is the loss of revenue incurred by the magazine if it chooses Scenario 2 instead of Scenario 1?

a. £400   b. £1,800   c. £2,800   d. £3,800   e. £5,600

Q29.4 The magazine sells the following adverts:

- 1 full colour quarter page advert
- 1 double column advert (5 cm) – black and white
- 3 single column adverts (4 cm) – black and white
- 1 single column advert (2 cm) – black and white

What is the total income made from these sales?

a. £1,850   b. £1,875   c. £2,125   d. £2,275   e. £2,325

Q29.5 What is the maximum income that the magazine can derive from one page of advertising?

a. £3,800   b. £4,560   c. £6,720   d. £10,080   e. £20,160

QR 30 Practice — A Matter of Time

Recently published statistics showed that, on some lines, trains run more slowly than 20 years ago.

The average journey times for three major lines were as follows:

Table showing average journey times in minutes

Journey	1987	2008
CANTERBURY EAST TO LONDON (VICTORIA)		
Canterbury East to Faversham (12 miles)	13	17
Faversham to Chatham (18 miles)	25	25
Chatham to Victoria (34 miles)	43	44
LEWES TO LONDON (VICTORIA)		
Lewes to Haywards Heath	15	20
Haywards Heath to Gatwick	13	14
Gatwick to East Croydon	17	17
East Croydon to Victoria	16	16
SOUTHEND TO LONDON (FENCHURCH STREET)		
Southend to Upminster	28	30
Upminster to Barking	9	8
Barking to Fenchurch Street	12	16

Source for timing: Thomas Cook European Timetables

Note: 1 mile = 1.6093 km

For the purpose of this exercise, you should assume that none of the trains stopped at any of the intermediary stations shown in the table above, i.e. assume that all trains ran non-stop from their city of origin to London.

Quantitative Reasoning – Practice

PRACTICE QUESTIONS

Q30.1 How much longer did the Lewes to London Victoria journey take in 2008 as compared to 1987?

    a. 5 min   **b.** 6 min   **c.** 25 min   **d.** 61 min   **e.** 66 min

Q30.2 What was the average speed of the Canterbury East to London Victoria train in 1987 over the whole line (to the nearest km/h)?

    a. 47 km/h   **b.** 58 km/h   **c.** 65 km/h   **d.** 76 km/h   **e.** 81 km/h

Q30.3 By what proportion did the journey time increase between Southend and London Fenchurch Street between 1987 and 2008?

    a. 9.00%   **b.** 9.26%   **c.** 10.00%   **d.** 10.20%   **e.** 10.26%

Q30.4 The train company's executives think that, in future, they can make the Canterbury East to London Victoria train journey as short as it used to be in 1987 by allowing their trains to run faster on the Faversham to Chatham portion of the route (with the times for the other two portions of the route remaining at 2008 levels).

At what speed would the train need to run on the Faversham to Chatham portion in order for the whole journey to last the same amount of time as in 1987?

    a. 43.2 km/h   **b.** 54.0 km/h   **c.** 69.5 km/h   **d.** 86.9 km/h   **e.** 89.6 km/h

Q30.5 The price of a Canterbury East to London Victoria ticket is £15.90. We are told that the price of a ticket on the Lewes to Victoria line is, on a pound per mile basis, the same as a Canterbury East to London Victoria ticket. Given that a ticket on the Lewes to London Victoria line costs £12.40, what is the distance between Lewes and London Victoria (to the nearest mile)?

    a. 50 miles   **b.** 55 miles   **c.** 61 miles   **d.** 66 miles   **e.** 82 miles

QR 31 Practice: Within Shopping Distance

A local authority has carried out a survey of the number of shops present within its boundaries. The data consists of the number of shops and the average turnover (in thousands of pounds) plotted against the distance from the county's central town.

PRACTICE QUESTIONS

Q31.1 How many shops were counted in total by the local authority?

a. 450   b. 550   c. 600   d. 650   e. 700

Q31.2 What is the total turnover of the shops located within a distance of 5 miles from the reference point?

a. £30,000   b. £120,000   c. £150,000   d. £30m   e. £150m

Quantitative Reasoning – Practice

Q31.3 Which part of the county has the highest total turnover?

   a. 0–1   b. 1–5   c. 5–10   d. 10–15   e. 20–25

Q31.4 What proportion of total turnover is held by the shops within a 10-mile radius from the reference point?

   a. 11.8%   b. 33.3%   c. 53.8%   d. 67.5%   e. 70.6%

Q31.5 In the zone within 1 mile of the reference point, all shops must pay a business tax based on their turnover.

The business tax is calculated as follows:

- 0.5% payable on the part of turnover up to £100,000
- 1% payable on the part of turnover above £100,000

Assuming that all shops within the zone have a turnover which is greater than £100,000, what is the average amount of tax collected per shop within the zone?

   a. £5,500   b. £6,000   c. £6,500   d. £7,500   e. £8,000

Q31.6 The council estimates that, with the recession, 20% of shops within a radius of 10 miles will close down whilst the number of shops beyond 10 miles will increase by 5%. What will be the number of shops left standing once the changes have taken effect?

   a. 300   b. 350   c. 595   d. 607   e. 650

Q31.7 A pensioner lives 12.5 miles away from the reference point. He can only drive a maximum of 7.5 miles in any direction. Assuming that all roads are straight lines, and all shops are along those straight roads, how many shops can this pensioner visit?

   a. 100   b. 150   c. 200   d. 325   e. Can't tell

QR 32 Practice: Shaken, not Stirred

A local bar offers the following cocktails (all quantities expressed in ml):

	Tequila	Cointreau	Lemon Juice	Orange Juice	Vodka	White Rum	Vermouth	Gin
Tequila Sunrise	50			100				
Journalist		5	5				25	50
Screwdriver				50	50			
Balalaika		25	25		25			
Martini							25	50
XYZ		25	25			40		
Vodkatini					50		25	
Velocity							50	25
Orange Bloom		25					25	50
Long Island	25		25		25	25		25

Pure alcohol content for each drink

Drink	% of pure alcohol
Tequila	38%
Cointreau	40%
Lemon Juice / Orange Juice	0%
Vodka	45%
White Rum	40%
Vermouth	15%
Gin	43%

PRACTICE QUESTIONS

Q32.1 What volume of vodka is required to make the following cocktails?

- 2 Screwdrivers
- 5 Balalaika
- 1 Long Island

a. 100 ml   b. 150 ml   c. 200 ml   d. 250 ml   e. 300 ml

Q32.2 What is the volume of pure alcohol contained within one Orange Bloom cocktail?

    a. 35.00 ml **b.** 35.25 ml **c.** 35.50 ml **d.** 35.75 ml **e.** 36.00 ml

Q32.3 At the start of the night the barman realises that he only has 4 litres of orange juice at his disposal, all of which gets used during the night. The bar till shows that during that night only 8 Tequila Sunrise cocktails have been sold and that no one was served orange juice on its own. How many Screwdrivers were sold that night?

    a. 32 **b.** 48 **c.** 56 **d.** 64 **e.** 72

Q32.4 Out of the five following cocktails, which one contains the smallest volume of alcohol?

    a. Martini **b.** Vodkatini **c.** Velocity **d.** Orange Bloom **e.** Journalist

Q32.5 Jane normally drinks one Balalaika at the start of the evening. Having got bored with it, she decides today to have an XYZ instead. What is the proportionate change in the volume of pure alcohol that she will consume when she switches to this new cocktail?

    a. −42.2% **b.** −22.4% **c.** +15.0% **d.** +22.4% **e.** +42.2%

Q32.6 During Happy Hour, the bar serves drinks in pitchers (jugs) of 1.5 litres. A group orders the following:

- 2 pitchers of Velocity
- 1 pitcher of Long Island

What volume of gin is required to make these?

    a. 1.15 litres **b.** 1.3 litres **c.** 1.5 litres **d.** 2.3 litres **e.** 4.1 litres

QR 33 Practice
Entente Cordiale

A courier needs to drive from London to Paris and back to deliver a package. The following diagram sets out the route, together with the availability of petrol stations, including prices and distances between each.

London	Dover	Calais	Paris
80 km	50 km ~~~	100 km	180 km	20 km

Price per litre
Diesel: 99p
Unleaded: 89p
Super: 93p

Price per litre
Diesel: €0.87
Unleaded: €1.25
Super: €1.47

Price per litre
Diesel: €0.95
Unleaded: €1.37
Super: €1.76

Between Calais and Dover, the car is loaded onto a ferry boat. The cost of a single ferry journey is £75. Including loading and offloading time, the ferry journey takes 2 hours each way.

Exchange rate: £1.00 = €1.20.
Capacity of the car's fuel tank: 45 litres.
The car runs on unleaded petrol.
1 litre of petrol enables the car to drive for 10 km.

Quantitative Reasoning – Practice

PRACTICE QUESTIONS

Q33.1 If the courier drives at an average speed of 110 km/h between London and Dover and at an average speed of 120 km/h between Calais and Paris, how long will it take him to travel from London to Paris, assuming that he does not stop at any petrol station?

    a. 3h 41 min   **b.** 3h 49min   **c.** 4h 41 min   **d.** 5h 41min   **e.** 5h 49min

Q33.2 The driver sets out from London with a full tank of fuel. He heads towards Paris with the intention of turning back as soon as he has delivered the package. He forgets to check his fuel gauge and runs out of petrol. At what distance from Paris will he stop?

    a. 10 km   **b.** 20 km   **c.** 30 km   **d.** 50 km   **e.** 70 km

Q33.3 The courier sets out from London with 20 litres of fuel in his tank. He fills his tank to full capacity every time he meets a petrol station and keeps the receipts to give to his boss. How much will his fuel receipts total for the single journey London to Paris?

    a. £43.29   **b.** £65.54   **c.** £72.78   **d.** £75.36   **e.** £81.76

Q33.4 The courier's car breaks down in Paris and he is offered a choice between two replacement cars for his return journey to London:

- Car A runs on diesel, using 1 litre of diesel per 15 km.
- Car B runs on super, using 1 litre of super per 10 km.

The driver leaves on a full tank (45 litres for both cars) and decides to refuel to full capacity at every petrol station. What is the difference in fuel spend between the two options?

    a. €22.05   **b.** €23.13   **c.** €24.21   **d.** €25.03   **e.** €26.05

Q33.5 The courier sets out from London in his usual car on a full tank of unleaded. On the way he stops at a petrol station to fill his fuel tank completely. The refuelling costs him €28.75 (or Pound Sterling equivalent). How many litres of unleaded did he buy?

    a. 8 litres   **b.** 23 litres   **c.** 25 litres   **d.** 27 litres   **e.** 41 litres

QR 34 Practice: Parking

A parking meter displays the following information:

PARKING FEES
This car park uses three separate charging time zones

Time Zone 1: Monday – Friday
9:00am – 1:00pm: 20p for each period of 10 minutes
1:00pm – 6:00pm: 30p for each period of 10 minutes

Time Zone 2: Saturday, Sunday & Bank Holiday
9:00am – 6:00 pm: 15p for each period of 20 minutes

Time Zone 3: 6:00pm – 9:00am any day
£1 standard fee regardless of the duration

IMPORTANT NOTES:

1 – Payment is made just as you exit the car park.

2 – Any period started should be paid for in full. For example, a driver staying in the car park for 15 minutes on a Monday afternoon should pay for a full 20 minutes (i.e. 2 x 10-minute periods).

3 – If a car is parked in the car park over several charging zones then a calculation will be made separately for each zone, each being subject to its own minimum charge. For example, a driver arriving at 12:59pm on a Monday and staying 20 minutes will be charged 20p for the period 12:59pm to 1:00pm and 60p for the period 1:00pm to 1:19pm, a total of 80p.

Quantitative Reasoning – Practice

PRACTICE QUESTIONS

Q34.1 A driver arrives at the car park at 9am on a Monday and stays in the car park for 37 minutes. How much will he be charged?

   a. 20p   b. 50p   c. 74p   d. 80p   e. £1

Q34.2 A driver enters the car park at 5:55pm on a Monday afternoon and leaves the car park at 6:15pm. How much will he be charged?

   a. 40p   b. 60p   c. £1   d. £1.15   e. £1.30

Q34.3 A driver parks his car on Monday morning at 9:00am and leaves it in the car park until Sunday evening 6:00pm. How much will it cost him?

   a. £59.10   b. £65.10   c. £71.10   d. £77.10   e. £83.10

Q34.4 A driver uses the car park all year round and contacts the council to obtain a weekly season ticket. The season ticket he requires is for commuters and only allows him to use the car park Monday to Friday between 8:30am and 6:00pm The cost of the weekly season ticket is £54. How much money will he save in comparison to paying full price for that period?

   a. £5   b. £10   c. £15   d. £20   e. £25

Q34.5 A driver comes into the car park at 12:58pm and leaves 4 minutes later at 1:02pm on a Monday lunch time after having dropped off his wife at the station. How much will he be charged?

   a. 10p   b. 20p   c. 30p   d. 40p   e. 50p

Q34.6 A driver only has £4.90 in his pocket to pay for car park fees. He enters the car park on Friday afternoon at 5pm. Until when can he stay in the car park?

   a. Friday 9:00pm
   b. Saturday 9:00am
   c. Saturday 11:00am
   d. Saturday 11:40am
   e. Saturday 1:40pm

QR 35 Practice: It Rings a Bell

The **Green Mobile Phone Company** offers the following tariffs:

Tariff Number	Monthly Fee	Talk minutes included	SMS texts included
1	£15	0	Unlimited
2	£20	200	Unlimited
3	£35	600	Unlimited
4	£35	700	250
5	£45	900	Unlimited
6	£55	1500	Unlimited

Talk minutes included in the tariffs include calls to all mobile phones on the Green network but not calls to mobile phones on other networks. Texts included in the tariffs include texts sent to any mobile phone on any network. Calls and texts made outside of the tariff are charged as follows:

- Calls to Green mobile numbers: 15p per minute
- Calls to other mobiles: 40p per minute
- Additional text messages (any network): 10p per text

The **H_2O Mobile Phone Company** offers the following tariffs:

Tariff Number	Monthly Fee	Talk minutes Included	SMS texts included
A	£15	100	100
B	£20	200	200
C	£25	300	300
D	£30	700	400
E	£35	800	500
F	£40	1000	500

Talk minutes included in the tariffs include calls to mobiles on all networks (and not just H_2O). Texts can be sent to any mobile phone on any network. Calls and texts made outside of the tariff are charged as follows:

- Mobile numbers: 30p per minute
- Additional text messages: 12p per text

PRACTICE QUESTIONS

Q35.1 A Green Mobile Phone Company customer has opted for Tariff 4. In January, he had the following consumption:

- 300 talk minutes to contacts on the Green Telephone network
- 300 minutes to contacts who are on the H_2O network
- 100 texts to contacts on the Green Telephone network
- 150 texts to contacts who are on the H_2O network

How much was his telephone bill?

a. £35   b. £75   c. £125   d. £155   e. £183

Q35.2 A potential mobile customer is wondering which company and tariff he should be using. All his friends and family are using the Green Mobile Phone Company and he reckons he will be spending 10.5 hours on the phone to them every month and text them 450 times per month. Which tariff would ensure the cheapest bill?

a. Tariff 3   b. Tariff 4   c. Tariff C   d. Tariff D   e. Tariff E

Q35.3 A customer on Tariff E is thinking of moving to Tariff F. What is the minimum number of minutes that he would need to talk on the phone each month in order to make the move worthwhile?

a. 716 min   b. 717 min   c. 800 min   d. 816 min   e. 817 min

Q35.4 A customer on Tariff 6 has five friends to whom he has spoken as follows in one month (he spoke to no one else). His bill for the month is £450. The bill shows that he used the following minutes:

Jane	Green	220 minutes
John	H_2O	Illegible
Kelly	Green	280 minutes
Mark	Green	1000 minutes
Roberta	Green	500 minutes

How many minutes did he speak to John for that month?

a. 633   b. 800   c. 937   d. 1,275   e. 2,133

QR 36 Practice
Voting Turnout

The following table summarises the number of voters eligible to vote in each of four constituencies (A, B, C and D), for each age range.

	18–24	25–34	35–44	45–54	55–64	65+
A	4000	5000	3500	4200	3500	7500
B	3500	3800	2800	2500	2000	1500
C	3600	2500	1500	500	3000	5000
D	2000	2500	3000	3500	4000	4500

The table below summarises the percentage of people who actually went out to vote for each age range.

	18–24	25–34	35–44	45–54	55–64	65+
A	50%	60%	20%	50%	40%	32%
B	10%	25%	25%	15%	35%	40%
C	30%	40%	35%	40%	50%	70%
D	15%	15%	25%	25%	80%	90%

PRACTICE QUESTIONS

Q36.1 In Constituency B, how many people aged 35–44 voted?

  a. 175   b. 350   c. 700   d. 1400   e. 2800

Q36.2 In Constituency A, how many people between the ages of 25 and 54 voted?

  a. 700   b. 2100   c. 3000   d. 5800   e. 6400

Q36.3 In Constituency C, how many people over age 55 did not vote?

  a. 1500   b. 2000   c. 2500   d. 3000   e. 3500

Q36.4 Across all four constituencies, what proportion of the over-65s did not vote?

  a. 10%   b. 30%   c. 43%   d. 52%   e. 67%

5 Quantitative Reasoning
Answers to Practice Questions

QR 1 – White Goods

Q1.1 – d: £411
The dishwasher costs £353, to which we must add £35 for delivery and £23 for installation. 353 + 35 + 23 = £411.

Q1.2 – c: £450
The cost of the fridge is:
412 (price) + 23 (delivery) + 0 (installation) + 15 (Saturday) = £450.

Q1.3 – d: £234
There are two ways of approaching the problem:

Method 1: Full calculation
Buying the combined fridge-freezer will cost Tessa:
586 (price) + 38 (delivery) + 15 (Saturday surcharge) = £639.

Buying the fridge and the freezer as two separate appliances will cost her:
412+383 (price) + 25+23 (delivery) + 2x15 (Saturday surcharge) = £873.
The saving is therefore 873 – 639 = £234.

Method 2: Working on savings for individual items:
Saving on price = 412 + 383 – 586 = £209
Saving on delivery = 25 + 23 – 38 = £10
Saving on Saturday supplement (1 instead of 2) = £15
Total saving = 209 + 10 +15 = £234

Q1.4 – c: £22
The installation cost is 416 – 349 – 30 – 15 (Saturday supplement) = £22.

Q1.5 – d: £305.10
Julia would spend (1 – 0.3) x £353 + 35 + 23 = £305.10.

Q1.6 – a: Washer dryer
To answer this question you can calculate the price after discount for all items and see which one matches the price paid. However, there is a risk that the answer may be the last item on the list and you will have wasted a lot of time. In this instance you can use the elimination process method:

If the price after discount is £401.60, then this will clearly exclude the dishwasher, the fridge and the freezer as they are too cheap to achieve that price after discount.

There remains the washer dryer and the fridge-freezer. The fridge-freezer has a price tag of £586. After the 20% discount, the price will be £468.80, well above the price paid. Therefore the only viable option is the washer dryer. Check: 452 x 80% + £25 + £15 = £401.60.

Q1.7 – a: £34.90
The maximum delivery charge they will be able to impose is 10% of the lowest priced item, i.e. 10% of £349 = £34.90.

Q1.8 – d: 55.2%
The fridge costs 412 + 23 = £435 in total. The additional cost of insurance is £4 per month, payable for 5 years (60 months), i.e. 60 x 4 = £240. This represents an increase of 240 / 435 = 0.552, i.e. 55.2%.

QR 2 – Field Areas

Q2.1 – a: 1:2000
The width of 500 m (i.e. 50,000 cm) is represented by 25 cm. The scale is therefore 25 / 50,000 = 1 / 2000.

Q2.2 – b: 10%
The current perimeter of the field is 2 x 1000 + 2 x 500 = 3000 m.
If we increase the length by 150 m but the width remains the same, then the perimeter will increase by 2 x 150 = 300 m, i.e. 10%.

Q2.3 – a: Greater
The area of the rectangular field is 1000 x 500 = 500,000 m^2. The perimeter of the field is 3000 m; therefore, if the field were square, its sides would measure 3000 / 4 = 750 m. The area of the square field would therefore be 750 m^2 = 562,500 m^2, i.e. greater than the area of the rectangular field.

Quantitative Reasoning – Practice

Q2.4 – e: 1000 km
Let's assume that the lawnmower travels left to right and then right to left, etc. (Note: you will get the same result if you assume that it travels up and down instead.) At each passage, the lawnmower will travel 1000 m = 1 km (i.e. the length of the field). It will do so as many times as there are strips of 50 cm (i.e. 0.5 m) in the width of the field (which is 500 m) i.e. 500 / 0.5 = 1000 times. The lawnmower will therefore travel 1000 x 1 km = 1000 km.

Q.2.5 – c: 50 cm²
Using a scale of 1:10000, the rectangle drawn on paper would have the following dimensions:
- Length: 1000 / 10000 = 0.1 m, i.e. 10 cm.
- Width: half the length, i.e. 5 cm.

The area is therefore: 10 x 5 = 50 cm².

QR 3 – Actual v. Reading Age

Q3.1 – e: 61.5%
The children with a reading age equal to or greater than their actual age will be those who appear on or above the diagonal line. There are 16 of them. The percentage is therefore 16 / 26 = 0.615, i.e. 61.5%.

Q3.2 – e: 3.5
The worst performing pupil is the child who is furthest away below the line. This is the child who has an actual age of 8 and a reading age of 4.5. He is 8 – 4.5 = 3.5 years behind.

Q3.3 – c: 5.583
There are three pupils with a reading age of 6. They are aged 5, 5.75 and 6. Their average age is therefore (5 + 5.75 + 6) / 3 = 5.583.

Q3.4 – d: 3
The current reading ages of the four children are 5.5, 5.75, 6 and 6.25. A year later, those will be 0.75 higher, i.e. 6.25, 6.5, 6.75 and 7. Therefore three of them will have a reading age below the age of 7.

QR 4 – Stamp Duty

Q4.1 – d: £43,750
The stamp duty on a property of £1m would be calculated as follows:

0 to £125,000: £0
£125,000 to £250,000: 2% x £125,000 = £2,500
£250,000 to £925,000: 5% x £675,000 = £33,750
£925,000 to £1 million: 10% x £75,000 = £7,500

Total: 0 + 2,500 + 33,750 + £7,500 = £43,750

Q4.2 – d: £1.552 m
We are told that the stamp duty payable up to a purchase price of £1.5 million is £93,750. John paid a total of £100,000 and therefore £100,000 – £93,750 = £6,250 is the amount paid within the 12% bracket. This means that the amount taxable at 12% was 6,250 / 0.12 = £52,083. The price of the house was therefore £1.5 million + £52,083 = £1,552,083.

Q4.3 – b: £30,000
On the portion of the price up to £2 million, there would be no difference as the same tax rates would apply under both regimes. However, under the new regime a tax of 15% instead of 12% would be payable on the remaining £1 million. The difference would therefore be 3% x 1m = £30,000.

Q4.4 – e: £247,549
If her budget is a total of £250,000 then the maximum price of the house will be in the £125,000 to £250,000 bracket.

The first £125,000 attracts no tax; therefore the remaining £125,000 of her budget will need to pay for the remainder of the house price and the stamp duty at 2% on that part.

125,000 / 1.02 = £122,549. This gives a total price of 125,000 + 122,549 = £247,549.

Note: You can also resolve this using a simple equation. If we define x as the property price, we have: $x + 2\% (x - 125,000) = 250,000$.

This gives $1.02x - 2,500 = 250,000$. So $x = 252,500 / 1.02 = £247,549$.

QR 5 – Restaurant Pricing

Q5.1 – c: £43.89
The cost of the ingredients is 158 / 1.2 / 3 = £43.89.

Q5.2 – e: £201.60
The party would pay: 50 x 3 x 1.2 (VAT) x 1.12 (service) = £201.60.

Q5.3 – b: £17.22
Without the wine, the total bill for the food is 172 – 48 = £124.
The cost of the ingredients per person is therefore:
124 / 1.2 (VAT) / 3 (cost multiplier) / 2 (number of people) = £17.22.

Q5.4 – e: £288
We know that the ingredients cost £32, therefore the price charged to customers for the food part of the meal will be 32 x 3 x 1.2 = £115.20. Since the drinks account for 60% of the total bill, then the food accounts for 40%. Therefore the total bill is: 115.20 / 0.4 = £288.

QR 6 – Distances & Journey Times

Q6.1 – e: 14h00min
The distance from Paris to Madrid is 1260 km. At a rate of 90 km/h this would take 1260 / 90 = 14 hours.

Q6.2 – d: 10h20min
The amount of actual driving will be 990 / 110 = 9 hours. During that time he will take 4 breaks (after 2, 4, 6 and 8 hours) of 20 minutes each, a total of 80 minutes, i.e. 1h 20 minutes. In total, the journey will therefore take 10h20min.

Q6.3 – c: 5.23%
The direct distance from Rome to Brussels is 1530 km.
The distance from Rome to Brussels via Geneva is:
930 (Rome → Geneva) + 680 (Geneva → Brussels) = 1610 km.
The increase is therefore 1610 / 1530 = 1.0523, i.e. 5.23%.

Q6.4 – e: £109.56
The distance between Geneva and Brussels is 680 km.
Suzie will therefore use 680 / 100 x 9 = 61.2 L of petrol, at a cost of:
61.2 x 1.3 = £79.56. Adding the £30 of toll fees gives a total of £109.56.

Q6.5 – b: 500 km
To calculate the distance between Paris and Amsterdam, you first need to convert the times into numbers you can calculate with.

2h36min = 2 x 60 + 36 = 156 min, i.e. 156/60 = 2.6 h.
2h40min = (2 + 2/3) h or 2.6666666 h.

The distance is therefore 100 x 2.6 + (2 + 2/3) x 90 = 500 km.

Q6.6 – c: 81 km/h
The distance between Madrid and Barcelona is 620 km, which he drove in a total time of 2h40min + 5h = 7h40min (or 7 + 2/3 hours = 7.67 h). Therefore his average speed during the whole journey was 620/7.67 = 81 km/h.

Note: To calculate the average speed over the whole journey, it doesn't actually matter what part of the journey was done at what speed. All that matters is the total distance and the total time.

Q6.7 – b: Geneva
We need to add the distance between Barcelona and Town X to the distance between Town X and Brussels. The quickest way to achieve that is to add up the numbers on each line across the Barcelona and Brussels columns. This can be done mentally fairly quickly, bearing in mind that it is not necessary to calculate the values for Amsterdam, Madrid and Rome, as they each contain a number greater than the total journey length.

	Barcelona	Brussels	Total
Amsterdam	1530	200	1730
Barcelona		1340	
Brussels	1340		
Geneva	810	680	1490
Madrid	620	1570	2190
Paris	1030	300	1330
Rome	1470	1530	3000

This tells us that the answer is Geneva.

Quantitative Reasoning – Practice

Q6.8 – c: 30min
The distance between Paris and Brussels is 300 km. If he drove the second half (i.e. 150 km) at a speed of 50 km/h then that leg of the journey will have taken him 150 / 50 = 3 hours. Add to that the 1h30min spent on the first leg of the journey, and you get a total driving time of 3h + 1h30min = 4h30min. Since the total journey lasted 5 hours, it means that he stopped for 30 minutes.

Q6.9 – a: 21h00min
The distance between Rome and Madrid is 2020 km / 1.6 = 1262.5 miles. At a speed of 60 mph, this can be driven in 1262.5/60 = 21.04166 h. This is equivalent to 21 hours + 2.5 minutes, i.e. 21 hours when expressed to the nearest 10 minutes.

Q6.10 – a: 3h45min shorter
The distance between Brussels and Geneva is 680 km but the Englishman thinks it is 680 miles. If he believes this will take him 10 hours then he is anticipating an average speed of 68 mph. In reality the distance is 680 km, i.e. 680 / 1.6 = 425 miles. At a speed of 68 mph this will take 425 / 68 = 6.25 hours, i.e. 3.75 hours (3 hours 45 min) shorter.

QR 7 – Sightseeing

Q7.1 – d: £150.80
The total price (not forgetting to allow for 2 lenses!) will be:
34x1.2 + 2x30 + 2x25 = £150.80.

Q7.2 – c: £84
The full price would be 36 + 2x38 = £112.
Applying a discount of 25% gives 0.75 x 112 = £84.

Q7.3 – e: 2:3
The total cost for single vision is: 26 + 2x15 + 2x20 = 96.
The total cost for single vision is: 34 + 2x30 + 2x25 = 144.
The ratio is therefore 96/144 = 2/3, i.e. 2:3.

Q7.4 – a: 7%
At For Your Eyes Only, varifocal glasses would cost:
36 + 2x38 + 2x30 = £172. This compares to £159.96 at the other shop. 159.96 / 172 = 0.93; hence the discount should be 1 – 0.93 = 0.07, i.e. 7%.

QR 8 – Amateur Science

In this question you might find it easier to work in dm instead of cm as you will get a direct conversion into litres.

Q8.1 – b: 24 L
Working in dm, the volume is 4 x 2 x 3 = 24 dm^3, i.e. 24 L. If you wanted to calculate in cm, you would need to divide the volume in cm^3 by 10^3 in order to reach the right result in litres, i.e. 40 x 20 x 30 / 1000 = 24.

Q8.2 – c: 108 g
12,000 cm^3 = 12 dm^3, i.e.12 L.
A concentration of 9 g/L will give 12 x 9 = 108 g of salt.

Q8.3 – d: 8%
The base of the tank has an area of 4 x 2 = 8 dm^2. Therefore, if the volume of water is 4 L, then the height of the water level is 4 / 8 = 0.5 dm, i.e. 5 cm. If the volume has increased to 5.4 cm during the freezing process then the increase in volume has been 5.4 / 5 = 1.08, i.e. 8%.

Q8.4 – b: 360 g
The volume of salted water (calculating in dm) is 4 x 2 x 1.5= 12 L. At a concentration of 30 g/L, the scientist would get 12 x 30g = 360 g of salt.

Q8.5 – b: 1.424 L
4,800 cm^3 is equal to 4.8 dm^3, i.e. 4.8 L. The average volume of oxygen per fish is therefore 4.8 x 0.89 / 3 = 1.424 L.

QR 9 – Eye In The Sky

Q9.1 – d: 427 m
The circumference of each wheel is calculated as π x D, with D being effectively the height of each wheel. So the average circumference can be calculated as: 3.14 x (208 + 165 + 135 + 112.5 + 60) / 5 = 427.354 m.

Q9.2 – b: 116.48 m
An increase of 12% on the Beijing wheel would give a new height of: 208 x 1.12 = 232.96 m. The radius of the new wheel would therefore be half of the height, i.e. 116.48 m.

Quantitative Reasoning – Practice

Q9.3 – a: 13.25 m
The distance between each consecutive capsule will be equal to the circumference divided by 32, i.e. 135 x 3.14 / 32 = 13.25 m.

Q9.4 – c: 29 cm/s
The circumference (which is the distance that each capsule will travel during a rotation) is 165 x 3.14 = 518.10 m. That distance is achieved over 30 minutes. Therefore in 1 second the capsule will have travelled:
518.10 / (30 x 60) = 0.2878, i.e. 29 cm.

Q9.5 – d: 9.3
The wheel executes 48 rotations per day, i.e. 48 x 350 = 16,800 per year. This represents 16,800 x 32 = 537,600 capsule loads.

The average number of tourists per capsule in each rotation is therefore calculated as: 5,000,000 / 537,600 = 9.3.

Q9.6 – e: 48
The circumference of the wheel would have been 3.14 x 208 = 653.12. The number of capsules would have been 653.12 / 13.607 = 48.

Q9.7 – c: The Berlin wheel will have twice as many capsules as the Singapore Flyer
If the Berlin wheel is twice as tall as the Singapore wheel then its circumference will be twice as long (because in the formula $\pi \times D$, you are doubling the value of D). If the distance between the capsules is the same in both wheels then one will be able to fit twice as many capsules on the Berlin wheel than on the Singapore Flyer. Looking at the other options:

- a: We have already ascertained that the answer is twice as many.

- b: If the two wheels rotate at the same speed then the Berlin wheel will take twice as long to do a full rotation because it has twice the distance to go.

- d: The circumference of the Berlin wheel will be 2π = 6.28 times the diameter of the Singapore Flyer.

- e: The answer is that it should have a speed which is twice that of the Singapore Flyer, and not half of it, since it has a perimeter that is twice as long.

1300 UCAT Practice Questions

QR 10 – Going Swimmingly

Q10.1 – d: £74.00
The total amount raised was 19 + 20.10 + 23.80 + 26 + 22.10 = £111.
If the money is distributed with a 2:1 ratio then the Red Triangle will get 2/3 of the total raised, i.e. 111x 2/3 = £74.

Q10.2 – c: C
For this question you can quickly eliminate two students:

- Students A and D both have 10 lengths but Student A has raised less than Student D and so can be eliminated.

- Students C and E both have 9 lengths but Student E has raised less than Student C and so can also be eliminated.

For the three remaining students, the amounts raised per length are:
- Student B: 20.10 / 8 = £2.51
- Student C: 23.8 / 9 = £2.64
- Student D: 26.00 / 10 = £2.60

The answer is therefore Student C.

Q10.3 – c: £15.60
Student D raised 26 / 10 = £2.60 per length. Therefore Student F will need to raise 2.60 x 6 = £15.60.

Q10.4 – b: £18.50
The total raised was 19 + 20.10 + 23.80 + 26 +22.10 = £111.
The difference in the cash received would therefore be:
111 x (1/2 – 1/3) = 111 x 1/6 = £18.50.

QR 11 – Insurance Claims

Q11.1 – d: 412
We are told that the number of claims in 2010 was 1920 and that this was a 20% increase on the previous year. Therefore, the number of claims in 2009 was 1920/1.2 = 1600. This compares to 2012 claims in the year 2015, i.e. an increase of 2012 – 1600 = 412.

Quantitative Reasoning – Practice

Q11.2 – e: 37.5%
The number of rejected claims in 2012 was 1733 – 1211 = 522.
In 2013, it was 1633 – 915 = 718.
The increase was therefore 718 / 522 = 1.375, i.e. 37.5%.

Q11.3 – d: 2014
In this question it is easier to deal with approved claims, since we are given all the relevant numbers, than with rejected claims. The year with the lowest percentage of rejected claims will be the year with the highest percentage of approved claims:

2011: 1435 / 2039 = 70.4%
2012: 1211 / 1733 = 69.9%
2013: 915 / 1633 = 56.0%
2014: 1532 / 1933 = 79.3%
2015: 1263 / 2012 = 62.8%

The answer is therefore 2014.

Q11.4 – d: 1769
Watch out; the question is asking for the expected number of <u>rejected</u> claims, and not the approved claims.

The expected total number of claims for 2030 is 2 x 2012 = 4024.
The percentage of approved claims in 2013 is 56.032%.
Therefore the expected number of rejected claims in 2030 is:
(1 – 0.56032) x 4024 = 1769.

QR 12 – New Employees

Q12.1 – d: 81
The second graph shows that 27% of the 300 recruits were allocated to sanitation. This represents 0.27 x 300 = 81 recruits.

Q12.2 – b: 24
The difference between sanitation and engineering is 27 – 19 = 8%.
This corresponds to 0.08 x 300 = 24 people.

Q12.3 – c: 33
The number of people allocated to construction was 0.33 x 300 = 99. If two-thirds of them had a BSc then one-third of them were recruited at GCSE or

A Level. Therefore the number of construction recruits with either GCSE or A Levels is 99/3 = 33.

Q12.4 – b: 15.7%
In 2015, the number of people recruited into admin was 0.04 x 300 = 12. Therefore in 2016, 3 x 12 = 36 people were recruited into admin, i.e. 24 more than in 2015. Since the number of recruits in all other categories was the same, then in total 300 + 24 = 324 people were recruited in 2016.

In 2015 (and therefore also in 2016 since we are told the number did not change from one year to the next), the number of people recruited in education was 0.17 x 300 = 51. This represents 51 / 324 = 0.157 = 15.7% of the 2016 population of recruits.

Q12.5 – d: 167%
The original number of admin recruits was 0.04 x 300 = 12. Adding an extra 20 recruits would mean an increase of 20 / 12 = 1.67, i.e. 167%.

Q12.6 – e: Can't tell
We know that 27% of all recruits are in sanitation and that 33% of all recruits have a BSc, but there isn't enough information to deduce what proportion of sanitation recruits have a BSc. It could be as little as 0% and as much as 100%.

Q12.7 – a: 9
Out of 300 recruits, 33%, i.e. 99, work in construction. The number of recruits without A Levels or a BSc (i.e. those who only have O Levels) is 30% of 300, i.e. 90. That means that at least 99 – 90 = 9 construction workers must have either A Levels or a BSc.

Q12.8 – c: 17.3%
The number of engineering recruits is 0.19 x 300 = 57, and so the number of non-engineering recruits is 300 – 57 = 243.

The total number of BSc recruits is 0.33 x 300 = 99. Out of those we know that 57 are in engineering, leaving 99 – 57 = 42 in non-engineering responsibilities. Therefore the proportion of non-engineering recruits with a BSc is 42 / 243 = 17.3%.

Quantitative Reasoning – Practice

QR 13 – Riding Lessons

Q13.1 – c: £764
Kathy will have spent 86 + (4 x 150) + 78 = £764.

Q13.2 – e: 35
If we deduct the annual fee from the total fee, we have 710 – 110 = £600 spent on actual tickets. We know from the range of the answers that she will have bought 31 to 35 tickets and, therefore, she will have bought at least 3 blocks of 10 tickets. The cost for those is 170 x 3 = £510.

This leaves 600 – 510 = 90 to purchase the remaining tickets, which happens to be the cost for a block of 5 tickets. Therefore she purchased a total of 35 tickets.

Q13.3 – a: 13.3%
Purchasing 5 tickets individually would cost 5 x 15 = £75, so there is a saving of £10 on the £65 cost of a 5-ticket block. The discount is therefore 10 / 75 = 0.133, i.e. 13.3%.

Q13.4 – d: 30
The annual fee for both children is 64 + 86 = £150, leaving 960 – 150 = £810 to purchase actual lessons. Purchasing 10 lessons for each child will cost 120 + 150 = £270. Therefore each child will have 810 / 270 = 3 lots of 10 lessons, i.e. 30 lessons.

QR 14 – Gravity

Q14.1 – c: 686 N
The weight is 70 x 9.8 = 686 N.

Q14.2 – d: 131%
The ratio will be 3.7 / 1.6 = 2.31. Therefore the <u>increase</u> is 131%.

Q14.3 – d: 215 N
A weight of 95 N on Pluto would give a mass of 95 / 0.62 = 153.23 kg. The weight on Jupiter would therefore be 153.23 x 1.4 = 214.52 N, i.e. 215 N to the nearest N.

Q14.4 – c: 26
There are 255 x 24 x 60 x 60 = 22,032,000 seconds in 255 days. Therefore the average speed was 563 / 22.032 = 25.55, i.e. 26 to the nearest km/s.

Q14.5 – a: 8:02 am
The trip takes 248,000,000 / 300,000 = 827 seconds, i.e. 827 / 60 = 13.8 minutes. The signal would therefore reach the Earth at 7:48 + 14 minutes = 8:02 am.

QR 15 – Exchange Rate

Q15.1 – e: £513.61
The currency exchange takes place in the UK bank, for which we are instructed that we should take the fee out of the Pound amount and then deduct the commission.

Therefore the equation that we need to solve, with X representing the amount in Pounds he needs to pay, is:

$850 =   (X - £6)   x   (1 – 0.015)   x   1.7
           Deduct fee   Commission   Conversion

This gives X = 850 / 0.985 / 1.7 + 6 = £513.61.

Note that the commission should be calculated as 0.985 of the Pound amount and not the amount divided by 1.015. If I have a sum of £100 on which I need to pay 1.5% commission, I will be left with £98.50 and not with 100/1.015 = £98.52.

Q15.2 – b: 2173.50
This is a similar calculation but this time from the US point of view. From the information given, the amount that should appear on his statement is calculated as follows, with X representing that amount:

X = [3,570   x   (1 + 0.035)   /   1.7]   +   £0   = £2173.50
      Purchase   Commission   Conversion   Fee

Q15.3 – d: £859.29
The first spending will be with regard to the £380 he exchanged before he left. Since the banks deduct both the commission and the fee from the original £380 given to the bank, he will simply have spent £380.

Secondly, he withdrew $780 in cash from an ATM in the US. The actual cost of this withdrawal is:

$780 x 1.025 / 1.7 + £9 (3 withdrawals at £3 each) = £479.29
Total = £859.29.

Q15.4 – b: Bank B
You can obviously calculate the cost for each bank, which would lead you to the answer quickly enough. However, it is possible to exclude some options simply by looking at the data. Looking at the rates we can conclude the following:

- Bank B and Bank C have the same fee but Bank B has a lower level of commission and is therefore cheaper.

- Bank B has a cheaper commission rate and cheaper fee than Bank D. Therefore Bank B is cheaper than Bank D.

This now leaves us with Bank A and Bank B as possible candidates.
The cost for Bank A is 3,400 x 1.035 / 1.7 + 0 = 2,070
The cost for Bank B is 3,400 x 1.03 / 1.7 + 1 = 2,061

The answer is therefore: Bank B.

Q15.5 – b: £11.12
By paying cash he will benefit from a commission rate of 2% instead of 3.2%, i.e. a saving of 1.2% or $24. This is equivalent to 24 / 1.7 = £14.12. However, he will be required to pay a £4 fee instead of a £1 fee, i.e. £3 more. Hence the total saving in Pounds is 14.12 – 3 = £11.12.

Q15.6 – d: 2.34%
By reducing its fee to zero, the bank will lose £4, which it needs to make up through higher commission. If the commission increase rate is R then we need to solve the following equation: £4 = R x 2000 / 1.7, which gives R = 0.0034; i.e. an increase of 0.34% increase. The new rate should therefore be 2.34%.

QR 16 – Amusement Park

Q16.1 – b: –13.29%
The income for the two years is as follows (in thousands of pounds)
2004: 27 x 3.55 + 20 x 6.10 = 217.85
2005: 24 x 3.55 + 17 x 6.10 = 188.90
The ratio is 188.90 / 217.85 = 0.8671 i.e. a decrease in sales by 13.29% (1 – 0.8671 = 0.1329). Note that we are asked to measure the change from 2004 to 2005; this is measured as a percentage of the 2004 income.

Q16.2 – b: 13.34%
Total income for 2006 is calculated as follows (in thousands):
44 x 3.35 + 24 x 4.00 + 32 x 5.35 + 17 x 6.65 + 12 x 2.00 + 14.3 x 4.00 = 608.85
Total income from group tickets for 2006 is calculated as follows (in thousands): 12 x 2.00 + 14.3 x 4.00 = 81.2.
Proportion of group tickets sales = 81.2 / 608.85 = 13.34%

Q16.3 – a: 7.84%
You could calculate all the ratios between 2005 and 2004 ticket sales; or you can look at the numbers carefully and solve the problem through logic. Looking at the 2004 and 2005 ticket sales, we can see that the Children Low Season loss has been of 4,000 tickets out of 51,000 in 2004, which is under 10%. For all other categories, the loss has been over 10%. The Children Low Season category is the category which has experienced the smallest loss. The percentage is 4,000 / 51,000 = 7.84%

Q16.4 – a: 4.81%
2004 income for Adult High Season tickets = 20,000 x 6.10 = 122,000.
Ticket price required for 2008 = 122,000 / 17,504 = £6.97.
Increase required = 6.97 / 6.65 = 1.0481, i.e. an increase of 4.81%

Note that although the price increase is calculated to match the 2004 income, the actual increase itself is expressed as a percentage of the previous years' price and not the 2004 price.

Q16.5 – c: £3.55
The income for 2007 for individual children was:
46,000 x £3.35 + 21,000 x £4.00 = £238,100.
This now has to be distributed between 46,000 + 21,000 = 67,000 tickets.
The price is therefore 238,100 / 67,000 = £3.55.

Quantitative Reasoning – Practice

Q16.6 – d: £72.00
The saving per adult in 2004 and 2005 is £5.10 – £4.05 = £1.05.
The saving per adult in 2006 and 2007 is £5.35 – £4.00 = £1.35.
Over four years, an adult will therefore save 2 x 1.05 + 2 x 1.35 = £4.80.
A group of 15 will therefore save 15 x £4.80 = £72.

Q16.7 – b: £2,760
The price per child was 70% of £2.00, i.e. £1.40.
The price per adult was 50% of £4.00, i.e. £2.00.
The total cost was therefore 900 x £1.40 + 750 x £2.00 = £2,760.

QR 17 – The Hunters and the Hunted

Q17.1 – a: 30,101 m^2
The area of the field is calculated as: (240 / 1.0936) x (150 / 1.0936).

Q17.2 – a: 12,514 yd^2
(1 – 1/6 – 2/7 – 1/5) x (240 x 150) = 12,514 yd^2

Q17.3 – a: 2
If Hunter A killed 2 pheasants then, since this is 3 times fewer than Hunter B, Hunter B has killed 6 pheasants, making a total of 8 pheasants killed.

Since they killed a total of 14 animals, this means they killed 6 rabbits between them.

We are told that Hunter A killed twice as many rabbits as Hunter B, therefore Hunter A killed 4 rabbits and Hunter B killed 2 rabbits.

Q17.4 – b: 901 rows
This is a simple interval problem. The trap to avoid is not to miss the final row. In 1 yard (i.e. 36 inches) we have 6 intervals of 6 inches each. In 150 yards, we therefore have 900 intervals of 6 inches each. The number of rows (i.e. lines delimiting the intervals) is therefore 901.

Q17.5 – b: 8min 34s
The full perimeter of the field measures (150 + 240) x 2 = 780 yd. This is equal to 780/1.0936 = 713.24 m or 0.71324 km. At a speed of 5 km/h, he will run the distance in 0.71324 / 5 = 0.14266 hours, i.e. x 60 = 8.559 minutes. This corresponds to 8 minutes and 0.559 x 60 = 34 seconds.

Q17.6 – a: 705m
The length of the field is 240 / 1.0936 = 219.459 m. The length of fence is therefore 2 metres less (1 metre on each side), i.e. 217.459 m

The width of the field is 150 / 1.0936 = 137.162 m. The length of fence is therefore 2 metres less (1 metre on each side) i.e. 135.162 m. The perimeter of the fence is therefore 2 x (217.459 + 135.162) = 705.242 m.

Q17.7 – e: 66 yd/min
At the time they meet, the combined distance they will have walked is: 240 + 150 + 240 = 630 yards. Hunter A will have walked 5 x 60 = 300 yards. This means that Hunter B will have walked 630 – 300 = 330 yards during those same 5 minutes. His speed is therefore 330 / 5 = 66 yd/min.

QR 18 – Diamonds are Forever

Q18.1 – e: $21,125
A weight of 2.6 g is equivalent to 2.6 / 0.2 = 13 carats.
A 13-carat diamond will cost 125 x 13^2 = $21,125.

Q18.2 – a: $7,000
Price of a 4-carat diamond = 125 x 4^2 = $2,000.
Price of a 7-carat diamond = 125 x 7^2 = $6,125.
Price of an 11-carat diamond = 125 x 11^2 = $15,125.
Saving = 15,125 – (2,000 + 6,125) = $7,000.

Q18.3 – b: $12,500
Price of a 2.5-carat rough diamond = 125 x 2.5^2 = $781.25.
Price of a 5-carat rough diamond = 125 x 5^2 = $3,125.
Profit = 20 x 781.25 – 3125 = $12,500.

Q18.4 – d: 7 carats
The new price would give the following equation:
$640 = (Price of 1 carat) x 4^2, i.e. price of 1 carat = $40.

This now gives us the equation 1960 = 40 x c^2, where c is the number of carats of the diamond. This gives c^2 = 1960 / 40 = 49, i.e. c = 7 carats.

Quantitative Reasoning – Practice

Q18.5 – d: $1,652m
The question is asking about 2007 values, whilst we are only given 2008 values with % change. It is important to remember that these percentages will be based on the 2007 value. So, for example, if Oct–Dec 2008 polished exports have a value of $428m, and the % change is –62.1% then we have (Oct–Dec 2008 value) = (Oct–Dec 2007 value) x (1 – 0.621).

Therefore Oct–Dec 2007 value for polished exports = 428 / (1 – 0.621) = 1129.29.
Similarly, Oct–Dec 2007 value for rough exports = 141 / (1 – 0.73) = 522.22.
Total exports for Oct–Dec 2007 = 1129.29 + 522.22 = 1651.51.

Q18.6 – c: –3.88%
The value of polished imports across 2008 was 594 + 3,787 = $4,381m.
The value across 2007 was 594 / (1 – 0.428) + 3,787 / (1 + 0.076) = $4,557.98m.

Ratio of 2008 over 2007 = 4381 / 4557.98 = 0.96117.
Change = 1 – 0.96117 = 0.03883, i.e. 3.88% decrease.

Q18.7 – b: $413m
The net export figure for the period Jan–Sep 2008 is calculated as:
(5,812 + 3,173) – (3,787 + 4,165) = 1,033.
An increase of 20% on the quarterly average will therefore give:
1,033 / 3 (there are 3 quarters in that period) x 1.20 = 413.20.

Q18.8 – c: $1,560m
This is simply calculated as the total polished exports over all quarters, divided by 4. This gives: (428 + 5812) / 4 = $1,560.

QR 19 – Printing

Q19.1 – c: £12,504
Litho printing:
- Initial set-up cost = £1000
- Printing: 126 x 1600 = 201,600 pages at 4.5p each = £9,072

Cover
- 1600 at £1.40 each = £2,240
- Lamination (Gloss) = 1600 at £0.12 each = £192

Total= £12,504

Q19.2 – c: £360
The cost of Option A is: 3000 x (£1.00 + £0.20) = £3,600
The cost of Option B is: 3000 x (£1.00 x 1.2 + £0.12) = £3,960
Cost difference = 3,960 – 3,600 = £360

Q19.3 – c: 3681
If the printing cost was £34,500 and the profit was £9,672, then the income he received from the bookshop is £9,672 + £34,500 = £44,172.

We know that the bookshop buys books at 75% of the RRP (£16), i.e. at £12 per book. So the bookshop purchased 44,172/12 = 3,681 copies.

Q19.4 – b: £2,000
The quote was for 300 pages x 2000 books = 600,000 pages. This would have been quoted at 5p per page, i.e. £30,000. The actual number of pages printed was 400 pages x 2000 books = 800,000 pages, which should be priced at 4p per page, i.e. a total of £32,000. The difference on the printing of the pages is therefore £2,000. Note that the number of covers is the same (2000); therefore the difference is purely on the pages.

Q19.5 – c: 4p
The cost of printing the cover for 50 books (3 colours, laminated gloss) is: 50 x (1.5 x 1.2 + 0.12) = £96. Since the total cost was £156, then this leaves £60 for the actual printing of the pages.

He wants to print 50 x 30 = 1500 pages. Therefore the cost per page is: 60 / 1500 = 0.04 i.e. 4p.

QR 20 – Fishy Business

Q20.1 – d: 6h 15min
The volume of the tank is 2,250 litres. At a rate of 6 litres per minute, it would take 375 minutes to fill, i.e. 6.25 hours, i.e. 6 hours and 15 minutes.

Q20.2 – b: 90 ml
The volume of water in the tank is 80% x 2250 = 1800 litres. We therefore need 1800 drops, i.e. 1800 x 0.05 = 90ml.

Q20.3 – c: 250 cm^3
The volume of water displaced by the fish is 0.5 x 200 x 150 = 15,000 cm^3. Dividing by 60 fish gives an average volume of 15,000 / 60 = 250 cm^3.

Quantitative Reasoning – Practice

Q20.4 – a: 81
The tank must not go over the 80% mark, and we know that 15% of the total volume is taken by the gravel. Therefore the water will occupy 65% of the volume, i.e. 65% x 2,250 =1462.50 litres.
We are allowed no more than 2.5cm of fish for 4.5 litres of water. Therefore the maximum length of fish allowed is 1462.50 / 4.5 x 2.5 = 812.50 cm. This represents 81 fish of 10 cm each. Note that we need to round down as having 82 fish into the tank would make us go over the limit allowed.

Q20.5 – c: 192
Each tile measures 12.5 cm, which means that we can fit exactly 16 tiles in the 2 m length of the tank; and exactly 12 in the 1.50 m width. The total number of tiles is therefore 12 x 16 = 192.

Q20.6 – c: 88.5 cm
The height of the tank is equal to its volume i.e. 2250 l (or 2,250,000 cm^3 or 2.25 m^3) divided by the two dimensions that we are given. This gives: 2,250,000 cm^3 / 200 cm / 150 cm = 75 cm. Adding 18% gives 88.5 cm.

Q20.7 – d: 6.4 kg
First we need to establish the volume of gravel needed for the tank. This will be given by the floor surface area of the tank multiplied by the desired height of gravel, i.e. (using cm) 150 x 200 x 3 = 90,000 cm^3

Second we need to establish how much volume the 5 kg bag can cover. This is equal to 10,000 cm^2 (i.e. 1 m^2) x 7 = 70,000 cm^3.

Therefore we need 9/7th of a bag to cover the tank floor.
9 / 7 x 5 kg = 6.4 kg.

Another way to solve is to say that the surface area of the tank is 3 m^2 (2 x 1.5). Covering the surface with 3 cm of gravel would use the same amount of gravel as covering 1 m^2 with 9 cm of gravel. This would use 9/7th of a bag.

Q20.8 – c: £3,917
The cubic tank has a volume of 30 cm x 30 cm x 30 cm =27,000 cm^3. The enthusiast's tank has a volume of 2,250 litres, which is equivalent to 2,250,000 cm^3. Its cost would therefore be 2250 / 27 x £47 = £3,917.

QR 21 – World News

Q21.1 – c: 68%
(98,700 + 130,000) / (98,700 + 130,000 + 110,000) = 0.675, i.e. 68%.

Q21.2 – e: £87,828
The income is calculated as:
156,000 x (0.37 x 0.50 + 0.63 x 0.60) = £87,828.

Q21.3 – d: £124,495
The income from Europe comes from Newspaper B and 37% of Newspaper C. In Year 4, the income was 156,000 x 0.60 + 37% x 167,000 x 0.50 = £124,495.

Q21.4 – d: 719,000
Total sales in Year 6 will be:
133,000 x (1 – 0.50) + 176,000 x (1 + 1.33) + 156,000 x (1 + 5/9)
= 719,247.

Q21.5 – d: Year 11
We know that the retail price remains at Year 5 level i.e. 60p. We need to calculate N, the number of years that it will take to have 30p x 1.1^N > 60p.

If you know about logarithms then you will find the answer quickly. However, logarithms are beyond the scope of the UCAT, so if you are not familiar with them, don't worry; you can simply start with 30 on your calculator and keep adding 10% until you get a result which is above 60.

Year 4: 30 x 1.1 = 33
Year 5: 33 x 1.1 = 36.3
Year 6: 36.3 x 1.1 = 39.93
Year 7: 39.93 x 1.1 = 43.923
Year 8: 43.923 x 1.1 = 48.3153
Year 9: 48.3153 x 1.1 = 53.14683
Year 10: 53.14683 x 1.1 = 58.461513
Year 11: 58.461513 x 1.10 = 64.3076643 is over 60p.

By simply typing "x 1.1" continuously into the calculator, you should get to the result within 20 seconds.

Q21.6 – d: 41.4%
In Year 3, a total of 110,000 + 190,000 + 135,000 = 435,000 copies were sold. Out of this, 110,000 (Newspaper B) and 37% x 190,000 = 70,300 (Newspaper C) = 180,300 copies were sold in Europe.
This represents 180,300 / 435,000 = 41.4%

Q21.7 – b: £79,127
For Years 1 to 3, the price is the same regardless of the continent (55p).
For Years 4 and 5, the weighted price is 37% x 50p + 63% x 60p = 56.3p.

The total income was therefore:
(98,700 + 100,000 + 190,000) x 0.55 + (167,000 + 156,000) x 0.563 = £395,634.

The average across the five years is therefore: 395,634 / 5 = £79,126.80.

QR 22 – D.I.Y.

Q22.1 – d: 481.72 ft²
Instead of converting all dimensions into feet, it is quicker to make the calculation in metres and to convert the result into ft² using the conversion rate 1 m² = (3.27)² ft², i.e. 10.6929 ft². The total surface area is equal to:
(3.2 + 1.2 + 1.8 + 3.3) x 3.6 + (3.5 x 3.1) = 45.05 m².
45.05 x 10.6929 = 481.72 ft².

Q22.2 – a: 1.86 cm²
On a scale of 1:200, each dimension must be divided by 200. The hall's surface on paper is therefore:
(3.20 + 1.20 + 1.80) / 200 x (1.20 / 200) = 0.000186 m²

Given that 1 m² = 100 dm² = 10,000 cm², this is equal to:
0.000186 x 10,000 = 1.86 cm².

Q22.3 – e: 1.50 m
The combined surface area of the rectangle made up of the bedroom and the bathroom is (3.20 + 1.20) x (3.60 – 1.20) = 10.56 m². The surface of the bathroom alone is therefore: 10.56 – 8.76 = 1.80 m². The length of the longer wall is therefore equal to 1.80 / 1.20 (the length of the shorter wall) = 1.50 m.

Q22.4 – d: 30.57 m²
The total surface of the walls, ignoring any of the openings, is calculated as the total length of the walls multiplied by the height of the walls (2.65 m):
(3.60 + 3.30) x 2 x 2.65 = 36.57 m².

The surface area occupied by the openings is:
(1.5 x 2) + (0.6 x 2) + (0.9 x 2) = 6 m².

The area occupied by the wallpaper is therefore 36.57 – 6 = 30.57 m².

Q22.5 – c: 32.4m
Top wall: 3.20 + 1.20 + 1.80 + 3.30 = 9.5 m
Right wall: 3.6 + 3.1 = 6.7 m

Bottom wall (L shaped): Horizontal walls add up to 9.5 m (i.e. same as top wall) + 3.1 m for the lounge's left wall = 12.6 m

Left wall: 3.6 m

Total: 32.4 m
The astute candidate will have spotted that in fact this is the same as twice the length of the top wall + twice the length of the right wall.

Q22.6 – b: £137.65
There are two ways to think about this problem, both of which lead to the same calculation.

Method 1 (using surface area)
The surface area occupied by the wooden floor should equal that of the room. The room's surface area is 3.5 x 3.1 = 10.85 m². One plank covers 1 x 0.10 = 0.10 m². Therefore we need 10.85 / 0.10 = 108.50 planks, i.e. we need to buy 5 packs (one not fully used). The cost is 5 x 27.53 = £137.65.

Method 2 (using length)
The lounge's length is 3.5 m, therefore one row of planks will consist of 3.5 planks. The lounge's width is 3.1 m. Since each plank has a width of 10 cm, we can fit 10 planks in one metre and there in 3.1 m we can fit 31 planks. The total number of planks required is therefore 3.5 x 31 = 108.5, i.e. 5 packs (one not fully used). The cost is 5 x 27.53 = £137.65.

Quantitative Reasoning – Practice

QR 23 – Going for a Ride

Q23.1 – a: 17min 30s
The distance from E to C is 12 km. If this is done in 20 minutes then the average travelling speed is 36 km/h. The distance between E and H is 10.5 km. At a speed of 36 km/h, this can be travelled in 10.5/36 = 0.291666 hour. Multiplied by 60, this gives 17.5 minutes i.e. 17 minutes 30 seconds.

Q23.2 – c: 8.0 km/h
The journey totals 47+3+9+8+7.5+3+6.5 = 84 km. If the cyclist rides this distance in 10 hours 30 minutes (i.e. 10.5 hours) then his average speed is 84 / 10.5 = 8.0 km/h.

Q23.3 – d: Town F
Mr Smith has 2h25 but will only be driving for 2h25 – 49 minutes = 96 minutes return, or 48 minutes for one single journey i.e. 48/60th of an hour. Driving at 70 km/h he will travel 70 x (48/60) = 56 km. Starting from point G, this will correspond to Town F.

Q23.4 – c: Town E
The cyclist will have travelled 40/60 x 18 = 12 km in 40 minutes. Starting from Town C, this will take him to Town E (9km + 3km).

Q23.5 – d: 20 km/h
The distance between Town D and Town H is 47 + 3 + 7.5 = 57.5 km. At a speed of 18.4 km/h, this would take 57.5/18.4 = 3.125 hours, i.e. 3 hours and 7.5 minutes.

Reducing the journey by 15 minutes would make it last 3.125 – 0.25 = 2.875 hours. Riding 57.5 km in that amount of time gives an average speed of 57.5 / 2.875 = 20 km/h.

Note that if you ever had to guess, you could easily dismiss answers a, b and c. If he wants to reduce his journey time, he will need to travel faster than 18.4 km/h and therefore only answers d and e are suitable.

Q23.6 – c: 1h 28min
The distance to travel from C to G is equal to 65 km. The tube will therefore take 65/30 hours (i.e. 2.16666 hours, or 130 minutes) + (1 minute x 3 intermediary stops) = 133 minutes, i.e. 2 hours and 13 minutes.

The car will travel 47 km at 94 km/h and 18 km at 72 km/h and will therefore take 47/94 + 18/72 = 0.75 hours, i.e. 45 minutes. The difference is therefore 88 minutes, or 1 hour 28 minutes.

Q23.7 – c: 36 times
Line FCH has a loop journey of 24.5 km. At 49 km/h, this will be achieved in 30 minutes.

The buses will therefore go through Town C twice every hour. Over the period 5am to 11pm (representing 18 hours), this represents 36 occasions.

QR 24 – Hot Chocolate

Q24.1 – d: 8.1 g
A drink made of 18 g of powder and 200 ml of whole milk contains 9.6 g of fat. 100 g of powder contains 8.4 g of fat, therefore 18 g of powder contains 18/100 x 8.4 = 1.512 g. The amount of fat in 200 ml of whole milk is therefore 9.6 – 1.512 = 8.088 g.

Q24.2 – a: 56 ml
The total fat content of 2.464 g contains fat from the chocolate (18/100 x 8.4 = 1.512). Therefore the milk/water mix contains 2.464 – 1.512 = 0.952 g of fat. Since we are told there is no fat in water, this can only come from the semi-skimmed milk. If 100 ml of semi-skimmed milk contains 1.7 g of fat, then to obtain 0.952 g, we need a volume of 0.952 x 100 / 1.7 = 56 ml.

Q24.3 – c: 7.0 pints
The box contains 360 g of chocolate (i.e. 20 x 18g).
He therefore needs 20 x 200 ml = 4,000 ml of milk which is equivalent to 4000/570 = 7.0 pints.

Q24.4 – c: 2 drinks
One chocolate drink made from water will have the same number of calories as the 18 g of chocolate powder used to make it, i.e. 372 x 18 / 100 = 66.96 kCal. The three water-based drinks together will therefore account for 3 x 66.96 = 200.88 kCal.

This leaves an allowance of 800 – 200.88 = 599.12 kCal for all other whole-milk-based drinks. We know from the table that each contains 200 kCal and therefore he is just short of being able to make 3 drinks. Since 3 drinks will just about push him over the limit, the answer is 2 drinks.

Q24.5 – c: 164g
The box contains 360 g of chocolate; therefore, at a rate of 18 g per drink, the client can make 20 drinks out of the whole box. For these 20 drinks he will require 20 x 200 ml of milk, i.e. 4 litres.

The protein included in the whole box (360 g) of chocolate amounts to 360/100 x 8.9 g = 32.04 g. The protein included in the 4 litres of semi-skimmed milk amounts to 40 x 3.3 g = 132 g.

The total amount of protein is therefore 164.04g.

Q24.6 – c: 9 kCal
This can be calculated using either of the two columns.
Column 1: (372 – 4 x 8.9 – 4 x 65.2) / 8.4 = 9
Column 2: (200 – 4 x 8.0 – 4 x 20.4) / 9.6 = 9

QR 25 – Time Traveller

Q25.1 – e: 6h 20min
The time in Los Angeles is 3 hours behind the time in New York. Therefore if a flight leaving New York at 11:30 (New York time) arrives at 14:50 (Los Angeles time), when the plane arrives in Los Angeles it will be 17:50 in New York (i.e. 3 hours more).

Therefore, when expressed in New York time, the flight times are 11:30 to 17:50 i.e. a duration of 6 hours and 20 minutes.

Q25.2 – c: 13h 35min
There are two ways of calculating the result:

The long way
Travel time from London to Paris = 10:15 – 7:50 = 2:25 – 1 hour difference = 1 hour 25 minutes.

Arrival at 10:15 in Paris means departure at 11:15 from Paris, hence waiting time of 1 hour.

Travel time from Paris to LA: 13:25 – 11:15 = 2:10 + time difference of 9 hours = 11 hours 10 minutes.

Total time travelled = 1:25 + 1:00 + 11:10 = 13 hours 35 minutes.

The short way
Essentially, since we are asked to calculate the total travelling time, it does not matter what happens between departure and arrival. Leaving at 7:50 from London makes him arrive in Paris at 10:15, where he can transfer to the 11:15 to LA, which arrives at 13:25.

The travelling time is therefore 13h 25min – 7h 50min = 5h 35min plus the time difference between London and Los Angeles (8 hours) = 13h 35min.

Q25.3 – d: 5,840km
The travel time between Paris and New York is 2 hours (difference between departure and arrival time) + 6 hours' time difference = 8 hours. Since the average speed is 730 km/h, the distance is 8 x 730 = 5,840km.

Q25.4 – e: 4h 15min
For this question, there is no need to deal with time differences at all, since the initial and final destinations are the same for both.

Jack flies via Paris using the 9:25 from London to Paris. He arrives in Paris at 11:50 and can then catch the 13:00 to LA, which arrives at 15:10.

John flies via New York using the 9:10 from London to NY. He arrives at 12:10 in NY, where he can then catch the 15:50 from NY to LA, which arrives at 19:10.

John therefore left 15 minutes earlier than Jack but arrived 4 hours later. He will therefore have travelled 4 hours 15 minutes more than Jack.

Q25.5 – d: 17:40
The last flight from NY to LA leaves at 20:10 therefore the new Paris to NY flight should arrive in NY at 19:40 (30 minutes before). Since the difference in time between the departure and arrival time is always 2 hours, this means that the plane should leave Paris at 17:40 local time.

Q25.6 – d: 68,474
All flights from Paris to Los Angeles take 11 hours and 10 minutes. Four daily flights represent 44 hours and 40 minutes of flight.

The fuel consumed is therefore: (44+40/60) x 730 x 2.1 = 68,474 litres.

Quantitative Reasoning – Practice

QR 26 – Conferencing & Banqueting

Q26.1 – d: £400
Although the number of participants is 7, the contract has a minimum of 8 participants required. Therefore the cost is £50 x 8 = £400.

Q26.2 – d: £799
The cost of each of the DDR items on a room basis is as follows:

Room: £250
Projector: £189
Flipchart: £15
30 coffee breaks (3 breaks x 10): 30 x £2.50 = £75
Orange juice (2 jugs) = 2 x £10 = £20
10 sit-down lunches: 10 x £20 = £200
Water: 10 bottles: 10 x £5 = £50
Total = £799

Q26.3 – e: 16
There are two ways of resolving this question:

Method 1 – Write an equation
The crossover point "P" where the DDR cost is equal to the RB cost is calculated as follows: 45 P = £250 + £15 + (2.50 x 3 + 20) x P.
i.e. 17.5 P = £265, hence P = 15.14.

At P = 15, the DDR cost is cheaper than the RB cost.
At P = 16, the DDR cost is greater than the RB cost.

Note: once you have identified which costs are fixed and which costs depend on the number of participants, you can also find the solution using trial and error, based on the options on offer.

Method 2 – Average cost calculation
Under a DDR contract, the cost per person is £45. Therefore we must find the number of participants which gives a cost of £45 under the RB contract.

If we take off the cost of food and drink (£20 + 3 x £2.50 = £27.50 per person), we are left with an average cost of £45 - £27.50 = £17.50 to pay for the room and the projector.

The total cost for the room and the flipchart is £250 + £15 = £265.
Therefore the limit is calculated as follows: 265 / 17.50 = 15.14.

Q26.4 – c: £44.04
The new rate is 45 / 1.175 x 1.15 = £44.04.

Q26.5 – d: £37.84
The average cost per person will be the £30 cost charged by the caterer + the cost of the room (including surcharge) split between 50 people, i.e. 30 + (350 x 1.12 / 50) = £37.84.

QR 27 – Milking It

Q27.1 – d: 5.089 kg
The daily production of milk is 15 x 8.75 = 131.25 litres, which weighs 131.25 x 1.034 = 135.7125 kg. 15% of this is cream, of which only 25% is butter. The weight of the butter is therefore 135.7125 x 0.15 x 0.25, i.e. 5.089 kg.

Q27.2 – c: 1,343.55
In April (i.e. 30 days), the weight of milk produced would have been:
30 x 15 x 8.75 x 1.034 = 4,071.375 kg. At £0.33 per kilogram, this would cost £1,343.55.

Q27.3 – c: 1.027 kg
If the volume of water added is 25% of the volume of raw milk, then in 1 litre of the new mix there are 800ml of milk and 200ml of water. This weighs: 0.8 x 1.034 + 0.2 = 1.0272kg

Q27.4 – c: 2,920.5 kg
On average, a cow will consume 19,800 / 160 / 15 = 8.25 kg per day during winter. He now has to feed 3 additional cows for 118 days, hence the hay required for that period will be 3 x 118 x 8.25 = 2,920.5 kg.

QR 28 – A Colourful Life

Q28.1 – b: 200ml
The volume of yellow paint contained in 2 litres of Amazon is 10% of 2 litres, i.e. 200ml.

Quantitative Reasoning – Practice

Q28.2 – c: 22%
The total volume of paint obtained is 500 ml.

The amount of red paint included in 100 ml of Crimson is 70% of 100 ml i.e. 70 ml. The amount of red paint included in 400 ml of Amazon is 10% of 400 ml, i.e. 40 ml.

In total, there is therefore 70 + 40 = 110 ml of red paint in a total volume of 500 ml. This is equivalent to 22%.

Q28.3 – e: 1.212 litres
A pot of 1 litre of Violet will contain:
- 400 ml of red
- 400 ml of blue
- 200 ml of yellow

Since we are only adding yellow paint to it, the volume of red and blue paints will not change.

Therefore, once we have obtained the Chocolate colour, it will be made up of 400ml of red, 400ml of blue and an unknown quantity of yellow.

We know that Chocolate contains 33% of both red and blue paint; therefore once the colour has been created, the 400ml of red will represent 33% of the final volume. The final volume is therefore 400 / 0.33 = 1,212 ml or 1.212 litres.

Q28.4 – c: 43.6%
The fact that the paints are mixed in equal quantities makes it easier to calculate. If we take a sample of 100 ml of each of the paints then the paint resulting from the mix will contain the following volume of blue paint: 33 + 80 + 45 + 40 + 20 = 218 ml out of a total volume of 500 ml.

The percentage is therefore 218 / 500 = 0.436 i.e. 43.6%.

QR 29 – Advertising Rates

Q29.1 – d: £720
The cost of a colour advert spanning two columns, with a height of 8 cm is: £75 x 8 x 1.2 = £720.

Q29.2 – c: £1,000
There are two options available:

- Option 1: Purchase 7 cm across 4 columns, which would cost £150 x 7 = £1,050.

- Option 2: Pay for a quarter page (7 cm is one quarter of the total 28 cm available). The cost would be £1,000. This is the cheapest option.

Q29.3 – b: £1,800
Scenario 1: The income generated is: 4 columns x 28 cm x £50 = £5,600.
Scenario 2: The income generated is £3,800.
The loss would therefore be £1,800.

Q29.4 – e: £2,325
Watch out for the minimum charge of 3 cm which will apply to the single column advert of 2 cm. The income gained from the adverts will be: (1000 x 1.2) + (75 x 5) + 3 x (50 x 4) + (50 x 3) (min charge) = £2,325.

Q29.5 – e: £20,160
The maximum income will be generated by selling all adverts on a single column basis, with all adverts having a height of 1 cm and being charged at a minimum rate of 3 cm, in full colour.

This is equivalent to 28 adverts per column, i.e. 112 adverts per page at a maximum cost of 3 x £50 x 1.2 = £180 each. The maximum income is therefore 112 x 180 = £20,160.

QR 30 – A Matter of Time

Q30.1 – b: 6 minutes
The additional journey time is 5 minutes for the first part of the journey (20 – 15) plus 1 minute for the second part of the journey (14 – 13). The final two parts took the same amount of time in both years.

Q30.2 – d: 76 km/h
The total distance was 12 + 18 + 34 = 64 miles.
This was travelled in 13 + 25 + 43 = 81 minutes (or 81/60 hours).
The average speed was therefore: 64 x 1.6093 / 81 x 60 = 76 km/h.

Quantitative Reasoning – Practice

Q30.3 – d: 10.20%
The journey time in 1987 on the Southend to Fenchurch Street line was 49 minutes. In 2008, it was 54 minutes. This represents an increase of 54 / 49 = 1.102, i.e. 10.2%

Q30.4 – d: 86.9 km/h
In 1987, the total journey time was 5 minutes less than in 2008. We are told that this time must be recovered on the Faversham to Chatham portion of the route and therefore this part of the journey (18 miles) will need to be done in 20 minutes instead of 25 minutes. 18 miles in 20 minutes is equivalent to 54 miles in an hour. Converting to kilometres (x 1.6093) gives a speed of 86.9 km/h.

Q30.5 – a: 50 miles
The number of miles on the Canterbury to Victoria Line is 64. Therefore the cost on a pound per mile basis is calculated as 15.90 / 64 = £0.2484375.

A ticket on the Lewes to Victoria line costs £12.40. Since the cost on a pound per mile basis is the same on both lines, the number of miles on the Lewes to Victoria line is 12.40 / 0.2484375 = 49.91 miles (rounded up to 50 miles).

QR 31 – Within Shopping Distance

Q31.1 – d: 650
The number of shops is obtained by looking at the grey bars and the left axis for each of the distances. It is equal to: 200 + 100 + 50 + 100 + 50 + 100 + 50 = 650 shops.

Q31.2 – e: £150m
We are asked for the total turnover (i.e. average turnover x number of shops) for shops within a 5-mile radius so both the 0–1 and the 1–5 categories need to be included. Expressed in thousands of pounds:

Total turnover for 0–1-mile radius = 600 x 200 = 120,000.

Total turnover for 1–5-mile radius = 300 x 100 = 30,000.

Total = 120,000 + 30,000 = 150,000. This is in thousands of pounds; hence the answer is £150m.

Q31.3 – a: 0–1
This is the type of question where it pays to look at the graph carefully. The section 0–1 has both the highest average turnover and the highest number of shops so it is the obvious answer.

Q31.4 – e: 70.6%
There is no substitute for doing all calculations here. To accelerate the process, you can, however, place together all data which have a common element:

Total turnover (in thousands)
= 200 x 600 + 100 x (300+400+200) + 50 x (600+200+100) = 255,000.

Turnover for shops within a 10-mile radius (i.e. the first three categories) in thousands = 200 x 600 + 100 x 300 + 600 x 50 = 180,000.

Percentage = 180,000 / 255,000 = 70.6%

Q31.5 – a: £5,500
First, we are told that all shops have a turnover over £100,000. So all of them will pay the 0.5% tax on the full £100,000 i.e. £500.

On average, the shops have a turnover of 600,000. So the portion above 100,000 will average 600,000 – 100,000 = 500,000 across all shops. A tax of 1% will correspond to an amount of £5,000.

In total the average tax is therefore £5,500 per shop.

Q31.6 – c: 595
The total number of shops within 10 miles is 200+100+50 = 350.
The total number of shops beyond 10 miles is 100+50+100+50 = 300.
Total number of shops after the change = 0.8x350 + 1.05x300 = 595.

Q31.7 – e: Can't tell
Because the zones are concentric around the reference point, two shops that are within the 10–15 zone could actually be up to 30 miles apart. The best we can conclude is that the pensioner will never be able to visit shops in zone 0–1, 20–25 and 25–30, but we can't conclude on how many shops he will actually have access to within the other zones.

Quantitative Reasoning – Practice

QR 32 – Shaken, not Stirred

Q32.1 – d: 250ml
The volume of vodka required is: 50x2 + 25x5 + 1x25 = 250 ml

Q32.2 – b: 35.25 ml
Alcohol volume = 25x40% + 25x15% + 50x43% = 35.25 ml

Q32.3 – d: 64
The 8 Tequila Sunrise cocktails will have used 800 ml of orange juice, leaving 3.2 litres for the Screwdriver cocktails (which is the only other cocktail that can be made with orange juice in this bar). This can make 3,200/50 = 64 Screwdriver cocktails.

Q32.4 – c: Velocity
As for all questions which look as if many calculations are required, you should try to identify ways of cutting down on the work required.

A quick scan of the table will identify that:

- All five options contain vermouth
- Most alcohols have an alcohol content of around 40% whereas vermouth only contains 15%. Therefore those containing proportionately more vermouth would contain less alcohol.
- Most of the cocktails in the list of options have a volume of 75 ml.

If you had to hazard a guess, Velocity would be a good candidate for the cocktail with the least volume of alcohol.

Check:
- Martini: 25x15%+ 50x43%= 25.25 ml
- Vodkatini: 50x45% + 25x15% = 26.25 ml
- **Velocity: 50x15% + 25x43% = 18.25 ml**
- Orange Bloom: 25x40% + 25x15% + 50x43%= 35.25 ml
- Journalist: 5x40% + 25x15% + 50x43% = 27.25 ml

Q32.5 – d: +22.4%
Volume of alcohol in Balalaika: 25x40% + 25x45% = 21.25 ml
Volume of alcohol in XYZ = 25x40% + 40x40% = 26 ml
Increase = 26 / 21.25 = 1.224 i.e. 22.4% increase

113

1300 UCAT Practice Questions

Q32.6 – b: 1.3 litres
We need to make 3 litres of Velocity and 1.5 litres of Long Island. A Velocity cocktail has a volume of 75 ml (50+25) and a Long Island cocktail has a volume of 125 ml. Therefore we need to make the equivalent of 3000/75 = 40 Velocity cocktails and 1500/125 = 12 Long Island cocktails.

This gives us a Gin volume of 40x25 + 12x25 = 1300 ml, or 1.3 litres.

QR 33 – Entente Cordiale

Q33.1 – d: 5h 41min
The UK leg of the journey is 130 km. The French leg of the journey is 300 km. The journey time is therefore: 130/110 + 300/120 + 2 hours (ferry) = 5.681818 hours i.e. 5 hours and 41 minutes.

Q33.2 – b: 20 km
The fuel tank has a capacity of 45 litres, which will enable the courier to drive a distance of 45 x 10 = 450 km.
The total distance from London to Paris is 430 km. Therefore he will be able to get to Paris safely but will run out of petrol 20 km thereafter.

Q33.3 – b: £65.54
The courier starts with a tank containing 20 litres of fuel. By the time he reaches the first petrol station, he will have travelled 80 km and therefore used 80/10 = 8 litres, leaving 12 litres in the tank. He therefore needs a top up of 45–12 = 33 litres. The cost is 33 x 89p = £29.37.

By the time he reaches the second petrol station, he will have travelled 150 km, using 15 litres. Refuelling will cost 15 x 1.25 / 1.20 = £15.62.

He then needs to travel 180 km and therefore use 18 litres of fuel to get to the final petrol station, where refuelling costs 18 x 1.37 / 1.20 = £20.55. The total spend equals £29.37 + £15.62 + £20.55 = £65.54.

Q33.4 – b: €23.13
The spend for Car A is calculated as follows:
(20/15) x 0.95 + (180/15) x 0.87 + (150/15) x (0.99x1.20) = €23.59.

The spend for Car B is calculated as follows:
(20/10) x 1.76 + (180/10) x 1.47 + (150/10) x (0.93x1.20) = €46.72.

The difference is €23.13.

114

Quantitative Reasoning – Practice

Q33.5 – b: 23 litres
There are only 3 possibilities for refuelling on the way:

- Between London and Dover: this would only be for 8 litres and would cost £7.12, well below the €28.75 that he paid.
- At the petrol station after Calais: this would be for 23 litres, calculated as (80+50+100)/10. It would cost 23 x €1.25 = €28.75 (the answer we are looking for).
- At the petrol station before Paris, this would be for 41 litres and would cost 41 x €1.37 = €56.17.

Another way to get to the answer is to spot that, roughly speaking, a litre of unleaded will cost between €1 and €1.4. A cost of €28.75 would therefore mean a refuelling of between 20 and 29 litres. This can only happen at the middle petrol station. At that petrol station the refuelling would need to be for 23 litres in view of the distance driven to get there and the consumption of 1 litre per 10km.

QR 34 – Parking

Q34.1 – d: 80p
A 37-minute stay will be charged as 40 minutes and will therefore cost 4 x 20p = 80p.

Q34.2 – e: £1.30
According to the system set out in Note 3, the first period of 5 minutes (5:55pm – 6:00pm) will be charged at 30p and the second part of the stay (6:00pm – 6:15pm) will be charged at the standard £1. Hence the total is £1.30.

Q34.3 – e: £83.10
The Monday – Friday 9am – 6pm stays will each cost:
- 9am to 1pm: 4 hours x 6 periods x 20p = £4.80
- 1pm to 6pm: 5 hours x 6 periods x 30p = £9.00

Total cost= £13.80 per day.

The Saturday and Sunday 9am - 6pm stays will each cost: 9 hours x 3 periods x 15p = £4.05 per day. We also need to account for 6 overnight stays i.e. £6 in total. Total cost = 5 days x £13.80 + 2 days x £4.05 + £6 overnight = £83.10.

Q34.4 – d: £20
The week-day cost from 9am to 6pm is £13.80 (see previous question for calculation). However, he can use the ticket from 8:30am to 9:00am, which would normally be charged at the standard £1 fee. The total for the day is therefore £14.80. Over 5 days, this costs 5 x 14.80 = £74, hence a saving of £20.

Q34.5 – e: 50p
Note 3 tells us that he will be charged a full 20p for the first 2 minutes and a full 30p for the next 2 minutes (since both are in different zones and therefore calculated separately with their own minimum charge).

Q34.6 – e: Saturday 1:40pm
Cost of Friday 5pm to 6pm = 6 x 30p = £1.80
Cost of overnight stay (Friday – Saturday) = £1. Cumulative total: £2.80
This leaves £2.10 to spend on the Saturday daytime. The cost of 15p per period, he can spend 2.10/0.15 = 14 periods of 20 minutes, i.e. 4 hours and 40 minutes in total. He must therefore have left the car park by Saturday 1:40pm.

QR 35 – It Rings a Bell

Q35.1 – d: £155
Tariff 4 includes 700 minutes (covering calls to the Green network only) and 250 texts (covering texts to all networks). Therefore his telephone bill for that month would be as follows:
- Monthly fee: £35
- 300 minutes to Green network: included
- 300 minutes to H_2O network: Not included – would be charged at 40p per minute i.e. a total of £120
- Total of 250 texts: included.

Hence the total bill would be £155.

Q35.2 – e: Tariff E
His usage corresponds to 630 minutes and 450 texts. Looking at the options proposed:

- Tariff 3 would be £35 but he would need to pay for an additional 30 minutes at 15p each i.e. an extra cost of £4.50. Total £39.50.

- Tariff 4 (also £35) would cover all his 630 minutes but would only cover 250 texts out of the 450 texts he expects to use (a shortfall of 200 texts). Therefore he would be liable for an additional £20. Total £55.

- Tariff C (£25) would result in having to pay for an additional 330 minutes and an additional 150 texts, i.e. £99 + £18 extra. Total £142.

- Tariff D (£30) would cover the minutes and all but 50 of the messages, i.e. an extra cost of £6. Total £36.

- Tariff E (£35) would cover everything.

Q35.3 – e: 817 min
Since both tariffs include the same number of texts, the move becomes worthwhile when the cost of Tariff E including any additional minutes becomes greater than the basic cost of Tariff F, which is £40.

Tariff F will become better than Tariff E when the cost of the additional minutes is greater than £5. The additional cost of 1 minute is 30p. Therefore he will need to speak for 5 / 0.3 = 16.67 minutes, which represents the cut-off point. He would therefore need to speak for an additional 17 minutes on top of the allowance of 800 minutes, i.e. a total of 817 minutes.

Q35.4 – b: 800
Tariff 6 has a monthly fee of £55. This leaves £450 – £55 = £395 for the cost of calls (texts are not charged separately under this tariff).

Out of the calls he made, 220 + 280 + 1000 + 500 = 2000 minutes are on the Green network, with the first 1500 minutes being included in the monthly fee. Therefore the 500 additional minutes will be charged, at a cost of 500 x 15p per minute, i.e. a total of £75.

This then leaves £395 – £75 = £320 for calls made to John. Minutes spent calling the H_2O network are charged at a rate of 40p per minute. The time spent calling John was therefore 320 / 0.40 = 800 minutes.

QR 36 – Voting Turnout

Q36.1 – c: 700
2800 x 25% = 700

Q36.2 – d: 5800
The number of people aged 25–54 in Constituency A who voted is:
60% x 5000 + 20% x 3500 + 50% x 4200 = 3000 + 700 + 2100 = 5800.

Q36.3 – d: 3000
The number who did not vote is (1 – 50%) x 3000 + (1 – 70%) x 5000
= 1500 + 1500 = 3000.

Q36.4 – c: 43%
The total population over 65 is 7500 + 1500 + 5000 + 4500 = 18,500.

Those who voted represent:
32% x 7500 + 40% x 1500 + 70% x 5000 + 90% x 4500 = 2400 + 600 + 3500 + 4050 = 10,550.

Therefore 18500 – 10550 = 7950 did not vote.
They represent 7950 / 18500 = 43%.

ABSTRACT REASONING

TIPS & TECHNIQUES

+

226
PRACTICE QUESTIONS & ANSWERS

6 Abstract Reasoning Format, Purpose & Key Techniques

FORMAT

The abstract reasoning part of the UCAT contains 55 items associated with shapes, which you must complete in 13 minutes (an additional minute is given so that you can read the instructions). Those items can take one of four possible types of question, which we describe in the following sections.

Typically, the exam will include:
- 50 items of Types 1 and 4 (a total of 10 exercises, each with 5 test shapes to allocate), and
- 5 items of Types 2 and 3 (each being a separate exercise).

Timewise, you should aim to spend approximately one minute on Type 1 and Type 4 exercises (so a total of 10 minutes) and 30 seconds on Type 2 and Type 3 exercises (so 2.5 minutes), hence a total of 12.5 minutes.

PURPOSE

The abstract reasoning test is designed to assess your ability to develop ideas, test them and change your approach if necessary. This is a skill that you will need to use and demonstrate throughout your medical career. For example:

- As a doctor you will often be presented with a set of symptoms and/or results which you will need to use to forge an opinion about possible diagnoses. An ability to recognise patterns in the data available to you will help you identify those diagnoses.

- Once you have determined a number of possible diagnoses (so-called "differential diagnoses"), you will need to test whether they are viable before discounting them or accepting them.

- Much of the data will come from a medical history that you will have taken from a patient and from the results of tests that you will have ordered. Some of the information will be relevant, but some of it won't. Your strength as a doctor will lie in your ability to sieve through the

Abstract Reasoning – Practice

information to use the relevant data and discard the irrelevant information.

- If you are involved in research, you may need to identify patterns in the data provided so that you can establish links between two or more parameters.

6.1 Type 1 Questions – Set A, Set B or Neither

You are given two sets of abstract shapes: Set A and Set B. All shapes within Set A are linked in one way; all shapes within Set B are linked in another way. Your first task is to determine the nature of the relationships between all shapes within each set. Once you have done so, you are given five test shapes and are asked to determine whether they belong to Set A, Set B or neither set.

EXAMPLE

SET A   SET B

In this example, you can clearly see that every single shape within each set contains two objects – a circle and another object – and that both overlap. However, in Set A, the circle crosses the other object on two separate edges, whereas, in Set B, the circle crosses the other object on the same edge.

It is worth noting that, although the relationship that unites all shapes in Set A is different to the relationship that unites all shapes in Set B, there is a similarity, i.e. both relationships refer to the manner in which the objects intersect. In the exam, this is a useful feature which will help you out for some of the more difficult exercises.

Once you have determined the relationships within each set, you can then proceed to the test shapes to decide which set they belong to, if any. For example:

Test shape 1
This test shape belongs to Set B because the circle crosses the shape on one edge only.

Test Shape 2
This shape belongs to neither set because the circle crosses the triangle on three different edges.

In some cases, the shapes will contain objects or features which are "distractors", i.e. they do not play any particular role and are simply there to confuse you. You will therefore need to recognise quickly which objects matter and which do not.

KEY TECHNIQUES

Typically, in the exam, you will only have one minute per Type 1 exercise, during which you will need to identify the relationships within each set and allocate each of the five test shapes to either set.

This gives you an average of 13 seconds per shape, which is very little; though in reality it will likely take you 30 seconds to identify the relationships leaving you with just 6 seconds per shape thereafter. It is therefore crucial that you have at your disposal a number of techniques that you can use to work out the correct relationships and that you are fully aware of the possible combinations that can come up in the exam; this will help you discard

Abstract Reasoning – Practice

the wrong relationships early on, and will assist you in recognising the more viable relationships at the earliest opportunity.

In this section, we have set out a number of techniques that you will need to practise when you do the abstract reasoning practice exercises and will help you save time at the exam:

Consider then validate or reject the simple/obvious relationships
Before you start making life complicated for yourself, make sure that you have considered the obvious. The possibilities are endless but here are some of the key relationships that you cannot afford to miss:

Type and size of the objects
- Are all objects within the shapes of the same type or different types?
- Are some objects of the same size or are they all different sizes?
- Is there one type of object which stands out in all shapes and could be a key object?
- Is there an object which consistently appears in each shape but with different colours and could be a key object?

Number of objects
- Is the number of objects the same in all shapes?
- Is the number of objects of one type the same in all shapes?
- Is there a relative relationship between two different types of objects (e.g. number of white objects = number of black objects + 1)?
- Is the number of objects of one type linked to a feature of another object (e.g. is the number of circles within each shape equal to the number of sides of another object within the shape)?
- If there are arrows, have you considered relationships which are linked not just to the number of arrows but also the number of arrow-heads (some arrows may be double ended)?

Number of sides
- Do all the objects have the same number of sides?
- Do all the objects have an odd or even number of sides?
- Do all the objects have a number of sides that is a multiple of 2, 3 or another number?
- Do the above relationships apply when taking all the shapes together as opposed to each object individually (e.g. is the sum of the number of sides for all objects within one shape the same)?

- Is the number of sides of one object linked to another object? For example, is the number of sides of Object 1 equal to the number of sides of Object 2 + 1?

Symmetries
- Are some objects a symmetrical image of other objects, either through line symmetry (i.e. mirror image) or rotational symmetry?

Number and type of angles
- Are all the angles under/over 90 or 180 degrees?
- Are there a fixed number of right angles?
- Does the number of right angles match the number of other objects within the shape?

Intersections
- Is the number of intersections the same in all shapes within the set?
- Do only certain types of objects intersect (e.g. those in a given colour, or those with a given number of edges)?
- Do the objects only intersect in a certain way (e.g. intersections are on straight edges but not on curved edges)?
- Do the objects that result from the intersection (i.e. the overlapping area) form a specific pattern which is the same across all shapes (e.g. they all have four sides, or they are coloured in the same way – striped, black, white)?

Colour of the objects
- Does the colour of the objects influence the counting of some of the key features (e.g. if you add the number of edges of the white shapes to double the number of edges of black shapes, do you get the same number)?
- Are some types of objects always of one particular colour (e.g. are all objects with four sides coloured in black)?

Position and direction of the objects
- Are some specific objects always in the same place? For example, is there always a triangle in the top right corner? If there is a circle in the shape, is it always in the centre of the shape or in a corner?
- Do some objects always point in the same direction? For example, are the triangles always pointing upwards? If an arrow is present, is it always pointing in the same direction?

Abstract Reasoning – Practice

- Is there always one type of object placed the same way relative to another object? For example, is there always a square to the right of a triangle? Or are the objects arranged in the same clockwise manner in each of the shapes?
- Are some objects inside others?
- Is one object overlapping another object in the same way in every shape? For example, is the black object always overlapping a white object? If yes, is it always the black or white object which is on top? Or it is always the object with the least number of sides which is on top?
- If the shapes contain a lot of arrows, are they all pointing in the same direction? Or perhaps they are pointing in all directions but one?

Consider relationships of dependence between objects
There are sets of shapes in which the status of one object will depend on another object, which acts as a key. For example:

In this set of shapes, there is always one white triangle and a number of black diamonds. It is therefore clearly a requirement that, in order to belong to this set, all shapes should have one and only one white triangle of this type, and that any diamonds present in the shape should be black and of the standard size of those present in the shape here.

However, you may have spotted too that some triangles are pointing upwards and others downwards. A quick count of the black shapes will reveal that, when the triangle points upwards, the number of diamonds is odd, whilst when the triangle points downwards the number of diamonds is even.

Another example:

In this set, there are several relationships, all of which are linked to the arrow:

- There is always one arrow next to two objects which feature one above the other and which are always white.
- If the arrow points upwards then the two objects are different, whilst if the arrow points downwards then the objects are identical.
- If the arrow is white then the objects do not overlap, whilst if the arrow is grey then the two objects overlap.

In this example, the fact that the same arrow presents in each shape under different guises should be a clue that it may be a key shape that dictates a number of relationships.

Watch out for distractors

Distractors are objects that are simply sitting there and have no particular relationship with the others, or are features which you may be paying attention to but in fact have no bearing on the relationship between the objects present in each shape.

In this set, the relationship is that:

- There is always one black object and one white object that are of the same type (two rectangles, two diamonds, etc.), with the white replica being smaller in size.
- There is always another object present, but the type of the object, its colour, its size, and position do not matter (i.e. no pattern can be established).

Abstract Reasoning – Practice

The good news is that distractors are not very common and, when they are present, they tend to be simple to spot. The main problem is that they will waste your valuable time and, in some cases, you will always be wondering whether there is something that you have missed. The most common distractors are as follows:

- The colours of the objects within the shape do not matter.
- The shapes of the objects do not matter.
- There are additional objects floating around which simply fill the space but are not part of any relationship.

Use both sets together to work out the relationships
In the exam, the two sets have exclusive relationships, i.e. the relationship common to all shapes within Set A is different to the relationship common to all shapes within Set B. However, the two relationships are usually related in a mirrored fashion. For example, you could have the following relationships:

Example 1
Set A: All objects within the shape have an odd number of edges. All those with curved edges are black; the others are white.
Set B: All objects within the shape have an even number of edges. All those with curved edges are white; the others are black.

Example 2
Set A: The shapes all contain triangles and circles. The number of circles is equal to the number of isosceles triangles within the shape. Colour is irrelevant.
Set B: The shapes all contain triangles and circles. The number of circles is equal to the number of triangles with a right angle.

Example 3
Set A: There are seven objects within each shape. All objects which overlap another are white; the others are black.
Set B: There are eight objects within each shape. All objects which overlap another are black. The others are white.

Example 4
Set A: If the arrow points upwards, then all circles are black. A striped triangle means that the circles are on the right. A striped arrow means that the circles are on the left.

Set B: If the arrow points downwards, then all triangles are white. A striped arrow means that the circles are on the right.

Looking at both sets together can enable you to find relationships more easily because you know that, if you identify a relationship in one set, you are likely to have a similar type of relationship in the other set (albeit using opposite parameters). It may also enable you to spot relationships that you would not necessarily have spotted by looking at one set only.

If you struggle, take a step back and look at the whole picture
There are times when your brain might simply not be looking in the right place, or where you will obsessively attempt to find relationships where there aren't any, which could cause frustration.

If you are struggling to find relationships which link all the shapes within one set, step back from the page/screen and look at it from a slight distance. You may see patterns that did not come to mind before, such as a dominant colour or a similarity between some shapes.

6.2 Type 2 Questions – Complete the series

In Type 2 questions, you will be given four frames in an order which forms a logical series. You will then be offered four frames to choose from, amongst which you will need to pick the one that completes the series.

EXAMPLE

In this example, you can see that each frame is made up of three shapes, each with a different colour. You may have noticed that:

- The colours are rotating clockwise.
- If you follow a particular colour, the number of sides of the shape in that colour increases by 1 as we move from frame to frame:

Abstract Reasoning – Practice

> Grey: Triangle (3 sides) → Square (4) → Pentagon (5) → Hexagon (6).
> White: Pentagon (5) → Hexagon (6) → Arrow (7) → Star (8).
> Black: Circle (1) → Heart (2) → Triangle (3) → Square (4).
>
> We would therefore expect the next shape to look like this:
>
> Or any shape where the colours are laid out in a similar fashion, with a white nonagon, a black pentagon, and a grey heptagon.

KEY TECHNIQUES

For Type 2 questions, you will have approximately 30 seconds to find the answer. You therefore need to acquire a range of techniques that will help you find the link between the frames quickly. In many ways, the features to look for are similar to those described for Type 1 exercises, but they will apply in a different way because you are now in a dynamic context because the shapes are evolving as you move through the series given to you.

Isolate individual features rather than deal with everything at once
It is always tempting to look at all the objects at the same time in an effort to identify a pattern. Instead, focus on one feature at a time. So, for instance, in the example given above, you would meet success quickly simply by following what happens to the black shape as you would see that it rotates and that the number of sides increases.

In exercises where the same shapes are repeated this often helps uncover the key to the exercises quickly.

Watch out for alternate series.
If you are given the series 1, 2, 3, 4 then it is not hard to see that the following number should be 5. Similarly, if the series is 2, 4, 6, 8 then you will swiftly conclude that the next number should be 10.

However, some patterns will work in alternate fashion. For example, you may be given a pattern of the style 1,3,2,4, in which case the next number along will be 3. That is because, if you look at every other item you will realise that you have in fact two series mixed together. The first and third shape will start a series going 1, 2, etc. whilst the second and fourth shape will start a series going 3, 4, etc.

Now, if all you were given were the two numbers 1, 2 then it would be hard to complete the series. Would it be 3 because you simply add 1 to the previous number? Or would it be 4 because you double the previous number? This is where the alternate series will help you. In this case, the alternate series goes 3, 4 and so you can see you simply add 1 to the previous number.

An alternative way of looking at it, if you really want to avoid thinking about alternate series, is to tell yourself that the relationship may vary from frame to frame. So if we are given the series 1, 3, 2, 4, then we can conclude that the pattern between frames is +2, -1, +2; therefore the next one will be -1.

Another form in which alternate series may play a role is in making shapes appear only in some frames. So, for example, you may find that every other frame has a white circle.

There is a limited number of possible relationships
There are only so many ways in which a particular shape can move or change from one frame to the other. Here are some of the common possibilities you need to watch out for:

Movement
- Is the shape moving clockwise or anti-clockwise? Is it alternating?
- Is the shape always moving by the same distance (i.e. a quarter turn or halfway along the frame) or is the distance itself subject to a series of its own (e.g. the shape moved by a quarter turn, then half a turn, then three-quarters of a turn, etc.)?
- If the movement does not seem regular, is it regulated by another object? For example, is the distance the object is moving dictated by the number of sides of another object?
- Is the position of the object relative to that of another object?

Number of sides and angles
- Is the number of sides of each shape changing in a regular pattern? Is it increasing or decreasing? (Watch out as different shapes may go in different ways.)
- Are the angles part of a pattern (look at normal angles as well as right angles)?

Abstract Reasoning – Practice

Rotations
- Are some of the shapes rotating on themselves or flipping?

Non-linear patterns
Some patterns may not follow the simple linearity or rotational rules. In some cases, there may be a visual element too. That may particularly be the case when each shape is divided into several sections which may behave independently. For example, consider the following pattern:

1	3
1	2

5	4
3	7

5	11
9	6

13	8
7	15

If you follow each individual square, you will get:
- For the top left square: 1, 5, 5, 13 – which doesn't make much sense.
- For the bottom right square: 2, 7, 6, 15, which may give you a feeling that the 15 is the sum of the previous 3 numbers, but that is a bit far-fetched.
- And so on.

So essentially it is hard to draw any immediate meaningful conclusion. However, if you now look at the same pattern using the following lines:

1	3
1	2

5	4
3	7

5	11
9	6

13	8
7	15

You will see two distinct patterns: 1,2,3,4,5,6,7,8 and 1,3,5,7,9,11,13,15.

Proceed by elimination
Look carefully at the possible answers given to you and proceed by elimination. It is possible that, if you were not given any options and simply had to guess the answer, you would come up with several possible answers. A quick look at the options given to you might reveal that one of your possible answers is not actually on offer.

It is also possible that an exercise contains three or four different rules that govern the series but that you only need two of them to be able to conclude which of the options on offer is the actual answer. Remember: the aim is not to identify all the relationships but to identify the correct answer.

6.3 Type 3 Questions – A is to B as C is to X

In this type of question, you are shown how one frame can become another through a given process. You are asked to identify that process and apply it to a given frame. The process is very similar to that followed for question types 1 and 2, except that you only have one frame to work from and so all the clues will be contained within it. As such, a lot of the features will be identical in the two frames you are given as an example, but there will have been some colour swapping and movement between the shapes concerned.

EXAMPLE

is to

as   is to

Here, in the top part, we have a black hexagon containing a white arrow pointing downwards and a grey hexagon with a black arrow pointing towards the top left. The relationship is that each hexagon moves to the place towards which the arrow they contain points. The new hexagon then takes the colour of the arrow it contained. So the black hexagon moves down and becomes white. The grey hexagon moves diagonally and becomes black. Note that in this case the original colours of the hexagons do not matter.

In the starting shape we are given we have a triangle with a black down arrow and a square with a left-pointing grey arrow. So the missing frame should be like this:

Abstract Reasoning – Practice

KEY TECHNIQUES

In Type 3 exercises, since you are only given one frame, there are no distractors, i.e. shapes that are just sitting there for no purpose. Therefore, you need to understand the purpose of each feature. Here are some common areas you need to investigate:

Colours
- Have shapes taken on the colour of another shape?
- Have the colours rotated?
- Are the colours linked to another feature (e.g. number of sides, number of angles)?

Arrows
- Are arrows dictating a movement?
- Are arrows dictating an increase or a decrease in the number of sides or angles (in that case you would only have up and down arrows)?
- What are the arrows pointing to?

Alternative representations
- Does the right-hand shape contain totally different objects to the left-hand shape? That would indicate that the same relationship is being represented in different ways and you should look at the number of intersections and sides. For example:

On the left you can see that we have a hexagon (six sides) intersecting with a triangle (three sides) in four different places. On the right we have an X-axis split into three units and a Y-axis split into six units, and a grey area which goes up four notches on the Y-axis.

Rotations and translations
- Have shapes changed orientation or position?
- Do objects with certain colours or certain shapes move in the same way?

6.4 Type 4 Questions – Which shape belongs to Set A/B?

This type of question is pretty much identical to Type 1 except that, instead of being given five shapes and being asked which set they belong to, if any, you are given four shapes and asked which of them belongs to Set A (or to Set B). The principles and techniques involved are exactly the same as for Type 1 questions.

PRACTISE, PRACTISE, PRACTISE

Abstract reasoning questions can be hard if you are not used to them. Some people get the answer straight away, whilst others need to think more to find it. However, there are only so many ways in which shapes can be arranged and, if you practise long enough, you will start seeing similar patterns reappear through various exercises. In this section you will find 100 exercises (226 practice questions), split as follows:

Type 1: 26 exercises, 130 questions
Type 2: 26 exercises, 26 questions
Type 3: 26 exercises, 26 questions
Type 4: 22 exercises, 44 questions

Give yourself time to find the answer. Even if you spend well over the allocated time, you will learn a lot just by trying. As you practise, your ability to identify patterns will increase and you will slowly be able to find the answers in an increasingly shorter period of time.

7 Abstract Reasoning Practice Questions

This section contains 100 exercises covering a total of 226 questions, split as follows:

Type 1 – 26 exercises – 130 questions
Type 2 – 26 exercises – 26 questions
Type 3 – 26 exercises – 26 questions
Type 4 – 22 exercises – 44 questions

These questions are designed to help you develop an awareness of the different techniques and tips mentioned in the previous section and to familiarise you with the different approaches that actual exam questions can take.

The answers to all questions, together with explanations, can be found from page 210 onwards.

Once you have practised on all test shapes questions, you should be ready to confront the mock exam which features at the back of this book and replicates the actual exam's format (which often consists of 50 shapes of Type 1 and Type 4, and 5 shapes of Type 2 and Type 3).

You may want to wait until you have practised all sections in this book before going ahead with the mock exam.

1300 UCAT Practice Questions

AR 1 Practice
Practice Exercise 1 – Type 1

Set A

Set B

To which of the two sets above do the following shapes belong?

Shape 1.1   Shape 1.2   Shape 1.3   Shape 1.4   Shape 1.5

☐ Set A   ☐ Set A   ☐ Set A   ☐ Set A   ☐ Set A

☐ Set B   ☐ Set B   ☐ Set B   ☐ Set B   ☐ Set B

☐ Neither ☐ Neither ☐ Neither ☐ Neither ☐ Neither

Abstract Reasoning – Practice

AR 2 Practice
Practice Exercise 2 – Type 1

Set A

Set B

To which of the two sets above do the following shapes belong?

Shape 2.1   Shape 2.2   Shape 2.3   Shape 2.4   Shape 2.5

☐ Set A   ☐ Set A   ☐ Set A   ☐ Set A   ☐ Set A
☐ Set B   ☐ Set B   ☐ Set B   ☐ Set B   ☐ Set B
☐ Neither   ☐ Neither   ☐ Neither   ☐ Neither   ☐ Neither

137

AR 3 Practice

Practice Exercise 3 – Type 1

Set A

Set B

To which of the two sets above do the following shapes belong?

Shape 3.1   Shape 3.2   Shape 3.3   Shape 3.4   Shape 3.5

☐ Set A   ☐ Set A   ☐ Set A   ☐ Set A   ☐ Set A
☐ Set B   ☐ Set B   ☐ Set B   ☐ Set B   ☐ Set B
☐ Neither ☐ Neither ☐ Neither ☐ Neither ☐ Neither

Abstract Reasoning – Practice

AR 4 Practice
Practice Exercise 4 – Type 1

Set A

Set B

To which of the two sets above do the following shapes belong?

Shape 4.1   Shape 4.2   Shape 4.3   Shape 4.4   Shape 4.5

☐ Set A   ☐ Set A   ☐ Set A   ☐ Set A   ☐ Set A
☐ Set B   ☐ Set B   ☐ Set B   ☐ Set B   ☐ Set B
☐ Neither   ☐ Neither   ☐ Neither   ☐ Neither   ☐ Neither

139

1300 UCAT Practice Questions

AR 5 Practice

Practice Exercise 5 – Type 1

Set A

Set B

To which of the two sets above do the following shapes belong?

Shape 5.1   Shape 5.2   Shape 5.3   Shape 5.4   Shape 5.5

☐ Set A   ☐ Set A   ☐ Set A   ☐ Set A   ☐ Set A
☐ Set B   ☐ Set B   ☐ Set B   ☐ Set B   ☐ Set B
☐ Neither   ☐ Neither   ☐ Neither   ☐ Neither   ☐ Neither

140

Abstract Reasoning – Practice

AR 6 Practice

Practice Exercise 6 – Type 1

Set A

Set B

To which of the two sets above do the following shapes belong?

Shape 6.1   Shape 6.2   Shape 6.3   Shape 6.4   Shape 6.5

☐ Set A   ☐ Set A   ☐ Set A   ☐ Set A   ☐ Set A
☐ Set B   ☐ Set B   ☐ Set B   ☐ Set B   ☐ Set B
☐ Neither ☐ Neither ☐ Neither ☐ Neither ☐ Neither

1300 UCAT Practice Questions

AR 7 Practice
Practice Exercise 7 – Type 1

Set A

Set B

To which of the two sets above do the following shapes belong?

Shape 7.1   Shape 7.2   Shape 7.3   Shape 7.4   Shape 7.5

☐ Set A   ☐ Set A   ☐ Set A   ☐ Set A   ☐ Set A
☐ Set B   ☐ Set B   ☐ Set B   ☐ Set B   ☐ Set B
☐ Neither   ☐ Neither   ☐ Neither   ☐ Neither   ☐ Neither

Abstract Reasoning – Practice

AR 8 Practice
Practice Exercise 8 – Type 1

Set A **Set B**

To which of the two sets above do the following shapes belong?

Shape 8.1 Shape 8.2 Shape 8.3 Shape 8.4 Shape 8.5

☐ Set A   ☐ Set A   ☐ Set A   ☐ Set A   ☐ Set A

☐ Set B   ☐ Set B   ☐ Set B   ☐ Set B   ☐ Set B

☐ Neither ☐ Neither ☐ Neither ☐ Neither ☐ Neither

1300 UCAT Practice Questions

AR 9 Practice

Practice Exercise 9 – Type 1

Set A

Set B

To which of the two sets above do the following shapes belong?

Shape 9.1   Shape 9.2   Shape 9.3   Shape 9.4   Shape 9.5

☐ Set A   ☐ Set A   ☐ Set A   ☐ Set A   ☐ Set A
☐ Set B   ☐ Set B   ☐ Set B   ☐ Set B   ☐ Set B
☐ Neither   ☐ Neither   ☐ Neither   ☐ Neither   ☐ Neither

144

Abstract Reasoning – Practice

AR 10 Practice — Practice Exercise 10 – Type 1

Set A

Set B

To which of the two sets above do the following shapes belong?

Shape 10.1   Shape 10.2   Shape 10.3   Shape 10.4   Shape 10.5

- [ ] Set A   - [ ] Set A   - [ ] Set A   - [ ] Set A   - [ ] Set A
- [ ] Set B   - [ ] Set B   - [ ] Set B   - [ ] Set B   - [ ] Set B
- [ ] Neither - [ ] Neither - [ ] Neither - [ ] Neither - [ ] Neither

1300 UCAT Practice Questions

AR 11 Practice — Practice Exercise 11 – Type 1

Set A

Set B

To which of the two sets above do the following shapes belong?

Shape 11.1   Shape 11.2   Shape 11.3   Shape 11.4   Shape 11.5

☐ Set A   ☐ Set A   ☐ Set A   ☐ Set A   ☐ Set A

☐ Set B   ☐ Set B   ☐ Set B   ☐ Set B   ☐ Set B

☐ Neither   ☐ Neither   ☐ Neither   ☐ Neither   ☐ Neither

Abstract Reasoning – Practice

AR 12 Practice — Practice Exercise 12 – Type 1

Set A

Set B

To which of the two sets above do the following shapes belong?

Shape 12.1   Shape 12.2   Shape 12.3   Shape 12.4   Shape 12.5

- [ ] Set A   [ ] Set A   [ ] Set A   [ ] Set A   [ ] Set A
- [ ] Set B   [ ] Set B   [ ] Set B   [ ] Set B   [ ] Set B
- [ ] Neither [ ] Neither [ ] Neither [ ] Neither [ ] Neither

1300 UCAT Practice Questions

AR 13 Practice

Practice Exercise 13 – Type 1

Set A

Set B

To which of the two sets above do the following shapes belong?

Shape 13.1　　Shape 13.2　　Shape 13.3　　Shape 13.4　　Shape 13.5

☐ Set A　　☐ Set A　　☐ Set A　　☐ Set A　　☐ Set A

☐ Set B　　☐ Set B　　☐ Set B　　☐ Set B　　☐ Set B

☐ Neither　☐ Neither　☐ Neither　☐ Neither　☐ Neither

Abstract Reasoning – Practice

AR 14 Practice

Practice Exercise 14 – Type 1

Set A

Set B

To which of the two sets above do the following shapes belong?

Shape 14.1 Shape 14.2 Shape 14.3 Shape 14.4 Shape 14.5

☐ Set A   ☐ Set A   ☐ Set A   ☐ Set A   ☐ Set A
☐ Set B   ☐ Set B   ☐ Set B   ☐ Set B   ☐ Set B
☐ Neither   ☐ Neither   ☐ Neither   ☐ Neither   ☐ Neither

149

1300 UCAT Practice Questions

AR 15 Practice — Practice Exercise 15 – Type 1

Set A

Set B

To which of the two sets above do the following shapes belong?

Shape 15.1   Shape 15.2   Shape 15.3   Shape 15.4   Shape 15.5

☐ Set A   ☐ Set A   ☐ Set A   ☐ Set A   ☐ Set A

☐ Set B   ☐ Set B   ☐ Set B   ☐ Set B   ☐ Set B

☐ Neither ☐ Neither ☐ Neither ☐ Neither ☐ Neither

150

Abstract Reasoning – Practice

AR 16 Practice
Practice Exercise 16 – Type 1

Set A

Set B

To which of the two sets above do the following shapes belong?

Shape 16.1 **Shape 16.2** **Shape 16.3** **Shape 16.4** **Shape 16.5**

☐ Set A   ☐ Set A   ☐ Set A   ☐ Set A   ☐ Set A
☐ Set B   ☐ Set B   ☐ Set B   ☐ Set B   ☐ Set B
☐ Neither   ☐ Neither   ☐ Neither   ☐ Neither   ☐ Neither

1300 UCAT Practice Questions

AR 17 Practice — Practice Exercise 17 – Type 1

Set A / **Set B**

To which of the two sets above do the following shapes belong?

Shape 17.1 | **Shape 17.2** | **Shape 17.3** | **Shape 17.4** | **Shape 17.5**

- [ ] Set A   [ ] Set A   [ ] Set A   [ ] Set A   [ ] Set A
- [ ] Set B   [ ] Set B   [ ] Set B   [ ] Set B   [ ] Set B
- [ ] Neither   [ ] Neither   [ ] Neither   [ ] Neither   [ ] Neither

152

Abstract Reasoning – Practice

AR 18 Practice — Practice Exercise 18 – Type 1

Set A

Set B

To which of the two sets above do the following shapes belong?

Shape 18.1   Shape 18.2   Shape 18.3   Shape 18.4   Shape 18.5

- [ ] Set A
- [ ] Set B
- [ ] Neither

- [ ] Set A
- [ ] Set B
- [ ] Neither

- [ ] Set A
- [ ] Set B
- [ ] Neither

- [ ] Set A
- [ ] Set B
- [ ] Neither

- [ ] Set A
- [ ] Set B
- [ ] Neither

1300 UCAT Practice Questions

AR 19 Practice

Practice Exercise 19 – Type 1

Set A

Set B

To which of the two sets above do the following shapes belong?

Shape 19.1   Shape 19.2   Shape 19.3   Shape 19.4   Shape 19.5

☐ Set A   ☐ Set A   ☐ Set A   ☐ Set A   ☐ Set A
☐ Set B   ☐ Set B   ☐ Set B   ☐ Set B   ☐ Set B
☐ Neither   ☐ Neither   ☐ Neither   ☐ Neither   ☐ Neither

Abstract Reasoning – Practice

AR 20 Practice
Practice Exercise 20 – Type 1

Set A

Set B

To which of the two sets above do the following shapes belong?

Shape 20.1   Shape 20.2   Shape 20.3   Shape 20.4   Shape 20.5

☐ Set A   ☐ Set A   ☐ Set A   ☐ Set A   ☐ Set A
☐ Set B   ☐ Set B   ☐ Set B   ☐ Set B   ☐ Set B
☐ Neither   ☐ Neither   ☐ Neither   ☐ Neither   ☐ Neither

1300 UCAT Practice Questions

AR 21 Practice

Practice Exercise 21 – Type 1

To which of the two sets above do the following shapes belong?

Shape 21.1   Shape 21.2   Shape 21.3   Shape 21.4   Shape 21.5

☐ Set A   ☐ Set A   ☐ Set A   ☐ Set A   ☐ Set A
☐ Set B   ☐ Set B   ☐ Set B   ☐ Set B   ☐ Set B
☐ Neither ☐ Neither ☐ Neither ☐ Neither ☐ Neither

Abstract Reasoning – Practice

AR 22 Practice

Practice Exercise 22 – Type 1

Set A

Set B

To which of the two sets above do the following shapes belong?

Shape 22.1 Shape 22.2 Shape 22.3 Shape 22.4 Shape 22.5

☐ Set A ☐ Set A ☐ Set A ☐ Set A ☐ Set A
☐ Set B ☐ Set B ☐ Set B ☐ Set B ☐ Set B
☐ Neither ☐ Neither ☐ Neither ☐ Neither ☐ Neither

157

AR 23 Practice

Practice Exercise 23 – Type 1

Set A

Set B

To which of the two sets above do the following shapes belong?

Shape 23.1   Shape 23.2   Shape 23.3   Shape 23.4   Shape 23.5

- [ ] Set A
- [ ] Set B
- [ ] Neither

- [ ] Set A
- [ ] Set B
- [ ] Neither

- [ ] Set A
- [ ] Set B
- [ ] Neither

- [ ] Set A
- [ ] Set B
- [ ] Neither

- [ ] Set A
- [ ] Set B
- [ ] Neither

AR 24 Practice

Practice Exercise 24 – Type 1

Set A

Set B

To which of the two sets above do the following shapes belong?

Shape 24.1 **Shape 24.2** **Shape 24.3** **Shape 24.4** **Shape 24.5**

☐ Set A   ☐ Set A   ☐ Set A   ☐ Set A   ☐ Set A
☐ Set B   ☐ Set B   ☐ Set B   ☐ Set B   ☐ Set B
☐ Neither   ☐ Neither   ☐ Neither   ☐ Neither   ☐ Neither

1300 UCAT Practice Questions

AR 25 Practice

Practice Exercise 25 – Type 1

Set A

Set B

To which of the two sets above do the following shapes belong?

Shape 25.1   **Shape 25.2**   **Shape 25.3**   **Shape 25.4**   **Shape 25.5**

☐ Set A   ☐ Set A   ☐ Set A   ☐ Set A   ☐ Set A

☐ Set B   ☐ Set B   ☐ Set B   ☐ Set B   ☐ Set B

☐ Neither ☐ Neither ☐ Neither ☐ Neither ☐ Neither

Abstract Reasoning – Practice

AR 26 Practice
Practice Exercise 26 – Type 1

Set A

Set B

To which of the two sets above do the following shapes belong?

Shape 26.1   Shape 26.2   Shape 26.3   Shape 26.4   Shape 26.5

☐ Set A   ☐ Set A   ☐ Set A   ☐ Set A   ☐ Set A
☐ Set B   ☐ Set B   ☐ Set B   ☐ Set B   ☐ Set B
☐ Neither   ☐ Neither   ☐ Neither   ☐ Neither   ☐ Neither

161

1300 UCAT Practice Questions

AR 27 Practice — Practice Exercise 27 – Type 2

Which figure completes the above series?

A B C D

AR 28 Practice — Practice Exercise 28 – Type 2

Which figure completes the above series?

A B C D

162

Abstract Reasoning – Practice

AR 29 Practice
Practice Exercise 29 – Type 2

Which figure completes the above series?

A   B   C   D

AR 30 Practice
Practice Exercise 30 – Type 2

Which figure completes the above series?

A   B   C   D

163

AR 31 Practice

Practice Exercise 31 – Type 2

Which figure completes the above series?

A B C D

AR 32 Practice

Practice Exercise 32 – Type 2

Which figure completes the above series?

A B C D

Abstract Reasoning – Practice

AR 33 Practice
Practice Exercise 33 – Type 2

Which figure completes the above series?

A B C D

AR 34 Practice
Practice Exercise 34 – Type 2

Which figure completes the above series?

A B C D

1300 UCAT Practice Questions

AR 35 Practice — Practice Exercise 35 – Type 2

Which figure completes the above series?

A   B   C   D

AR 36 Practice — Practice Exercise 36 – Type 2

Which figure completes the above series?

A   B   C   D

166

Abstract Reasoning – Practice

AR 37 Practice
Practice Exercise 37 – Type 2

Which figure completes the above series?

A B C D

AR 38 Practice
Practice Exercise 38 – Type 2

Which figure completes the above series?

A B C D

1300 UCAT Practice Questions

AR 39 Practice
Practice Exercise 39 – Type 2

Which figure completes the above series?

A   B   C   D

AR 40 Practice
Practice Exercise 40 – Type 2

Which figure completes the above series?

A   B   C   D

Abstract Reasoning – Practice

AR 41 Practice
Practice Exercise 41 – Type 2

Which figure completes the above series?

A B C D

AR 42 Practice
Practice Exercise 42 – Type 2

Which figure completes the above series?

A B C D

169

1300 UCAT Practice Questions

AR 43 Practice — Practice Exercise 43 – Type 2

Which figure completes the above series?

A B C D

AR 44 Practice — Practice Exercise 44 – Type 2

Which figure completes the above series?

A B C D

170

Abstract Reasoning – Practice

AR 45 Practice
Practice Exercise 45 – Type 2

Which figure completes the above series?

A   B   C   D

AR 46 Practice
Practice Exercise 46 – Type 2

Which figure completes the above series?

A   B   C   D

1300 UCAT Practice Questions

AR 47 Practice
Practice Exercise 47 – Type 2

Which figure completes the above series?

A B C D

AR 48 Practice
Practice Exercise 48 – Type 2

Which figure completes the above series?

A B C D

172

Abstract Reasoning – Practice

AR 49 Practice
Practice Exercise 49 – Type 2

Which figure completes the above series?

A   B   C   D

AR 50 Practice
Practice Exercise 50 – Type 2

Which figure completes the above series?

A   B   C   D

173

1300 UCAT Practice Questions

AR 51 Practice
Practice Exercise 51 – Type 2

Which figure completes the above series?

A   B   C   D

AR 52 Practice
Practice Exercise 52 – Type 2

Which figure completes the above series?

A   B   C   D

Abstract Reasoning – Practice

AR 53 Practice
Practice Exercise 53 – Type 3

is to

as

is to

Which figure completes the statement?

A   B   C   D

AR 54 Practice
Practice Exercise 54 – Type 3

is to

as

is to

Which figure completes the statement?

A   B   C   D

175

1300 UCAT Practice Questions

AR 55 Practice
Practice Exercise 55 – Type 3

is to

as

is to

Which figure completes the statement?

A   B   C   D

AR 56 Practice
Practice Exercise 56 – Type 3

is to

as

is to

Which figure completes the statement?

A   B   C   D

176

Abstract Reasoning – Practice

AR 57 Practice — Practice Exercise 57 – Type 3

is to

as

is to

Which figure completes the statement?

A   B   C   D

AR 58 Practice — Practice Exercise 58 – Type 3

is to

as

is to

Which figure completes the statement?

A   B   C   D

1300 UCAT Practice Questions

AR 59 Practice — Practice Exercise 59 – Type 3

is to

as

is to

Which figure completes the statement?

A B C D

AR 60 Practice — Practice Exercise 60 – Type 3

is to

as

is to

Which figure completes the statement?

A B C D

178

Abstract Reasoning – Practice

AR 61 Practice
Practice Exercise 61 – Type 3

is to

as

is to

Which figure completes the statement?

A B C D

AR 62 Practice
Practice Exercise 62 – Type 3

is to

as

is to

Which figure completes the statement?

A B C D

1300 UCAT Practice Questions

AR 63 Practice
Practice Exercise 63 – Type 3

is to

as

is to

Which figure completes the statement?

A   B   C   D

AR 64 Practice
Practice Exercise 64 – Type 3

is to

as

is to

Which figure completes the statement?

A   B   C   D

180

Abstract Reasoning – Practice

AR 65 Practice
Practice Exercise 65 – Type 3

is to

as

is to

Which figure completes the statement?

A B C D

AR 66 Practice
Practice Exercise 66 – Type 3

is to

as

is to

Which figure completes the statement?

A B C D

1300 UCAT Practice Questions

AR 67 Practice
Practice Exercise 67 – Type 3

is to

as

is to

Which figure completes the statement?

A B C D

AR 68 Practice
Practice Exercise 68 – Type 3

is to

as

is to

Which figure completes the statement?

A B C D

182

Abstract Reasoning – Practice

AR 69 Practice
Practice Exercise 69 – Type 3

is to

as

is to

Which figure completes the statement?

A   B   C   D

AR 70 Practice
Practice Exercise 70 – Type 3

is to

as

is to

Which figure completes the statement?

A   B   C   D

183

1300 UCAT Practice Questions

AR 71 Practice
Practice Exercise 71 – Type 3

is to

as

is to

Which figure completes the statement?

A B C D

AR 72 Practice
Practice Exercise 72 – Type 3

is to

as

is to

Which figure completes the statement?

A B C D

184

Abstract Reasoning – Practice

AR 73 Practice
Practice Exercise 73 – Type 3

is to

as

is to

Which figure completes the statement?

A   B   C   D

AR 74 Practice
Practice Exercise 74 – Type 3

is to

as

is to

Which figure completes the statement?

A   B   C   D

185

1300 UCAT Practice Questions

AR 75 Practice — Practice Exercise 75 – Type 3

is to

as

is to

Which figure completes the statement?

A   B   C   D

AR 76 Practice — Practice Exercise 76 – Type 3

is to

as

is to

Which figure completes the statement?

A   B   C   D

Abstract Reasoning – Practice

AR 77 Practice
Practice Exercise 77 – Type 3

is to

as

is to

Which figure completes the statement?

A B C D

AR 78 Practice
Practice Exercise 78 – Type 3

is to

as

is to

Which figure completes the statement?

A B C D

AR 79 Practice

Practice Exercise 79 – Type 4

Set A | Set B

79.1 Which of the following belongs to Set A?

A   B   C   D

79.2 Which of the following belongs to Set B?

A   B   C   D

Abstract Reasoning – Practice

AR 80 Practice
Practice Exercise 80 – Type 4

Set A

Set B

80.1 Which of the following belongs to Set A?

A   B   C   D

80.2 Which of the following belongs to Set B?

A   B   C   D

1300 UCAT Practice Questions

AR 81 Practice
Practice Exercise 81 – Type 4

Set A

Set B

81.1 Which of the following belongs to Set A?

A   B   C   D

81.2 Which of the following belongs to Set B?

A   B   C   D

190

Abstract Reasoning – Practice

AR 82 Practice

Practice Exercise 82 – Type 4

Set A

Set B

82.1 Which of the following belongs to Set A?

A   B   C   D

82.2 Which of the following belongs to Set B?

A   B   C   D

191

1300 UCAT Practice Questions

AR 83 Practice
Practice Exercise 83 – Type 4

Set A

Set B

83.1 Which of the following belongs to Set A?

A B C D

83.2 Which of the following belongs to Set B?

A B C D

192

Abstract Reasoning – Practice

AR 84 Practice
Practice Exercise 84 – Type 4

Set A

Set B

84.1 Which of the following belongs to Set A?

A B C D

84.2 Which of the following belongs to Set B?

A B C D

193

AR 85 Practice — Practice Exercise 85 – Type 4

85.1 Which of the following belongs to Set A?

A   B   C   D

85.2 Which of the following belongs to Set B?

A   B   C   D

Abstract Reasoning – Practice

AR 86 Practice
Practice Exercise 86 – Type 4

Set A

Set B

86.1 Which of the following belongs to Set A?

A   B   C   D

86.2 Which of the following belongs to Set B?

A   B   C   D

AR 87 Practice

Practice Exercise 87 – Type 4

Set A

Set B

87.1 Which of the following belongs to Set A?

A   B   C   D

87.2 Which of the following belongs to Set B?

A   B   C   D

Abstract Reasoning – Practice

AR 88 Practice
Practice Exercise 88 – Type 4

Set A

Set B

88.1 Which of the following belongs to Set A?

A B C D

88.2 Which of the following belongs to Set B?

A B C D

197

1300 UCAT Practice Questions

AR 89 Practice
Practice Exercise 89 – Type 4

Set A

Set B

89.1 Which of the following belongs to Set A?

A B C D

89.2 Which of the following belongs to Set B?

A B C D

Abstract Reasoning – Practice

AR 90 Practice
Practice Exercise 90 – Type 4

Set A   **Set B**

90.1 Which of the following belongs to Set A?

A   B   C   D

90.2 Which of the following belongs to Set B?

A   B   C   D

199

1300 UCAT Practice Questions

AR 91 Practice — Practice Exercise 91 – Type 4

Set A

Set B

91.1 Which of the following belongs to Set A?

A B C D

91.2 Which of the following belongs to Set B?

A B C D

Abstract Reasoning – Practice

AR 92 Practice
Practice Exercise 92 – Type 4

Set A

Set B

92.1 Which of the following belongs to Set A?

A   B   C   D

92.2 Which of the following belongs to Set B?

A   B   C   D

1300 UCAT Practice Questions

AR 93 Practice

Practice Exercise 93 – Type 4

Set A

Set B

93.1 Which of the following belongs to Set A?

A B C D

93.2 Which of the following belongs to Set B?

A B C D

Abstract Reasoning – Practice

AR 94 Practice
Practice Exercise 94 – Type 4

Set A

Set B

94.1 Which of the following belongs to Set A?

A B C D

94.2 Which of the following belongs to Set B?

A B C D

1300 UCAT Practice Questions

AR 95 Practice
Practice Exercise 95 – Type 4

Set A

Set B

95.1 Which of the following belongs to Set A?

A   B   C   D

95.2 Which of the following belongs to Set B?

A   B   C   D

204

Abstract Reasoning – Practice

AR 96 Practice
Practice Exercise 96 – Type 4

Set A

Set B

96.1 Which of the following belongs to Set A?

A   B   C   D

96.2 Which of the following belongs to Set B?

A   B   C   D

205

1300 UCAT Practice Questions

AR 97 Practice

Practice Exercise 97 – Type 4

Set A

Set B

97.1 Which of the following belongs to Set A?

A   B   C   D

97.2 Which of the following belongs to Set B?

A   B   C   D

206

Abstract Reasoning – Practice

AR 98 Practice
Practice Exercise 98 – Type 4

Set A

Set B

98.1 Which of the following belongs to Set A?

A　　B　　C　　D

98.2 Which of the following belongs to Set B?

A　　B　　C　　D

207

1300 UCAT Practice Questions

AR 99 Practice
Practice Exercise 99 – Type 4

Set A

Set B

99.1 Which of the following belongs to Set A?

A   B   C   D

99.2 Which of the following belongs to Set B?

A   B   C   D

208

AR 100 Practice

Practice Exercise 100 – Type 4

Set A | **Set B**

100.1 Which of the following belongs to Set A?

A   B   C   D

100.2 Which of the following belongs to Set B?

A   B   C   D

8 Abstract Reasoning
Answers to Practice Questions

AR1 – Practice Exercise 1 – Type 1

Set A: The total number of edges across all objects in any one shape is equal to 13. For example, in the first shape, there are five circles (1 edge each, total 5 edges), one triangle (3 edges) and a pentagon (5 edges).

Set B: The total number of edges across all objects in any one shape is equal to 9. For example, in the first shape, there is one triangle (3 edges), two circles (2 edges) and one square (4 edges).

Answers:
Shape 1.1: Neither. 10 edges.
Shape 1.2: Set A
Shape 1.3: Neither. 14 edges.
Shape 1.4: Set A
Shape 1.5: Neither. 7 edges.

Comments:
Other questions that you should have asked yourself to check possible relationships (other than the basic ones) include:

- Does anything specific happen when an object is black? For example, is there always an odd or even number of objects in the shapes? Or are some objects in a specific location or of a specific size? It isn't the case here.

- Does the fact that some objects intersect matter? The intersections seem random here.

The fact that the objects in each shape are in very different combinations suggests that the relationships are not linked to the objects themselves. When you are presented with shapes which are very different, it is a good idea to check the number of sides to check a possible link. You only need to check three shapes to establish whether a pattern is present; if you find the same number then proceed to count the sides for the other shapes.

Abstract Reasoning – Practice

AR2 – Practice Exercise 2 – Type 1

Set A: There is at least one circle in each shape. All other objects have only straight edges (e.g. triangles, pentagons, squares).

Set B: There is also at least one circle in each shape, but also one object which has both straight and curved edges. There is also always one additional object with straight edges.

Answers:
Shape 2.1: Neither. All objects have straight edges, but there is no circle.
Shape 2.2: Set B
Shape 2.3: Neither. No straight-edged shape and no mixed shape either.
Shape 2.4: Neither. No circle.
Shape 2.5: Neither. No circle.

Comments:
The presence of a circle in each shape should be straightforward to detect at a glance. So is the presence of the mixed objects in Set B as they are in large format. This should lead you to think quickly that Set B must have at least one circle and one of the mixed objects.

At this point you must investigate whether there is a relationship with any other shapes. What we can say for Set B is that once we have excluded the circles and the big mixed object, we are left with either triangles or squares: all objects with straight edges.

You must also investigate further whether there is any relationship with the black colouring, but since Set B has two shapes which contain the same objects with a slightly different arrangement it is unlikely.

The relationship in Set A would be set to balance that in Set B in that we also have one circle at least and one object with straight edges, but no mixed object. Remember to use that "mirror" approach to derive the relationship in one set from that of the other set. It will save you a lot of time.

AR3 – Practice Exercise 3 – Type 1

Set A: Arrows point in all directions except towards the right.
Set B: Arrows point in all directions except towards the left.

1300 UCAT Practice Questions

Answers:
Shape 3.1: Neither. The relationship is that there should be arrows pointing in <u>all directions except right (Set A) or left (Set B)</u>. In 3.1, there are no downward-pointing arrows. This illustrates the need to derive the most specific relationship that you can find, i.e. in this case, not only the fact that there are no arrows pointing left or right but also the fact that there must be arrows pointing in all other directions.
Shape 3.2: Set A
Shape 3.3: Set A
Shape 3.4: Neither. Arrows pointing in all directions.
Shape 3.5: Set B

Comments:
When dealing with arrows, there are a limited number of options that you can consider. Direction is the most obvious one and in this case would give you the answer. Other relationships that you would need to investigate include:

- Is the number of arrows, either in total or in a given direction, constant? For example, is there always the same number of arrows pointing upwards? In this case, the answer is no.

- Is there some relationship between two sets of arrows within a shape? For example, it could be that in one set the number of arrows pointing upwards is twice the number of arrows pointing downwards (with a reverse mirror relationship for the other set). Here, the answer is no.

- Are some arrows in the same location (e.g. all arrows pointing to the left are towards the right-hand side of the shape)? This is not the case here.

AR4 – Practice Exercise 4 – Type 1

Set A: The rotational symmetry has an order of 2 (i.e. all objects look the same when rotated by half a turn).
Set B: The rotational symmetry has an order of 4 (i.e. all objects look the same when rotated by a quarter of a turn).

Answers:
Shape 4.1:   Neither. If the moon is rotated, it needs to do a full turn to look the same again.

Abstract Reasoning – Practice

Shape 4.2: Set A
Shape 4.3: Set A. (Note: if it did not have the line crossing in the middle, it would belong to Set B.)
Shape 4.4: Neither. The rotational order is 5, i.e. it needs to rotate by a fifth of a turn to look the same.
Shape 4.5: Neither. The arrow needs to do a full turn to look the same again.

Comments:
When you have single objects, the relationship is often linked to symmetry, to angles or number of sides. There are essentially two types of symmetry:

- Rotational symmetry (as above)
- Reflectional (or line) symmetry (i.e. you can fold along a line and obtain a mirror image).

All objects in Set A have two lines of reflectional symmetry except the parallelogram drawn under the rectangle, which is not line symmetrical. The only other symmetry left is therefore rotational.

In Set B, all objects have four lines of reflectional symmetry; however, this is a feature of objects that have a rotational symmetry order of 4 and therefore it amounts to the same relationship. So if this is the relationship that you have derived, then it is equally valid and will lead to the same result.

AR5 – Practice Exercise 5 – Type 1

Set A: All black objects can fit together within the white circle. This is not true of the grey objects.

Set B: All grey objects can fit together within the white circle. This is not true of the black objects.

Answers:
Shape 5.1: Neither. The two black objects do not fit within the circle and neither does the grey object.
Shape 5.2: Set A
Shape 5.3: Set B
Shape 5.4: Neither. All black objects fit within the circle but so does the grey object.
Shape 5.5: Neither. Both the black object and the grey object fit within the circle.

Comments:
This question is one which is best resolved by stepping back from the screen and looking at the two sets as a whole. Visually, you may be able to spot that the colour grey dominates Set A, and that the black colour dominates Set B.

Another clue is that the white circle appears in absolutely every single shape. Because of this it cannot be a distinguishing factor between Set A and Set B and therefore is likely to play some form of pivotal role. It may also simply be a distractor, but its omnipresence is worthy of investigation.

AR6 – Practice Exercise 6 – Type 1

The relationships rest on the number of white, black, and grey areas, irrespective of whether they are inner circles or outer rings.

Set A: Has a total number of 5 white sectors, 1 grey and 2 black.
Set B: Has a total number of 3 white sectors, 3 grey and 2 black.

Answers:
Shape 6.1: Set B
Shape 6.2: Set B
Shape 6.3: Neither. 4 white sectors.
Shape 6.4: Set A
Shape 6.5: Neither. 4 white sectors.

Comments:
Other relationships that you would need to investigate but do not occur here include:

- Is there a specific colour or combination which appears in the same place (e.g. the top left corner outer ring is always white)?

- Do the same combinations reoccur (e.g. are black outer rings always associated with a black inner ring)?

- Do the circles follow in a certain order clockwise (e.g. is an outer-white-ring/ inner-grey-circle combination always followed by an outer-black-ring/ inner-white circle)?

Abstract Reasoning – Practice

- Is there a link between the numbers of each coloured circle (e.g. is the number of outer white rings always equal to or a multiple of the number of inner black rings)?

- Are the rings set out in mirror images or reverse mirror images (i.e. with grey remaining grey but black becoming white and vice versa)?

AR7 – Practice Exercise 7 – Type 1

The relationship in each set is linked to the result when one multiplies the number of hours shown by the hour hand by the number of minutes shown by the minute hand.

Set A: The number of hours multiplied by the number of minutes is 60 (12x5, 2x30, 6x10, 4x15, 3x20 and 5x12).

Set B: The number of hours multiplied by the number of minutes is 120 (6x20, 4x30, 5x24, 3x40, 8x15 and 12x10).

Answers:
Shape 7.1: Neither. 3x5 = 15.
Shape 7.2: Neither. 3x45 = 135.
Shape 7.3: Neither. 3x30 = 90.
Shape 7.4: Set B
Shape 7:5: Neither. 9x60 = 540.

Comments:
Exercises involving clocks will either be linked to the number of minutes/seconds (in which case you simply need to manipulate the numbers given to derive a relationship) or to the angles between the two hands.

AR8 – Practice Exercise 8 – Type 1

All shapes contain the same objects to make up two "eyes" and a "mouth".

Set A: Each large circle contains 7 objects.
Set B: Each large circle contains 6 objects.

Answers:
Shape 8.1: Set B
Shape 8.2: Set A

Shape 8.3: Set A
Shape 8.4: Set A
Shape 8.5: Set A

Comments:
In this exercise, the fact that the objects within the large circle are set out to look like a face may make you lose sight of some of the more basic relationships such as the number of objects. Instead your brain will be looking naturally for a relationship based on symmetry or other factors linked to appearance, which may not be relevant. The lesson here is: do not ignore the obvious.

AR9 – Practice Exercise 9 – Type 1

The relationships are linked to the ability to link similar objects using a straight line without encountering another object.

Set A: The circles (regardless of their colour) are the only objects in each shape which can be linked by a straight line without encountering an object of a different type (e.g. triangle or square).

Set B: The triangles (regardless of their colour) are the only objects in each shape which can be linked by a straight line without encountering an object of a different type (e.g. circle or square).

Answers:
Shape 9.1: Neither. The squares can also be linked by an uninterrupted line.
Shape 9.2: Neither. The squares can also be linked by an uninterrupted line.
Shape 9:3: Set A
Shape 9:4: Set A
Shape 9:5: Set A

Comment:
The difficulty in this exercise is that there is a superposition of two concepts:

- You must be able to draw a straight line between similar objects.
- The circles or triangles must be the only objects for which this is possible.

Abstract Reasoning – Practice

If you identify only a partial relationship and miss out the fact that no other shapes can be linked by a straight line then you will get some of the answers wrong (though not all). Therefore, once you have found a relationship that, you feel, works, it is worth spending a few seconds extra to see whether it can be refined.

AR10 – Practice Exercise 10 – Type 1

Set A: The large object is white and the number of black circles is equal to the number of sides in the large object <u>minus</u> one. The remaining object is also white and can be of the same type or different type to the large object.

Set B: The large object is black; the number of white squares is equal to the number of sides <u>plus</u> one. The remaining object is white and is of the same type as the large object.

Answers:
Shape 10.1: Set A
Shape 10:2: Neither. The big object is white and has 4 sides. Therefore the shape would require 3 black circles and not 5 in order to fit within Set A.
Shape 10.3: Neither. For the shape to fit within Set B, the small white circle would need to be a small parallelogram instead.
Shape 10.4: Neither. Two big objects stand out.
Shape 10.5: Set B

Comments:
Too often, candidates look for relationships which are more complex than they really are. In many cases, a simple count of the number of sides is worth doing. To save time, simply count the sides in two shapes in each set to determine a possible pattern. If a pattern seems to emerge then count the rest.

AR11 – Practice Exercise 11 – Type 1

Both sets contain a white 'key' object in the top left corner. It is the position of the other copies of this object that are important, either horizontally, vertically or on the diagonal. The other objects are irrelevant.

Set A: Grey copies of the key object are two spaces away from the key object whilst black copies are three spaces away.

Set B: Grey copies of the key object are one space away from the key object whilst black copies are two spaces away.

Answers:
Shape 11.1: Set B
Shape 11.2: Set B
Shape 11.3: Neither. The black copy is one step away. It would need to be two or three steps away to belong to any set.
Shape 11.4: Set B
Shape 11.5: Neither. The black copy is one step away, as is the grey copy. The black copy would need to be two steps away for the object to belong to Set B.

Comments:
Look out for shapes with objects which are well aligned. In such cases, the relationships are often linked to their relative positions. In such cases, try to select the shapes which have some obvious features (such as the second shape of the first column in Set A, where you can clearly see that the two grey squares are two places away from the white object. This may give you an idea. In many cases, it can be difficult to determine a relationship based simply on one of the sets.

Use the fact that the relationships in both sets are of a similar nature to get ideas. For example, you may spot that in Set B the grey object is always close to the white object. Ask yourself whether there is a similar relationship in Set A. Once you have established the relationship between white and grey objects, ask yourself whether there may be a similar relationship for the black objects.

AR12 – Practice Exercise 12 – Type 1

Both sets have the same different shapes laid out in the same clockwise order, i.e. triangle, diamond, circle, heart, moon and square. The two sets differ in the relationships between the colours.

Set A:
- The Square and the Circle are always the same colour.
- The Triangle and the Heart are always of opposite colour (i.e. when one is black, the other one is white).

Abstract Reasoning – Practice

Set B:
- The Triangle and the Heart are always the same colour.
- The Square and the Circle are always of opposite colour (i.e. when one is black, the other one is white).

Answers:
Shape 12.1: Neither. The objects are in the wrong order.
Shape 12.2: Set B
Shape 12.3: Set A
Shape 12.4: Set B
Shape 12.5: Neither. Triangle, Heart, Square and Circle are all of the same colour.

Comments:
When the same objects are present in all shapes, you should watch out for the following:
- Is the object in one particular position always of the same colour or a particular type, e.g. is the top right corner shape always white or always a square? (This is not the case here.)
- Is there a relationship between two objects, e.g. a black triangle always matches with a white heart? (This is the case here in Set A.)
- Are the objects laid out in a certain order? (Watch out in particular for clockwise orders – this is the case here.)

AR13 – Practice Exercise 13 – Type 1

The relationships are linked to the order in which the series of dots rotates and their colours depending on the quarter in which they sit. The colour of the background is determined by the colours of the dots.

Set A:
The quarters may or may not contain dots. However, if they do, then the top left quarter only contains one, the top right quarter contains two, the bottom right quarter contains three and the bottom left quarter contains four.

All the dots within one quarter must be of the same colour, but they can have different colours between quarters. If the dots are all of the same colour then the background is of that colour. If the dots are of different colours then the background is grey.

Set B:
The number of dots also rotates clockwise but starting from the top right quarter instead of the top left quarter. All dots must be of the same colour. The background is of the opposite colour (i.e. black if the dots are white, and white if the dots are black. Grey is not an option in Set B).

Answers:
Shape 13.1: Set B
Shape 13.2: Neither. The colour pattern matches the requirement for Set A but the position of the dots does not. Also the position of the dots is correct for Set B but the colour pattern is not.
Shape 13.3: Set B
Shape 13.4: Set A
Shape 13.5: Set A

Comments:
In these shapes, it will get you nowhere to count the circles. The presence of several circles and the mix of colours make it difficult for the eye to pick up relationships quickly. If you are struggling to find a relationship within 30 seconds, you may want to back away from the page/screen to detach yourself from the detail. You will often find that it enables you to pick up some clues much more easily, such as – in this case – the fact that the circles are set out in a clockwise 1, 2, 3, 4 pattern, always starting from the same quadrant.

AR14 – Practice Exercise 14 – Type 1

The relationship is simply linked to the number of triangles versus the number of circles.

Set A: The number of triangles is equal to the number of circles.
Set B: The number of triangles is equal to the number of circles + 2.

Answers:
Shape 14.1: Neither. No triangles in the shape.
Shape 14.2: Set A
Shape 14.3: Neither. Number of triangles is lower than number of circles.
Shape 14.4: Neither. Number of triangles is lower than number of circles.
Shape 14.5: Set B

Abstract Reasoning – Practice

Comments:
Many of the shapes in this exercise are set out in a way that is designed to draw your attention towards false relationships such as a possible symmetry. In reality, the relationships are much simpler, being based on a basic count of objects. Do not let yourself be distracted by appearance unless you see a clear pattern emerging.

Also note that there are very few shapes with grey. In Set A, there is only one object which is grey. This is not enough to establish a pattern and therefore the colour of the objects has to be a distractor.

AR15 – Practice Exercise 15 – Type 1

In each shape, there are a total of six different types of objects. One type of object is represented 5 times (the black ones) and the other five types are represented only 4 times (appearing in various colours).

Set A: The 5 black objects are set out in an "X" pattern. The corner objects are all white (this is the only type of object which has all four white). All other objects present under different colours, with no particular pattern.

Set B: The 5 black objects form a "T" pattern (either straight or at an angle). The corner objects are the same and are all grey. This is the only type of object which has all four grey. All other objects present under different colours, with no particular pattern.

Answers:
Shape 15.1: Neither. The shape does have 5 black objects in a "T" pattern as well as 4 similar grey objects in the corners, suggesting that it would belong to Set B. However, the other objects would need to be in sets of four of each of the other unused objects (i.e. hearts, diamonds, squares, and flags). This particular shape only has circles and triangles.
Shape 15.2: Set B
Shape 15.3: Neither. The "X" pattern is contained within Set A, but the four corners are not all from the same white object since the top left corner is taken by one of the black objects.
Shape 15.4: Set A
Shape 15.5: Neither. The objects in the black "T" shape are not all the same.

Comments:
In this exercise, there are a lot of objects to count and look at: far too many to manage in just a couple of minutes. When you have busy shapes, step away from the sets and look at them from a distance. You will spot patterns more easily. Here, like in the exam, some shapes are clearer than others e.g. those with fewer colours. Look at these first and compare them to another easier shape. Once you have an idea of a possible relationship, see if it works for the other shapes.

When there are too many objects, you may also find it easier to step back to determine a possible visual pattern (such as the X or T patterns here). If your eyes are too close to the page/screen, you run the risk of paying too much attention to some of the useless detail. In these shapes, there are a lot of distractors when all that matters are the corner objects and the black objects.

AR16 – Practice Exercise 16 – Type 1

Set A: The total number of sectors is odd. There are always more black sectors than white sectors.

Set B: The total number of sectors is even. There are always more white sectors than black sectors.

Answers:
Shape 16.1: Set B
Shape 16.2: Set A
Shape 16.3: Neither. One sector of each colour so no dominance.
Shape 16.4: Neither. Odd number of sectors, with dominance of white.
Shape 16.5: Neither. Odd number of sectors, with dominance of white.

Comments:
On first visual inspection, you may be able to determine quickly that Set A has a black dominance and that Set B has a white dominance. You should then count the sectors and count the sides to determine any other possible relationships. In this case you would be able to determine the odd/even relationships. Note that it is not the number of objects which counts here, but the number of sectors (so for example, the white circle with a cross within it would count as four sectors and not one object).

Abstract Reasoning – Practice

AR17 – Practice Exercise 17 – Type 1

The relationships are linked to the relative positions of the arrows and the circles, the colour of the circles in the corners and the nature of the remaining objects.

Set A: The arrows always present in pairs with one being slightly lower than the other. They are always located in one corner, with a black circle present in the diagonally opposite corner.
- If the arrows both point upwards, then the remaining objects all have straight edges only.
- If the arrows both point downwards then the remaining objects all have curved edges only.
- If the arrows point in opposite directions, then the remaining objects all have a mix of curved and straight edges.

Set B: The arrows always present in pairs with one being slightly lower than the other. They are always located in one corner, with a circle present in the free corner located on the same vertical line.
- If the arrows both point upwards, then the circle is white and the remaining objects all have curved edges only.
- If the arrows both point downwards, then the circle is black and the remaining objects all have straight edges only.
- If the arrows point in different directions, then the circle is grey and the remaining objects have both straight and curved edges.

Answers:
Shape 17.1: Set A
Shape 17.2: Neither. No set has the circle on the same horizontal line as the arrows.
Shape 17.3: Neither. The black circle is not in a corner.
Shape 17.4: Neither. The white circle cannot be opposite the arrows.
Shape 17.5: Neither. For Set B, the black circle requires arrows pointing downwards. In any case, even if the arrows pointed down, we would need to have all straight-edged objects in order to satisfy the relationship for Set B.

Comments:
The main difficulty in this exercise is that you must exclude the circle to understand the relationships. If you exclude the circle (which is present in all the shapes) then you can see more easily that each shape has objects

223

of different natures: straight, curved, or mixed edges. The other difficulty is that, other than the colour of the circle in Set B, the colour of the other objects does not matter. This confuses things visually.

When you have objects in common between all shapes, they will either be used as a key object (i.e. they will influence other objects) or they will be used as distractors. In Set A, the black circle is a distractor, i.e. it is simply sitting there, always black, and always in a corner. The arrows, however, are linked to the other objects. In Set B, the colour of the circle is linked to the directions of the arrows and therefore both are pivotal objects.

AR18 – Practice Exercise 18 – Type 1

Set A: The total number of edges equals 16 when counting black objects as double.

Set B: The total number of edges equals 20 when counting white objects as double.

Answers:
Shape 18.1: Set A. 8 sides x 2 = 16
Shape 18.2: Set B. 2 x 5 + 2 x 5 = 20
Shape 18.3: Neither. The total number of sides is 12 + 6 = 18. Since both of the objects are of a different colour then one of the numbers will need to be doubled, which will take the number of sides way over 20.
Shape 18.4: Set B. Total number of edges = 12 + 8 = 20 in black.
Shape 18.5: Set B. 7 edges in the arrow x 2 = 14. Adding 2 x 3 sides = 6 sides for the triangles gives 20.

Comments:
If counting sides does not lead you to any immediate conclusion, do not forget to allow for the colour element. In most cases (and indeed in the exam itself), the most likely relationship is that one colour will count double. If a straight count or a count based on one colour being doubled does not lead you to any conclusion, then move on.

Abstract Reasoning – Practice

AR19 – Practice Exercise 19 – Type 1

Set A: All large objects which have a right angle are black. Those with no right angle are grey. The number of white diamonds is equal to the number of right angles present in the coloured objects within the shape.

Set B: All large objects which have a right angle are grey. Those with no right angle are black. The number of white diamonds is equal to the number of angles which are not right angles in the coloured objects within the shape.

Answers:
Shape 19.1: Neither. The black objects all have right angles, which would suggest Set A. However, the number of white diamonds is equal to the number of angles which are not right angles instead of the number of right angles.
Shape 19.2: Set A
Shape 19.3: Set A
Shape 19.4: Neither. One right angle and the object is black suggests Set A. However, there are two diamonds instead of one.
Shape 19.5: Set B

AR20 – Practice Exercise 20 – Type 1

There is always one arrow on the left-hand side, with two other objects (one black, one grey) on its right, one being above the other.

Set A:
- If the arrow points upwards, then the grey object is higher than the black object. If the arrow points downwards then the black object is higher than the grey object.
- A white arrow means that the two objects overlap, with the bottom object being above the top object.
- A shaded arrow means that the two objects do not overlap.

Set B:
- If the arrow points upwards, then the black object is higher than the grey object. If the arrow points downwards then the grey object is higher than the black object.
- A white arrow means that the two objects overlap, with the black object being on top of the grey object.
- A shaded arrow means that the two objects do not overlap.

225

Answers:
Shape 20.1: Neither. A white arrow means objects should overlap.
Shape 20.2: Set A
Shape 20.3: Neither. The black object would need to be on top of the grey object in order for the shape to belong to Set B. To belong to Set A, the black object would need to be above the grey object, with the black object being on top.
Shape 20.4: Set B
Shape 20.5: Neither. The arrow is on the right instead of the left.

Comments:
Objects which feature on their own within each of the shapes are often the main drivers for the relationships within shapes. For example, in this case, the arrow is dictating through both its orientation and its colour the order and colour of the other objects.

If you identify an object which is likely to play such pivotal role, it is often best to avoid looking at all the shapes at the same time. For example, rather than looking at Set A in its entirety, start looking at the shapes which have white arrows (regardless of their orientation) and see what they have in common. Then look at the shapes which have an arrow pointing upwards (regardless of colour) and see what they have in common.

Bearing in mind that the relationships in Set A and Set B are often related, look at shapes with similar features in both sets. For example, looking at the shapes which have an upwards pointing arrow both in Set A and Set B will help you easily determine that, in Set A, the grey object is always above the black object whilst, in Set B, the reverse applies.

AR21 – Practice Exercise 21 – Type 1

Each shape has two objects: one black, one white.

Set A: The white object always has 4 more sides than the black object.
Set B: The black object always has 2 more sides than the white object.

Answers:
Shape 21.1: Neither. The white shape has 2 more sides than the black shape.
Shape 21.2: Set B

Abstract Reasoning – Practice

Shape 21.3: Neither. It does have 10 white edges and 6 black edges which would suggest Set A. However, it contains 3 objects instead of the 2 contained in all shapes within Set A.
Shape 21.4: Neither. Difference between numbers of sides is only one.
Shape 21.5: Set A

Comments:
The seemingly random nature of the objects (including the fact that some have angles and others don't and that some are totally separate and others within one another) suggests that the relationships is linked to the number of sides rather than any other feature.

AR22 – Practice Exercise 22 – Type 1

Each shape has one three-arrow object, one triangle and two circles. In all shapes:

- The set of arrows is always in a corner.
- The triangle is always in the middle alongside an edge.
- If the triangle is white then the two circles are side to side.
- If the triangle is striped then the two circles are not touching.
- If the triangle is grey then the two circles overlap.

Set A: The set of arrows points in three directions except one. The triangle is located in the middle of the edge towards which no arrow points. So, for example if the three arrows point left, down, and right, then the triangle will be in the middle of the top edge of the shape. The location of the circles within the shape is random.

Set B: The triangle is located in the middle of the edge towards which the middle arrow points. So, for example if the three arrows point left, down, and right, then the triangle will be in the middle of the bottom edge of the shape. The circles are always located along the edge opposite the triangle.

Answers:
Shape 22.1: Set A
Shape 22.2: Set B
Shape 22.3: Set B
Shape 22.4: Neither. The triangle is striped but the circles touch.
Shape 22.5: Neither. The arrows are in the middle of the bottom side.

Comments:
All objects are of a similar nature in all shapes, the only distinguishing factors being the orientation of the arrows and the location of the objects. When large arrows are present within a shape, they are often used as a pivotal object, i.e. an object that guides the others. Since arrows are primarily used for directions, it makes sense to look at the position of the other objects in relation to the directions in which the arrows are pointing.

Since all circles are grey, they are only involved either because of their location or because of their overlapping nature. By looking at the shapes which have similarly arranged circles (e.g. just touching or overlapping) then you should be able to spot their link to the colour of the triangles.

AR23 – Practice Exercise 23 – Type 1

All black objects are the same and all white objects are the same.

Set A:
- The number of black objects equals the number of arrowheads.
- The number of white objects equals the number of straight lines.
- The objects are spread randomly within the shape.

Set B:
- The number of black objects equals the number of arrowheads.
- The number of white objects equals the number of straight lines + 1.
- The white and black objects are separated by the straight lines forming a boundary.

Answers:
Shape 23.1: Set A
Shape 23.2: Neither. The number of black objects is greater than the number of arrowheads.
Shape 23.3: Neither. The numbers of white and black objects satisfy the relationship for Set B. However, the objects are randomly set out instead of being separated on each side of the boundary.
Shape 23.4: Set B
Shape 23.5: Neither. The shape would meet the criteria for Set B if the two white objects were on the same side of the line.

Abstract Reasoning – Practice

Comments:
When a shape contains many arrows, the relationships are either linked to the directions of the arrows (e.g. they are all pointing in the same direction) or they are used as a pivotal shape with the other objects in the shape being linked, as is the case here, to the number arrows or arrow heads.

Look out for shapes that have similar features as they provide valuable clues. For example, two shapes in Set A have 3 white ovals but have 1 and 2 black diamonds respectively. The only difference between the two is the number of arrow heads. Similarly, in Set B, the top two shapes both have 2 black diamonds but the second shape has many more white ovals (which can be linked to the more complex set of straight lines).

AR24 – Practice Exercise 24 – Type 1

In both sets there is only one black object and the number of other objects is equal to the number of sides (and therefore angles) in the black object.

Set A: The black object has an even number of sides. All other objects (white or grey) have an odd number of sides. The number of grey objects equals the number of right angles in the black object. All other objects are white (and therefore their number equals the number of angles in the black object which are not right angles).

Set B: The black object has an odd number of sides. All other objects (white or grey) have an even number of sides. The number of white objects equals the number of right angles in the black object. All other objects are grey (and therefore their number equals the number of angles on the black object which are not right angles).

Answers:
Shape 24.1:   Set A
Shape 24.2:   Neither. All objects have an even number of sides.
Shape 24.3:   Neither. The grey objects have a mix of even and odd number of sides (e.g. triangle and diamond).
Shape 24.4:   Set B
Shape 24:5:   Set A

Comments:
The presence of a large black object should alert you to the fact that it plays a pivotal role (the exercise would be too easy if there simply had to be a

1300 UCAT Practice Questions

large black object!). Number of sides and angles usually play a sizeable role in the relationships within each set.

AR25 – Practice Exercise 25 – Type 1

Each set consists of three objects: one arrow and two other objects of a similar nature, though not always of the same colour or size. The size and colour of the objects is dictated by the colour of the arrow.

In all cases, the three objects are located in all but the bottom left corner and the object in the bottom right corner is always white. The shape of the object in the top right corner is taken as the shape of the object below it, rotated according to the direction of the arrow. So an arrow pointing to the right means that the object in the top right corner is equal to the object in the bottom right corner rotated 90 degrees clockwise, whilst a left-pointing arrow indicates a rotation of 90 degrees anti-clockwise. A "U-turn" arrow means that the object is rotated 180 degrees.

Set A:
- A white arrow means that the two other objects have the same colour and same size.
- A black arrow means that the two objects have the same size but the top object is black.
- A striped arrow means that both objects are white but the top object is of smaller size than the bottom object.

Set B:
- A white arrow means that both objects are white but the top object is of a smaller size.
- A black arrow means that the top object is black and is of greater size than the bottom object.
- A striped arrow means that both objects are white and of the same size.

Answers:
Shape 25.1: Set A
Shape 25.2: Neither. The star is not rotated.
Shape 25.3: Set A
Shape 25.4: Set B
Shape 25.5: Neither. The black object is smaller than the white object, which fits the profile of neither set in the presence of a black arrow.

Abstract Reasoning – Practice

Comments:
The presence of an arrow in each shape (with different orientations and colours) indicates that it is likely to play a central role in defining the other shapes. You can see clearly that the other two objects are of the same type but in different positions and colours.

To facilitate your task of identifying the relationship within each shape, avoid looking at all the shapes at the same time. Take all the shapes which have an arrow pointing towards the right and see whether you can identify a trend. Similarly look at all the shapes which have a white/striped arrow and see if you can spot similarities.

When several parameters come into play (e.g. colour and orientation), fix one of these parameters by selecting all the shapes that satisfy it (e.g. by selecting all white arrows) and see how the other parameter influences the shapes.

AR26 – Practice Exercise 26 – Type 1

Each shape contains two dominoes, one of which is black and the other one white. The relationships are linked to the orientation of the dominoes and the total number of dots on each domino.

Set A:
In each domino, the higher number of dots is at the top and the lower number of dots is at the bottom. The domino with the lower total number of dots is black.

Set B:
In each domino, the higher number of dots is at the bottom and the lower number of dots is at the top. The domino with the higher total number of dots is black.

Answers:
Shape 26.1: Set A
Shape 26.2: Neither. Higher number of dots is not always at the top or the bottom.
Shape 26.3: Set B
Shape 26.4: The higher number of dots is at the bottom, suggestive of Set B. However, the domino with the lower total number of dots is black.

Shape 26.5: Neither. The higher number of dots is at the top and at the bottom respectively.

Comments:
In the same way that, when you have clocks, the answer usually has to do either with the angle between the two hands or with the result of adding up or multiplying the numbers pointed to by the two hands, when you have dominoes the relationships are fairly limited. You would need to look at the following:

- Where the larger or smaller number of dots are positioned.
- The total number of dots of each domino, across the top or the bottom and on the diagonals.
- The relationship between two sets of dots (e.g. is the top number of dots always one more than the bottom number of dots?).

AR27 – Practice Exercise 27 – Type 2

Answer: B
The triangle rotates anti-clockwise and alternates between grey and black.
The white circle alternates between top and bottom of the frame.
The square rotates clockwise and alternates between black and white.

AR28 – Practice Exercise 28 – Type 2

Answer: D
All circles are moving downwards by one space as shown on the diagram below. Those reaching the bottom reappear at the top.

With regard to the "Morse code", the pattern at the top represents the black dots and the pattern at the bottom represents the white dots read in descending order. One dot is represented by a short line and two consecutive dots are represented by a long line.

So for example, using the left frame above: ●○●●○○●

Abstract Reasoning – Practice

AR29 – Practice Exercise 29 – Type 2

Answer: A
The number of sides of the outside shape increases by 2 between each frame: 1 – 3 – 5 – 7. So we expect the next one to have 9 sides.

The number of sides of the inside shape decreases by 1 between each frame: 5 – 4 – 3 – 2. So we expect the next one to have 1 side.

The inside shape alternates between white and black.

AR30 – Practice Exercise 30 – Type 2

Answer: C
The chess board is being unveiled through a clockwise rotation (in a snail configuration). The number of squares added increases by one as we move from one frame to the next.

AR31 – Practice Exercise 31 – Type 2

Answer: B
The circles form a "snake" which rotates anti-clockwise to fill the square. The starting frame has four circles already in place and thereafter, between each frame, the snake advances by three places.

The snake is made up of circles, which alternate black and white, with the number of circles of one colour being one more than the number of circles of the previous colour.

Only the relevant circles appear in the square. So for example, in the second frame, we have 1 black, followed by 2 whites, followed by 3 blacks. Thereafter, in the snake, there are 4 whites but since we are only advancing 3 circles at a time, only one of the 4 white circles is visible. When we move to the third frame, all of those 4 white circles are visible.

233

1300 UCAT Practice Questions

In the fourth square the tail of the snake has 3 black circles showing out of a possible 5. So the next step will have the remaining two black circles and one white circle.

```
   6 whites      5 blacks    4 whites  3 blacks  2 w   1b
  ○○○○○○ ● ● ● ● ● ○ ○ ○ ○ ● ● ● ○ ○ ●
                                            | Frame 1
                                    | Frame 2
                            | Frame 3
                    | Frame 4
  Not visible | Frame 5
```

AR32 – Practice Exercise 32 – Type 2

Answer: C
The black dots are moving horizontally, going to the next line when they reach the end of a line, and going back to the top when they reach the bottom right corner.

Between Frame 1 and Frame 2, the black dots move by one position; between Frame 2 and Frame 3, they move by two positions; between Frame 3 and Frame 4 they move by three positions. The next frame will therefore involve a move by four positions.

AR33 – Practice Exercise 33 – Type 2

Answer: C
If you ignore the colours and the white circle, you can see that the triangles are switching places in this way: the top one goes to the bottom and the bottom two move up one place. Therefore, the only possible answers suitable are C and D.
If we number the triangles 1 (bottom), 2 (middle) and 3 (top), the white circle follows the pattern: 2, 1, 3, 2 and so the next place for it will be 1 (essentially it goes down one level at each frame. This excludes D and therefore the answer is C.

This is confirmed by the fact that the pattern of the black colour is 3, 2, 1, 2 and so we expect the next one to be 3 (i.e. it goes down and up), which would also exclude D.

234

Abstract Reasoning – Practice

The difficult part of this question is that you need to dissociate the shape from the colour, i.e. it is not the black triangle which is moving in a unified way. Both the triangular shape and the black colour are moving but in different ways.

AR34 – Practice Exercise 34 – Type 2

Answer: B
Ignoring the shapes, if you follow the movement of the colours, you can see that they are all rotating by one place clockwise between frames. Therefore, the colour pattern of the frame we are looking for will be the same as in the first frame. This limits the answer to B or C.

If you look carefully at the shapes, you will see that some repeat between frames. In particular, the bottom left shape of one frame is the same as the top right shape of the following frame. Similarly, the top left shape of one frame is the same as the bottom right shape of the following frame. The objects appearing on the left-hand side of the second frame are taken at random and are used as "seeds" for the next frame.

Using Frame 4 as a starting point, we are therefore looking for a frame which has a circle in the top right corner and a diamond in the bottom right corner i.e. Frame B.

AR35 – Practice Exercise 35 – Type 2

Answer: C
The circle moves clockwise from one corner to the next. This excludes Frame B. It also alternates between black and white; the next one therefore has to be black, which excludes Frame B again and Frame D.

To identify the place of the black square, you must look at every other frame. Between Frame 1 and Frame 3, the black square has moved clockwise by half the length of a side. Between Frame 2 and Frame 4, the black square has moved anti-clockwise by half the length of a side. Therefore, in the following frame, the black square should be in the bottom right corner, i.e. half a length further clockwise compared to Frame 3. This is the case in Frames C and D. But since Frame D has already been excluded, then Frame C is the answer.

AR36 – Practice Exercise 36 – Type 2

Answer: D
The circle moves clockwise to every other corner. It should therefore end up on the right-hand corner, thus ruling out Frame C.

The triangle moves anti-clockwise by a number of corners which increases by one each time. So it moves by 1 corner between the first two frames, and then by 2, and then by 3. We therefore expect it to have moved by 4 in the frame we are looking for. This places it in the top right corner, thus ruling out Figure A. Note that the triangle always retains the same orientation, i.e. its base remains horizontal.

The only difference between Frames B and D is the orientation of the line. We can see that, in each frame, the triangle is pointing towards the opposite side. The line is close to and parallel to the opposite side and starts opposite the triangle.

AR37 – Practice Exercise 37 – Type 2

Answer: B
The large square swings from left to right with an angle which increases by 45 degrees from one frame to the next. So between Frame 1 and Frame 2, the square tilts 45 degrees to the left. Then 2 x 45 = 90 degrees to the right between Frame 2 and Frame 3, then 3 x 45 = 135 degrees to the left. Therefore, the next frame should see the square 4 x 45 = 180 degrees to the right. This places the black band on the right-hand side of the square and points to Frames B and D.

In all frames, the black square is straight, which points to Frame B as the answer. This is also confirmed by the fact that the grey circle is rotating clockwise within the large square and should therefore end up in the top left corner of the large square when looking at it with the black band as its bottom.

Abstract Reasoning – Practice

AR38 – Practice Exercise 38 – Type 2

Answer: D

There are many ways to get to the right answer. Here are the relationships one can find in this exercise. You will need only some of them to reach the right answer.

The two lines at a right angle rotate clockwise but, since all the possible options place them in the same position, they are nothing to be concerned about. More importantly we can see that the diamond and circle at their extremities swap places every time we move on to the next frame. As such we should expect the next frame to have a diamond in the top right corner and a circle in the bottom left corner, which excludes Frame C.

The square located at the intersection of the two lines follows the pattern: black – grey – absent. So, since it is black in the fourth frame, we would expect it to be grey in the next frame, ruling out Frame B (which has no square).

The arrow always points to the right and follows the pattern: black – hashed – white – hashed. So we expect it to go back to black thereafter. This rules out Frame A.

The pentagon is always in the corner opposite the square and always points towards the diamond at the end of the lines. This rules out Frame A.

The circle in the pentagon follows the pattern: grey – black – white – grey and so we expect the next one to be black, ruling out Frame B.

AR39 – Practice Exercise 39 – Type 2

Answer: B
There are four distinct areas which are changing independently. If you write the number of black circles in each, you will get the following:

        2 1   4 3   6 2   8 4
        8 1   6 3   4 5   2 7

If you align the numbers according to their position in the matrix, you get:

Top left: 2 – 4 – 6 – 8 (and so the next one has to be 10)
Top right: 1 – 3 – 2 – 4 (and so the next one has to be 3 (+2 then -1)
Bottom left: 8 – 6 – 4 – 2 (and so the next one has to be 0)
Bottom right: 1 – 3 – 5 – 7 (and so the next one has to be 9)

AR40 – Practice Exercise 40 – Type 2

Answer: C
The number of areas defined by the objects increases by 1 between frames. So the next frame has to have 5 areas, which rules out A and B.

The number of black dots equals the number of right angles in the frame. Frame D has 6 right angles but only 2 dots, whilst Frame C has 4 dots and right angles.

AR41 – Practice Exercise 41 – Type 2

Answer: B
The object in the frame is made up of a series of shapes piled up one on top of the other. As we move from one frame to the next, the shape at the front moves to the back and therefore the one which was second becomes first. By looking at the front shape in each frame we can determine that the order in which the shapes are piled up is as follows:

○ on top of △ on top of ⬠ on top of ♡

Abstract Reasoning – Practice

There is also a bar [⎯⎯⎯⎯⎯], which is next in line and therefore will come to the front at the next frame. On that basis, we can eliminate Frames A and D.

In any case, Frame A does not make sense because as the white dot has been relegated to the back, it would be behind the heart and not in front of it. Frame D also makes no sense as it shows that the shapes are ordered as pentagon then triangle then heart; this does not follow the pattern established earlier.

Frame C is wrong because, if the bar is at the front, then it should have the dot behind it (which would not be visible as the bar would hide it) and then the triangle. Therefore, it does not make sense to see the pentagon straight behind the bar.
Frame B is the correct answer because it shows the following pattern:

Bar – (Dot – not visible) – Triangle – Pentagon – Heart which matches the pattern above. Bear in mind that if the bar is at the front then the dot will be hidden behind it, which explains why it is absent from the picture.

AR42 – Practice Exercise 42 – Type 2

Answer: B
Each of the arrows is moving by an increasing multiple of 45 degrees. So the black arrow rotates by 1 x 45 degrees, and then 2x then 3x. In the next frame, it should therefore have rotated by 4 x 45 = 180 degrees, so we expect it to point downwards.

The white arrow follows the same pattern but lagging by one frame (i.e. its first rotation is 0 x 45 degrees). So we expect it to have rotated by 3 x 45 degrees and therefore it should be pointing upwards.

AR43 – Practice Exercise 43 – Type 2

Answer: D
The line is rotating by 3 x 45 degrees clockwise. The white circle is rotating by a decreasing multiple of 45 degrees (3x, 2x, 1x) and therefore the next frame would have a rotation of 0 x 45, i.e. it will not move between Frame 4 and Frame 5. The black square is moving back and forth horizontally,

moving by half a length between each frame. Therefore, in Frame 5, it is expected to be centred.

AR44 – Practice Exercise 44 – Type 2

Answer: D
In Frame 2, the cross in the middle extends one arm to the right to reach the second circle. In Frame 3, it rotates 90 degrees anti-clockwise and extends further to reach the third circle. In Frame 4, the longer arm stays in place whilst a new half-length arm forms to the right. Therefore, we can expect that in the next frame, the new arm with extend to the full length and the whole thing will rotate 90 degrees anti-clockwise.

AR45 – Practice Exercise 45 – Type 2

Answer: B
Imagine that the line drawn in the middle is a graph starting from coordinates (0,0). Imagine also that each of the circles on the two axes represents coordinates 1, 2, 3, 4 and 5. As you move along the graph to the next point in along the frames, the black circles on the axes give you the coordinates for that point. For example, for Frame 1:

The fourth frame corresponds to the point in the top right and so, if we follow the graph, the next frame should deal with the point in the top left. This has coordinates (1,5).

AR46 – Practice Exercise 46 – Type 2

Answer: C
This exercise is more complex than the others because it introduces a slightly different mechanism, sometimes called an "engine". What this means is that an action is being performed on an object so that it becomes a different object. The nature of that action is dictated by another object called the "engine". In this exercise the "engine" is the three dots in the

Abstract Reasoning – Practice

middle and the pattern the dots display dictates what happens to the other two objects in the frame.

Those dots change from one frame to the next in a particular pattern. If we number them 1, 2 and 3, the pattern for the black dots is [1], then [1, 2], then [1,2,3], then [2,3] and so logically the next frame should have [3].

The fact that all possible options give you the dots in the same configuration is a clue that they may have a particular use. Similarly, you will notice that the arrow is always on the left and pointing downwards. That is another clue that is designed to draw your attention to the fact that something is going on.

If you study the shapes in each frame carefully, you will see that there are only two types of shapes – circles and squares – and that the bottom shape of one frame becomes the top shape of the next frame. Therefore, this excludes Frame A as we would expect the top shape to be a large white circle.

The dots (buttons) have the following functions (you can deduce it by looking at what makes the shapes vary within each frame):

- First button: Change size
- Second button: Change colour
- Third button: Change shape

So in Frame 1, only the first button is activated and so the small black circle at the top becomes a large black circle at the bottom.

In Frame 2, buttons 1 and 2 are activated and so both the size and the colour will change. Hence the large black circle becomes a small white circle.

In Frame 3, all three buttons are activated, which means that the size, the colour, and the shape will change. Hence a small white circle will become a large black square.

In Frame 4, buttons 2 and 3 are activated, meaning that the colour and the shape will change. So the large black square becomes a large white circle.

Since the next frame has only button 3 (i.e. the shape change) activated then the large white circle should become a large white square.

AR47 – Practice Exercise 47 – Type 2

Answer: B
As we move from one frame to the next, one circle is removed. They are removed from a corner in a clockwise order. So the next frame should have the circle in the bottom left removed.

AR48 – Practice Exercise 48 – Type 2

Answer: A
Starting from the gap featuring at the top in Frame 1, each time we move to the next frame, the star which is four places along (ignoring spaces) is removed.

Next one to be removed   Last one removed

AR49 – Practice Exercise 49 – Type 2

Answer: D
From one frame to the next, two shapes are swapped. The shapes which should be swapped are determined by a clockwise rotation.

Between Frames 1 and 2, the two shapes on the left-hand side are swapped (i.e. the two black circles, hence why the two shapes look the same).

Between Frames 2 and 3, the two top shapes are swapped.

Between Frames 3 and 4, the right-hand side shapes are swapped.

Therefore, the next frame should be computed using a swap of the two bottom shapes (i.e. the two black circles again, hence why the next frame should be the same as Frame 4).

AR50 – Practice Exercise 50 – Type 2

Answer: B
Each frame contains a large and a small shape which intersect. The shape of the overlapping area becomes the large shape in the following frame.

The small object is random. Since in Frame 4 the overlapping area is a short arrow then Frame B is the only option which satisfies the relationship.

AR51 – Practice Exercise 51 – Type 2

Answer: A
The black dot is moving anti-clockwise by an increasing multiple of 2. So:
- Between Frames 1 and 2 it has moved by 2 places.
- Between Frames 2 and 3 it has moved by 4 places.
- Between Frames 3 and 4 it has moved by 6 places.

The grey dot is moving clockwise in relation to the black dot by 2 spaces. Be careful: we are talking about the relative position of the grey dot to the black dot here, and not its absolute position. So:

- Between Frames 1 and 2 there are 2 spaces between the black and grey dot (when counting clockwise from the black dot).
- Between Frames 2 and 3 there are 4 spaces between the black and grey dot (when counting clockwise from the black dot).
- Between Frames 3 and 4 there are 6 spaces between the black and grey dot (when counting clockwise from the black dot).

In the next frame, we therefore expect the back dot to have moved by 8 places anti-clockwise and the grey dot to be 8 positions behind it when counting clockwise.

AR52 – Practice Exercise 52 – Type 2

Answer: C
To solve this exercise, you need to read the frames one after the other following the diagonals as follows:

You will then identify two separate patterns:

Pattern 1 – starting from the bottom: 1 – 3 – 5 – 0 – 2 – 4 – 6 – 1 i.e. moving up by 2 each time and starting back at 0 to continue the series (hence 5 is followed by 0 (skipping 6), and 6 is followed by 1 (skipping 0)).

Pattern 2 – starting from the top: 6 – 5 – 4 – 3 – 2 – 1 – 0 – 6 i.e. moving down by 1 and starting back at 6 when 0 has been reached.

So the next diagonal going down should be 5 – 4.
And the next diagonal going up should be 3 – 5.

AR53 – Practice Exercise 53 – Type 3

Answer: C
The large black shape rotates clockwise.
The white dot rotates anti-clockwise.
The arrow remains as is.
We are therefore looking for a horizontal shape, with an arrow pointing upwards and a white dot on the left, i.e. shape C.

AR54 – Practice Exercise 54 – Type 3

Answer: D
The colours of the shapes in the right-hand frame are the same as in the left-hand frame, except that the two shapes on the upward diagonal have been swapped.

The two shapes which were on the left-hand side in the left-hand frame have rotated 45 degrees clockwise.

The two shapes which were on the right-hand side in the left-hand frame have rotated 45 degrees anti-clockwise.

AR55 – Practice Exercise 55 – Type 3

Answer: B
The colours of the circles in the left-hand shape dictate the colours of the squares on the right-hand side. The circles on the diagonal are coloured Grey, White, White, Grey, White, and Black, therefore the squares in the right-hand shape are coloured in the same order going first down the left column and then down the right column.

Abstract Reasoning – Practice

The colours of the squares in the left-hand shape dictate the colours of the circles in the right-hand shape.

The correct answer is therefore B, which has a totally black square as it contains a black circle on a black background.

AR56 – Practice Exercise 56 – Type 3

Answer: A
In the right-hand frame, the type of shape contained within the white domino is the same as that contained within the white shape. And the same goes for the black shape and the black domino. So on the left-hand side we have white triangles in a black shape and black diamonds in a white shape. The same will apply for the dominoes in the right-hand frame.

The number of objects appearing in the top part of each domino in the right-hand frame is equal to the number of objects contained within the shape of the opposite colour on the left-hand side. So:

2 triangles in black pentagon → 2 diamonds at top of the white domino.
3 diamonds in white trapezium → 3 triangles at top of the black domino.

The number of objects appearing in the bottom part of each domino in the right-hand frame is equal to the number of sides of the shape of the opposite colour on the left-hand side. So:
Black pentagon → 5 diamonds at the bottom of the white domino.
White trapezium → 4 triangles at the bottom of the black domino.

1300 UCAT Practice Questions

AR57 – Practice Exercise 57 – Type 3

Answer: B
The shape becomes its mirror image, i.e. it flips vertically.

AR58 – Practice Exercise 58 – Type 3

Answer: B
The shape rotates 45 degrees and moves along by half the length of a side clockwise. Another shape which is its mirror image appears, filling the opposite side of the shape and the overlapping area is coloured black. The square should therefore appear standing on one of its corners at the bottom of the shape, i.e. Frame B.

AR59 – Practice Exercise 59 – Type 3

Answer: B
The left-hand frame has a grey square (4 sides) containing a black pentagon (5 sides). The right-hand frame has a black pentagon (5 sides) containing a grey trapezium (4 sides). So, essentially, the relation is reversed i.e. the number of sides and the colour of the external shape become the features of the new internal shape and vice-versa. The actual shapes used do not matter so long as the number of sides matches.

We should therefore expect the new frame to involve a white triangle containing a white hexagon, i.e. Frame B.

AR60 – Practice Exercise 60 – Type 3

Answer: D
To go from the left-hand frame to the right frame you simply need to enhance each object within the frame by adding its mirror image and reversing the order.

246

Abstract Reasoning – Practice

In addition, the shapes are reversed in their order. So the external shape becomes the internal shape, and vice-versa. The middle shape remains in the middle.

So if the left-hand frame contains: Square > Rectangle with length = 2 x width> triangle with right angle, we are most likely looking for the following pattern:

Square > Square > Rectangle, i.e. Frame D.

Note: depending on how you double up a shape, you could end up with a different result.

For example, ◺ could become ◁ , thus leading to several possible answers.

However, the list of possible options will only contain one of those possible answers, meaning there is a unique answer amongst those proposed.

AR61 – Practice Exercise 61 – Type 3

Answer: C
Folding the pattern on the left-hand side will make the same box as folding the pattern on the right-hand side. There are many ways of thinking about this exercise and those of you with spatial awareness may be able to just "see it". But for the many others, here is one way of solving the problem:

The three grey squares are in a row therefore it cannot be Frame A. Indeed, in Frame A, the three grey squares all have one corner in common and so cannot unfold in a straight line. In the other three frames however, the grey squares are all in consecutive squares on the side when you fold the box.

If you fold the left-hand box, you will see that the two white squares are on adjacent sides. In Frames B and D, however, they will end up on opposite sides (top and bottom). Therefore, Frame C is the only option left.

AR62 – Practice Exercise 62 – Type 3

Answer: C
The shape on the right-hand side is obtained by making the large shape on the left-hand side fit into the shape that it contains, and then excluding the overlapping area. So in the case of the example given, the trapezium is being squeezed into the square as shown. This leaves two standing triangles (shown in white).

Squeezing an equilateral triangle into a square would give the shape shown here in white, thus Frame C.

AR63 – Practice Exercise 63 – Type 3

Answer: C
This exercise is a little trickier than it looks. At first, you look at the left-hand frame with three arrows and one missing and notice that they are all pointing in different direction. There is an empty circle and the arrow pointing right seems to be the missing item (it would make a complete set of arrows, all pointing in a different direction: left, right, up, down). However, when you look at the left-hand frame that you are supposed to be working on, it suddenly strikes you that, with two arrows pointing right and one pointing in a diagonal, this cannot be the relationship we are looking for.

The relationship is that every circle is being pointed at by an arrow. The missing arrow should therefore be pointing towards the circle that is not yet being pointed at. In the left-hand frame, the two circles on the right-hand side are being pointed at by the two horizontal arrows on the left. The bottom left circle is being pointed at by the diagonal arrow in the top right corner. So, we now need an arrow pointing towards the top left circle. Hence, Frame C is the answer.

AR64 – Practice Exercise 64 – Type 3

Answer: A
The four dots on the left-hand side on the board are moving around the board according to the sequence of arrows located on the same row as those circles. Each arrow represents a move by one square in a particular direction. If there is a dot, then it means that there is no movement.

Abstract Reasoning – Practice

However, if a dot moves to different row, then its colour will also change to match the colour of the dot which was originally on that row. This is why, in the example given, the dots on row 2 are both black and the dots on row 3 are both grey.

With the frame that we are given, we would therefore expect all dots on row 1 to be black (hence Frame B can be excluded) and all dots on row 3 to be hashed (hence Frame C can be excluded).

The only difference between the two remaining frames (A and D) is the location of the two white dots. We can see from the second row that the white dot should be static. Hence Frame A is the answer.

AR65 – Practice Exercise 65 – Type 3

Answer: B
Each line is represented by a circle. Each intersection between two lines is represented by the fact that the circles are touching. So for example:

is represented by the pattern:

because one line (represented by the middle circle) is being intersected by two other lines (represented by the two other circles). The actual placing of the circles does not matter. Only the fact that they touch each other matters. The answer is therefore Frame B.

Frame A is not the answer because it would mean that one line is being intersected by four other lines, which is not the case. Frame C has overlapping circles which have no meaning. Frame D has four circles arranged in a circular pattern, which implies the lines would form a quadrilateral shape; this is not the case either.

AR66 – Practice Exercise 66 – Type 3

Answer: C
To solve this exercise, you need to imagine the large hand of a clock moving according to the following principles: an arrow pointing to the top represents a whole hour, an arrow to the right represents a quarter of an hour,

an arrow to the bottom represents a half hour and an arrow to the left represents three-quarters of an hour.

You simply need to add them all up. In the example, you have two full hours plus one quarter plus one half. Therefore, the arrow would in total have moved by three-quarters of an hour, hence the arrow pointing to the left in the right-hand frame.

Using the new frame, we have 1/4 + 1/4 + 3/4 + 1 so the clock hand will have moved by 1/4 in total. So the answer is an arrow pointing to the right, hence Frame C.

AR67 – Practice Exercise 67 – Type 3

Answer: D
The frame contains four shapes made up of quarters which are either black, grey, or white. The shapes rotate clockwise by a number of places equal to the number of black quarters. For example, the top left shape has 3 black quarters and therefore moves by 3 places clockwise. Hence it ends up at the bottom left corner. If a shape contains a grey quarter, then the shape will rotate around its own centre by 90 degrees.

3 black quarters
=
Moves by 3 places clockwise

1 grey quarter
=
Rotates clockwise by 90 degrees

In the frame we are given, the diamond with 3 black quarters and 1 grey quarter sits in the bottom right corner. It should therefore move to the top right corner and rotate by 90 degrees. This points to Frames A and D.

Similarly, the shape with 3 black quarters and 1 white quarter sits in the top left corner and should therefore end up in the bottom left corner unrotated. Out of Frames A and D, only Frame D satisfies this condition.

A quick check will also demonstrate that the other two shapes in Frame D satisfy the relationship.

Abstract Reasoning – Practice

AR68 – Practice Exercise 68 – Type 3

Answer: B
The grid contains a number of shapes. To create the right-hand grid from the left-hand one, all you need to do is move the shapes along horizontally by a number of spaces equal to the number of sides the shapes have. So a circle will move by one space, a moon will move by two spaces, a triangle will move by 3 spaces, etc. If you reach the bottom of the grid then you start back at the top left corner.

Looking at the new frame we are given, there is a triangle in the second square on the bottom line. If we move it by three spaces, it will end up in the top left corner. This points to Frames A and B.

The only difference between Frames A and B is the position of the other triangle. In the original frame, that triangle sits in the third square on the first row. Therefore, moving it by three spaces will land it in the second box of the second row. This points to Frame B.

AR69 – Practice Exercise 69 – Type 3

Answer: D
The shapes in the left-hand frame contain parts which can fold or unfold. A grey-shaded part will unfold, whilst a black-shaded part will fold. So, for example, the top-left-corner shape is a rectangle with two grey strips. If you unfold them, you obtain a larger rectangle. Because those two strips can now be folded they appear black.

Along the same line, the capsule-type shape in the top right corner has a black part. If you fold that black part over the other half, you get half a capsule with a grey tinge since it can be unfolded.

For the new frame, the easiest starting point is the triangle in the top right corner, made up of one white and three black triangles. All three black triangles will fold in onto the central triangle, leaving only one single small triangle which will need to be coloured grey since it can fold out. Hence this leaves only Frames B and D.

We can then look at the single grey triangle in the bottom-left corner of the new frame. If we unfold it, we have a black triangle and a white triangle (onto which the other triangle was folded over). So the answer is Frame D.

AR70 – Practice Exercise 70 – Type 3

Answer: B
The two circular shapes in the right-hand frame represent views from the object in the left-hand frame both from above and from underneath.

In the new frame we are given, if you look from above, the only two shapes visible will be the white triangle (which will appear as a white circle) and the grey area, which will appear as a larger grey disk. So we are expecting a large white circle in a larger grey disc, i.e. Frames B or D.

Looking from underneath, we will see a black circle within a white circle, within a black circle, within a grey circle. In fact, both Frames B and D have that option, except that in Frame B the proportions are equal, whereas in Frame D there is a large bias towards the black area. The way in which the objects are set up in the left-hand frame suggests the areas should be of roughly similar proportions (certainly there is no way the black area should be that wide since the white triangle is not far off its border), so Frame B is the answer.

AR71 – Practice Exercise 71 – Type 3

Answer: A
The lines in the right-hand frame are of a length equal to the distance between two identical objects on the left-hand side. So, in the example given, the two hearts are at opposite ends of the frame; therefore, they will be represented by a line which stretches to nearly the whole width of the frame. Similarly, the two black dots are very close together and will therefore be represented by a very short line.

However, you will see that, in the possible answers given, the lines are the same from one frame to the other, albeit they appear in a different order in each frame. It therefore means that their order has to be determined by another relationship.

In this exercise, the order in which the lines appear is linked to the number of sides that the object it represents has. The top line will be for the object with one side (i.e. a circle or ellipse). The second line will be for the object with two sides (in this case a heart or a moon), etc. until you reach the bottom (fifth) line, which will represent an object with five sides.

Abstract Reasoning – Practice

The answer can therefore be found as follows:

Object	Length of matching line
• (1 side)	Full length
ℂ (2 sides)	Half length
△ (3 sides)	Very short
□ (4 sides)	Full length
⌂ (5 sides)	Half length

This combination matches Frame A

AR72 – Practice Exercise 72 – Type 3

Answer: C
The direction of the arrow within a frame determines whether the number of sides increases (arrow up) or decreases (arrow down) by 1. So, for example, a square with an arrow pointing downwards will become a triangle.

The shapes with the arrows pointing upwards will switch colour whilst those with the arrows pointing downwards will keep their original colour.

In the new frame, we therefore expect:

- The white triangle to become a black quadrilateral (which excludes Frame A since it is white).
- The black trapezium to become a white pentagon (which now excludes Frame B).
- The white circle to become blank since the down arrow will leave it with zero sides (which now excludes Frame D).

AR73 – Practice Exercise 73 – Type 3

Answer: B
Each object is made up of two shapes which are either intersecting or with one contained within the other. In addition, there are a number of circles at some of the vertices.

The rules are as follows:
- The number of circles at the vertices determines the number of sides of the object which features inside the large white circle in the

right-hand frame. So, if an object has three white circles then the large white circle on the right will include a triangle.

- The number of lines which stick out of the large circle is determined by the two main shapes in the object on the left. If the two objects intersect then you multiply the number of their sides. If one object contains the other one, then you add up the numbers of their sides. E.g. if a triangle intersects with another triangle (top right-hand corner) then you should have 3 x 3 = 9 lines sticking out. If a triangle contains an ellipse (bottom left-hand corner) then you should have 3 + 1 = 4 lines sticking out.

With the new frame we are therefore looking for the following:

Top left:
- Triangle intersecting with a heart: 3 x 2 = 6 lines (which rules out Frames C and D)
- 2 circles = 2-sided shape (nothing ruled out).

Top right
- Arrow (7 sides) containing an ellipse: 7 + 1 = 8 lines (which rules out Frame D)
- No circle = empty shape (which rules out Frame C).

Bottom left
- Arrow intersecting with an ellipse: 7 x 1 = 7 lines (which rules out Frames C and D).
- 4 circles = 4-sided shape (which rules out Frame D).

Bottom right
- 2 ellipses intersecting: 1 x 1 = 1 line (which rules out Frames A and C).
- No circles = empty shape (which rules out nothing).

AR74 – Practice Exercise 74 – Type 3

Answer: D
The shape on the left can be folded to make the box on the right.

We can immediately exclude Frame B because it has a white circle on a white background, which is not the case in the object on the left.

Abstract Reasoning – Practice

Frame A can also be excluded because if we folded the object so that the front facing side had the white dot and the right-hand side was plain grey, then the top would have the black dot and the black side would be underneath, not above.

Frame C can also be excluded because the plain white and the plain grey sides should be on opposite sides, and not adjacent.

AR75 – Practice Exercise 75 – Type 3

Answer: C
Circles move by two steps at a time and triangles move by one step at a time. Shapes on the inside move clockwise whilst shapes on the outside move anticlockwise.

AR76 – Practice Exercise 76 – Type 3

Answer: C
Imagine a set of scales tipping to the left or the right depending on the weights of the objects sitting at either side. In the example frame, we have two sets of scales; the top one will tip towards the right whilst the bottom one will remain stable. The lines in the right-hand frame represent those movements.

In the new frame, the top set of scales will remain stable (one object on each side) and the bottom set of scales will tip towards the right.

AR77 – Practice Exercise 77 – Type 3

Answer: B
The shapes are arranged/superposed in an order determined by how long the line linking them to the black dot is. The top shape is that linked by the shortest line and the bottom shape is that linked by the longest line.

AR78 – Practice Exercise 78 – Type 3

Answer: C
All shapes gather in the middle. If there is an overlap, the white shape sits on top. The whole thing then rotates by 90 degrees.

AR79 – Practice Exercise 79 – Type 4

In both sets there are two central shapes which either overlap or sit one next to the other. In some cases, there is a larger shape which contains them. The number of sides of the larger shape that contains the two central objects is dictated by the positioning of the two central shapes.

Set A: If the two central shapes sit next to each other then you add the number of their sides together; however, if they overlap then you subtract one from the other. For example:

- The top left corner frame has two triangles sitting next to each other, 3 + 3 = 6; hence they are contained within a hexagon.
- The frame below has a hexagon and a heart. 6 - 2 = 4; hence they are contained in a square.
- The bottom left frame has two overlapping quadrilaterals, 4 - 4 = 0 hence there is no object around them.

Set B: This is essentially the reverse relationship to Set A i.e. if the two central shapes overlap, then you add the number of their sides together; however, if they are next to each other, then you subtract one from the other.

Answers:
79.1: Frame B (5 - 1 = 4)
79.2: Frame A (2 + 4 = 6)

AR80 – Practice Exercise 80 – Type 4

The objects overlap with the following rules ('>' means 'on top of'):

Set A: Grey > Hashed > Black > White
Set B: White > Black > Hashed > Grey

The shapes of the objects are irrelevant.

Answers:
80.1: Frame B
80.2: Frame A

Abstract Reasoning – Practice

AR81 – Practice Exercise 81 – Type 4

The three graduated bars contain a grey area which represents a number, e.g. 4 sections highlighted = 4.

Set A: Subtract the number of the second bar from the number in the first bar to obtain the number in the third bar. The dot is black if the result is odd and white if the result is even.

Set B: Add the number from the first 2 bars to obtain the number in the third bar. The dot is white if the result is odd and black if the result is even.

Answers:
81.1: Frame C
81.2: Frame D

AR82 – Practice Exercise 82 – Type 4

Each frame consists of a circle, a square and another shape which varies.

Set A: The black dot sits in the area common to the square and the circle only. The white dot sits in the area common to all three shapes.

Set B: The black dot sits in the area common to the circle and the third shape. The white dot sits in the area common to the square and the third shape.

Answers:
82.1: Frame B
82.2: Frame C

AR83 – Practice Exercise 83 – Type 4

Each frame contains a large circle with a letter and small black circle with a number.

Set A: When the letter only has straight edges then the number is odd. If it has at least one curved edge, then the number is even.

Set B: When the letter only has straight edges then the number is even. If it has at least a curved edge, then the number is odd.

The colour of the large circle is irrelevant, as are the positions of the two circles.

Answers:
83.1: Frame C (Straight edges with odd number)
83.2: Frame B (Straight edges with even number)

AR84 – Practice Exercise 84 – Type 4

Each frame contains two white shapes and two black shapes. Their position is irrelevant.

Set A: The two white shapes are symmetrical along both a vertical and a horizontal axis. The two black shapes are symmetrical only along a vertical axis.

Set B: The two black shapes are symmetrical along both a vertical and a horizontal axis. The two white shapes are symmetrical only along a horizontal axis.

Answers:
84.1: Frame C
84.2: Frame D (Note that Frame B is not suitable because all four shapes are symmetrical along both the vertical and horizontal axes, where the white shapes in Set B should be symmetrical along their horizontal axis only.)

AR85 – Practice Exercise 85 – Type 4

Set A: The ellipse is pointing towards the cross.
Set B: The ellipse is pointing towards the circle.

Answers:
85.1: Frame A
85.2: Frame B

AR86 – Practice Exercise 86 – Type 4

Draw a line between the two black dots.

Set A: The line that links the two black dots will cross an odd number of black lines.

Set B: The line that links the two black dots will cross an even number of black lines.

Answers:
86.1: Frame C
86.2: Frame B

AR87 – Practice Exercise 87 – Type 4

Set A: Each frame contains a string made up of:
- Successive black circles with one white circle on either side.
- At one end, a circle which is either grey or hashed.
- At the other end, a shape with a number of sides equal to the number of black circles in the string. If the circle at the other end is grey, then the shape has a large size; if the circle at the other end is hashed then the shape has a small size. The shape is always white.

Set B: Each frame contains a string made up of:
- Successive white circles with one black circle on either side.
- At one end, a circle which is either grey or hashed.
- At the other end, a shape with a number of sides equal to the number of white circles in the string. If the circle at the other end is grey, then the shape is white; if the circle at the other end is hashed then the shape is black. The size of the shape is irrelevant.

Answers:
87.1: Frame B
87.2: Frame A

AR88 – Practice Exercise 88 – Type 4

Each shape contains three squares coloured black, grey, or white, and two white shapes, one contained within the other. The difference in the number of sides between the two shapes is dictated by the rank of the square coloured black. So, if the first square is black, then one shape will have one more side than the other. If the second square is black, then one shape will have two more sides than the other. And if the third square is black, then one shape will have three more sides than the other.

Set A: If the two non-black squares are grey, then the shape with the higher number of sides will be on the outside. If they are white, then the shape with the lower number of sides will be on the outside.

Set B: If the two non-black squares are grey, then the shape with the lower number of sides will be on the outside. If they are white, then the shape with the lower number of sides will be on the inside.

Answers:
88.1: Frame B
88.2: Frame B

AR89 – Practice Exercise 89 – Type 4

Set A: The shape in the middle has the same number of sides as it takes to go from the grey needle to the white needle **clockwise in increments of 45-degree turns**. So for example, in the top-left shape, the distance is 1 x 45 degrees, hence the middle shape is a circle (1 side). In the top-right shape, the distance is 4 x 45 degrees, hence the middle shape is a square (4 sides).

A full circle represents 8 x 45 degrees, so a quarter turn (2 x 45 degrees) could be represented either by a shape with 2 sides or a shape with 10 sides (as is the case in the bottom right shape).

Set B: The shape in the middle has the same number of sides as it takes to go from the grey needle to the white needle **anti-clockwise in increments of 90-degree turns**.

A full circle represents 4 x 90 degrees so a quarter turn of 90 degrees could be represented either by a shape with 1 side or a shape with 5 or 9 sides.

Answers:
89.1: Frame B (6 clockwise 45-degree turns needed to go from the grey to the white needle = 6 sides in middle shape)

Abstract Reasoning – Practice

89.2: Frame D (1 anti-clockwise 90-degree turn needed to go from the grey to the white needle = 1 or 5 or 9 sides in the middle shape. In this case, it is a pentagon)

AR90 – Practice Exercise 90 – Type 4

The shapes are organised in a 4 x 4 grid. The actual shapes and colours are random.

Set A: There is one row only which contains four shapes. None of the columns contains four shapes.

Set B: There is one column only which contains four shapes. None of the rows contains four shapes.

Answers:
90.1: Frame C
90.2: Frame B

AR91 – Practice Exercise 91 – Type 4

Each frame consists of a chain of shapes (circles and squares), each linked to the next by some form of arrow. The chain starts in the top left square area. The arrows can be single-ended or double-ended; they can also be straight (⟶), curved (⤳) or square (⌐⟶)

For both sets, if you follow the chain from the top left square area to the end:
- A straight arrow will always lead to a white shape.
- A curved arrow will always lead to a black shape.
- A square arrow will always lead to a grey shape.

Note: This only works if you start the chain at the top left corner of the shape, i.e. in the square area. It will not work if you go back up the chain.

Set A:
- If the arrow is single ended, then the shape remains the same.
- If the arrow is double ended, then the shape changes.

Set B:
- If the arrow is single ended, then the shape changes.
- If the arrow is double ended, then the shape remains the same.

Answers:
91.1: Frame D
92.2: Frame B

AR92 – Practice Exercise 92 – Type 4

Each frame consists of a central shape which can be either black or white, surrounded by a number of shapes of the opposite colour.

Set A:
- If the central shape is white, then the shapes that surround it have 1 side fewer than the central shape (e.g. in the top left corner, the central shape is a square, so 4 sides, and the surrounding shapes are triangles, so 3 sides).
- If the central shape is black, the shapes that surround it have 1 side more than the central shape (e.g. in the bottom right corner, the central shape is a rectangle, so 4 sides, and the surrounding shapes are pentagons, so 5 sides).

Set B: This is the reverse of Set A's relationship:
- If the central shape is white, then the shapes that surround it have 1 side more than the central shape.
- If the central shape is black, the shapes that surround it have 1 side fewer than the central shape.

Answers:
92.1: Frame D – the central white square (4 sides) is encapsulated by 2 three-quarter circles (3 sides): ◖.
92.2: Frame D – the central white D shape (2 sides) is surrounded by 3 'triangles' (so 3 sides), some of which have a curved edge.

AR93 – Practice Exercise 93 – Type 4

Each frame contains four "flags", each containing three vertical bars. The bars are coloured black, white, grey, or hashed. Looking at the flags in a clockwise rotation, you will notice the following relationships:

Abstract Reasoning – Practice

Set A:
A black band of one flag becomes a white band in the next flag.
A white band in one flag becomes a grey band in the next flag.
A grey band in one flag becomes a hashed band in the next flag.
A hashed band in one flag becomes a black band in the next flag.

Or as a diagram: BLACK → WHITE → GREY → HASHED → BLACK

Set B:
BLACK → GREY → WHITE → HASHED → BLACK

Answers:
93.1: Frame B
93.2: Frame A

Note: The above relationships are valid if you look at the flag clockwise. You will get to the right result, too, if you look at the flags in a different order, as long as it is always the same order. For example, for Set A, you could also say that, if you look at the flags anti-clockwise, then the relationship is BLACK → HASHED → GREY → WHITE → BLACK. That will also lead you to Frame B.

AR94 – Practice Exercise 94 – Type 4

In both sets:
- The shapes used within each frame are all identical, whatever the shape might be.
- If there is an even number of shapes, then the shapes are white. If there is an odd number of shapes, then the shapes are black.

In addition:

Set A: When the individual shapes are put together, they form an object which is of the same shape as its components. So for example, the four white triangles at the top left form a bigger triangle of the same proportions. Similarly, the nine black diamonds form a bigger diamond of the same proportions, etc.

Set B: When the individual shapes are put together they form an object which is different to its components (e.g. the six triangles form a hexagon, the five black squares form a cross).

263

Answers:
94.1: Frame D (4 white rectangles form a larger rectangle)
94.2: Frame B (2 white rectangles form a square). Note that Frame C is not the correct answer because, although it is made up of three right-angled triangles and it is coloured black, the triangles do not have the same size.

AR95 – Practice Exercise 95 – Type 4

Each frame contains three shapes, one inside the other.

Set A:
- The outside shape has a smaller number of sides than the middle shape, which has, itself, a smaller number of sides than the inside shape.
- Shapes with an even number of sides are white; those with an odd number of sides are black.

Set B:
- The outside shape has a greater number of sides than the middle shape, which has, itself, a greater number of sides than the inside shape.
- Shapes with an even number of sides are black; those with an odd number of sides are white.

Answers:
95.1: Frame D
95.2: Frame A

AR96 – Practice Exercise 96 – Type 4

In both sets, there are four points of intersection between shapes.

Set A: The intersections involve several shapes (e.g. in the top left frame, a circle, a triangle, and a diamond are needed).

Set B: Only two shapes are needed to achieve the four intersections.
All shapes which are loose (i.e. who do not intersect with others) are distractors.

Abstract Reasoning – Practice

Answers:
96.1: Frame A
96.2: Frame A

AR97 – Practice Exercise 97 – Type 4

In both sets, the number of white dots is equal to the number of vertices in the black shape. The white dots are positioned in the same arrangements as the actual vertices of the black.

Set A: The line drawn between the white dots will not cross one of the black shape's sides.

Set B: The line drawn between the dots will cross at least one of the black shape's sides.

Answers:
97.1: Frame C
97.2: Frame D

AR98 – Practice Exercise 98 – Type 4

Each shape has two bulging parts separated by a "neck". It also has two black and two white dots adhering to its side, either on the inside or on the outside.

Set A:
- If the two black dots are on the same side of the neck, then they are positioned on the inside of the shape. If they are on opposite sides of the neck, then they are positioned on the outside of the shape.
- If the two white dots are on the same side of the neck, then they are positioned on the outside of the shape. If they are on opposite sides of the neck, then they are positioned on the inside of the shape.

Set B:
- If the two black dots are on the same side of the neck, then they are positioned on the outside of the shape. If they are on opposite sides of the neck, then they are positioned on the inside of the shape.
- If the two white dots are on the same side of the neck, then they are positioned on the inside of the shape. If they are on opposite sides of the neck, then they are positioned on the outside of the shape.

Answers:
98.1: Frame B
98.2: Frame A

AR99 – Practice Exercise 99 – Type 4

In this exercise, treat the letters as shapes, not as letters.

Set A: The two shapes in the top row are symmetrical with regard to the horizontal axis only. The two shapes in the bottom row are symmetrical with regard to the vertical axis only.

Set B: The two shapes in the top row are symmetrical with regard to the vertical axis only. The two shapes in the bottom row are symmetrical with regard to both the horizontal and the vertical axis.

Answers:
99.1: Frame B
99.2: Frame A

AR100 – Practice Exercise 100 – Type 4

Set A: All shapes can be drawn without lifting the pencil or going over the same line again.

Set B: The shapes cannot be drawn in one single line without lifting the pencil or going over an existing line.

Answers:
100.1: Frame D
100.2: Frame B

VERBAL REASONING

TIPS & TECHNIQUES

+

200
PRACTICE QUESTIONS & ANSWERS

9 Verbal Reasoning Format, Purpose & Key Techniques

FORMAT

The verbal reasoning test consists of 11 text passages, which deal with a wide range of topics. Those topics are generic and do not necessarily relate to medicine. The text passages usually contain 200 to 350 words and may take different forms including newspaper articles, instruction manuals or even complaint letters. For each of the 11 text passages, you are given 4 questions that can follow 2 different formats:

Format 1 – True/False/Can't tell
You are given a statement and are asked to determine whether that statement is "True", "False", or "Can't tell" based on the information provided in the text.

Format 2 – Multiple choice
You are given a question of the type: "Which of the following answers can be deduced from the text?" or "Which of the following statements is the author most likely to agree [or disagree] with?" You must choose the answer from 4 possible options.

The time given at the exam to answer all 44 questions is 22 minutes (1 minute to read the instructions and 21 minutes to answer). You therefore have just under 2 minutes per text or 30 seconds per question.

PURPOSE

The purpose of the verbal reasoning test is to determine whether you are able to comprehend information and interpret it in a meaningful way. In medicine, this is an important skill that you will need to use in many contexts. For example:

- Throughout your medical career, you will be required to read journals and interpret the findings presented in research papers. In some cases, you will need to draw the lessons from such papers so that you can apply them to your own clinical practice. It is therefore crucial that you draw the right conclusions.

Verbal Reasoning – Practice

- The study of medicine and putting it into effective practice involves the learning and understanding of what factors cause or affect a disease, for which you will need to ensure that you are able to draw the correct conclusions from the information at your disposal. For example, a study may uncover the fact that most patients with lung cancer are also regular drinkers; however, this does not necessarily mean that alcohol causes lung cancer. Indeed, it could be that most people who smoke also happen to drink.

- As a doctor, you will gain much information from talking to your patients. It is particularly important that you make decisions based on the information available to you rather than by jumping to the wrong conclusions either because you have misunderstood what you were being told or because you made assumptions.

The verbal reasoning test is therefore primarily a logic test as well as a test of your ability to interpret information based on known facts.

EXAMPLE

TEXT
Some common foods can interfere with medications. Grapefruit juice is specifically in the line of fire. Drinking it could indeed dangerously worsen the side effects of some drugs because it facilitates their absorption into the system. In particular, the interaction of grapefruit juice with simvastatin and, to a lesser extent, with atorvastatin (two anti-cholesterol drugs) can lead to severe muscular problems. With transplant anti-rejection drugs, such as tacrolimus and cyclosporin, the kidneys are endangered. Finally, with cisapride, prescribed for severe gastric reflux, there are risks of severe cardiac arrhythmia.

Question: **Patients taking simvastatin are likely to experience more severe side effects than patients taking atorvastatin.**

Answer: CAN'T TELL. The text states that grapefruit juice interacts with atorvastatin to a lesser extent than with simvastatin. This does not mean simvastatin gives more severe side effects than atorvastatin. The text only deals with the effect of grapefruit juice on someone taking those drugs but does not deal with the side effects of the two drugs in normal circumstances. As such, we cannot conclude whether the statement is true or not.

KEY TECHNIQUES

In the verbal reasoning test, there are a number of difficulties that you must be aware of and that you must practise to overcome:

Practise reading the text quickly and efficiently
Since you have under 2 minutes to read the text and answer all 4 questions, you will not have enough time to read any 300-word text in detail. You should therefore practise gathering all important information quickly.

Very often, a question will refer to information contained in a specific paragraph or sentence of the text only and not the whole text. In the example discussed on the previous page, the question could be answered simply by looking at the sentence *"In particular, the interaction of grapefruit juice with simvastatin and, to a lesser extent, with atorvastatin (two anti-cholesterol drugs) can lead to severe muscular problems"*. Therefore, when you read the text for the first time, you may want to simply scan through it to identify the different topics that it addresses. For example, the text on the previous page may be categorised as follows:

- Generalities on grapefruit juice
- Cholesterol drugs
- Transplant drugs
- Gastric drugs.

When you read the question, you can then refer to the relevant portion of text in more detail. This way, you only read in detail what you really need to read, which can save you a lot of time considering that many of the texts contain information that is never used in the questions.

You may still encounter questions which require information to be gathered from different paragraphs and may therefore take up a lot of time to answer; but the time you will have saved on the more straightforward questions should enable you to spend a bit more time on these.

Focus on the text and ignore what you know through other means
Some texts may deal with issues with which you are familiar or may be based on facts or assumptions that contradict information that you know through other sources. In some cases, the text might give information that you know to be inaccurate. Whatever your prior knowledge, the text is the only source of information that you should consider.

Learn to interpret keywords that are likely to influence the answers
Both the text and the questions may contain phrases which could be easily overlooked when read quickly (such as "may", "might", "would", "could", "can", "only", "the most", "the least", "commonly") and could switch the answer from "True" or "False" to "Can't tell". In particular:

- "Can" means that it is possible for an event to take place, even if it is not frequently. For example, sharks can eat human beings. It does not mean that they do it often; it does not mean that all sharks do it; and it does not mean either that it has ever happened. "May", "might" and "could" also mean that an event is possible without any reference to frequency or probability. For example, prolonged exposure to sun rays may lead to skin cancer. It is simply possible (i.e. it has probably happened to some people but that is as far as you can conclude).

- "Commonly" and "frequently" suggest that an event is not an unusual occurrence. It does not mean that it happens all the time or to everyone, though it implies that it would happen in a majority of cases (i.e. over 50%). It is simply something that one should be expecting to happen in many instances under common conditions. For example, high cholesterol is commonly associated with either poor diet or family history, i.e. these would be considered two important factors that would affect most people.

- "Many" suggests a large number but not necessarily a majority. For example, many newborn babies are male. It does not mean that the majority of newborn babies are male. "Many" therefore relates to a number rather than a proportion. "Most" or "the majority", however, refer to a proportion. Depending on the context, "most" may mean either that it applies to over 50% of the population or sometimes an overwhelming majority, i.e. "most people who replied to the survey were from London" suggests a large percentage, though one cannot really say for sure. The use of "most" also suggests that some people do not fall into that category.

- "Unlikely" refers to something that has a probability which is too low to be considered seriously. For example, you are unlikely to be eaten by a shark in the Mediterranean if none of the sharks in that sea have ever bitten anyone or if these sharks are vegetarian, but it is not completely impossible. It is just highly improbable.

- "Cannot" and "impossible" refer to events that can never happen, i.e. it is simply not possible. For example, men cannot fly without the help of technology. In practice, there are very few things that are truly impossible; so if a question is asking you to comment on the fact that a particular event cannot take place, double-check that the answer should not be "can't tell" instead. In particular, the fact that something has never happened before or has an extremely low chance of occurring does not mean that it is impossible. You see that a lot in court cases; for example, the probability that three babies by the same mother die of cot death has an extremely low probability but one can't tell for sure that it cannot happen.

- "Average" is a word that occurs often in the texts used in the exam. Usually the text will give an average and the statement in the question will ask you whether the average figure can be applied to any particular individual. For example, the text could say: "The average unemployment rate across all UK counties was 3% in 2007." The question would then state "Unemployment in Surrey was 3% in 2007", which we cannot confirm either way since the only figure we are given is an average across the country.

Questions containing "average" can cause a particular problem. For example, in the example above, consider the question "Some counties had an unemployment rate under 3% in 2007." One could reasonably state that, since the figure of 3% is an average, some counties would have a rate below 3% and others a rate above 3%, and that therefore the statement is true. However, there is also a (very remote) possibility that all counties have an unemployment rate of exactly 3%, in which case the average would still be 3% but the statement would be false. It is of course highly improbable but still possible. In the absence of conclusive information, I would suggest that you opt for "can't tell" as this would be the absolutely correct answer.

Practise the key logic rules
The verbal reasoning test is a test of comprehension and logic, i.e. can you deduce the right information from what you are given. There are three logic rules which are often used in the exam to create questions:

▶   Rule 1: If A → B, then you always have (non-B) →(non-A).
▶   Rule 2: If A → B, then (non-A) does not always imply (non-B).
▶   Rule 3: If A → B, then B does not always imply A.

Verbal Reasoning – Practice

Consider the following statement: "All shoes made by the ABC Company are made of real leather." We can conclude from this statement that shoes which are not made of real leather cannot come from the ABC Company (Rule 1). However, we cannot conclude from the statement that all shoes which are not made by the ABC Company are not made of real leather (Rule 2); indeed the statement does not exclude the fact that other companies may also make shoes with real leather. Nor can we conclude that any shoes which are made of real leather are made by the ABC company (Rule 3); indeed the statement does not deal at all with other companies.

Differentiate link and causation
The text may present facts which seem related, may be linked but do not necessarily have a direct cause and effect relationship. For example, consider this text: "Scientists have found that the vast majority of patients who contracted a liver disease had also been heavy smokers throughout their life." This indicates that there is a relationship between smoking and liver disease but you should be careful not to over-extrapolate. Consider the following statements:

Q: Smoking causes liver disease.
A: Can't tell. Based on the text, this is a possibility, but it is also possible that smoking is associated with other behaviours which lead to liver disease. For example, it may be that all heavy drinkers also happen to be heavy smokers.

Q: Smokers are more likely to develop liver disease than non-smokers.
A: Can't tell. It depends on the ratio of smokers and non-smokers in the general population. So, for example, let's say that 90% of those with liver disease were found to be heavy smokers, but that, in the general population, 90% were heavy smokers anyway; then the statistics would not be that meaningful. However, if only 20% of people in the overall population smoked, this would indicate that smokers are more likely to develop liver disease (although, as we have seen above, this may not necessarily be caused by the smoking itself, but other associated factors).

Such reasoning forms the basis of numerous questions in the test and provides an opportunity for the examiners to confuse you with statements which appear true but are in fact ambiguous. With a little bit of practice, you will acquire the necessary mental agility to be able to manipulate these concepts confidently and quickly in the exam.

Answer all questions and don't be afraid of the "Can't tell" option

The UCAT is not negatively marked, i.e. you are not penalised for a wrong answer, so it is important that you tick an option, even if you are unsure. By ticking any box, you have one chance out of three to get it right. By ticking none, you are guaranteed to score nil on that question. If you struggle with one question, it may be worth leaving it and coming back to it later on. You may get a bright idea in the meantime and, by taking a step back, you may read the text in a different light next time round.

Candidates usually find it difficult to tick the "Can't tell" answer. Psychologically they may feel uncomfortable at not being able to settle on a definite answer and may be constantly worried about missing something obvious. Overall, it is easier for an examiner to write questions that have an ambiguous answer than to write questions that have a definite answer and do not appear too obvious. On balance, therefore, there ought to be more questions to which the answer is "Can't tell" than the other two options. If you are really stuck on an answer, I would therefore suggest that you tick the "Can't tell" box as it may have a higher probability of being the right answer (the fact that you are struggling with it in the first place may actually be an indication that the answer cannot actually be concluded from the text).

Beware of time wasting on Format 2 questions

Format 2 questions (i.e. those where you have to choose between 4 different statements) will take longer to solve because you may need to check whether each statement is true or not. This could take valuable time. Do not go systematically through all the answers if you can avoid it. Read all four options quickly and select the one that you instinctively think may be the answer. Test it against the text. Then proceed to your next best guess.

Read the question properly

This is particularly important for Format 2 questions. Some questions will be asking you to find the answer that can be deduced from the text or which the author is most likely to agree with. This will require you to pick the only option out of the four that is true. Other questions may ask you for the answer that cannot be deduced from the text, in which case, all the statements presented will be true other than the one you are looking for (which will either be "false" or "can't tell"). Other questions still will ask you for the statement that the author is most likely to disagree with, in which case you are looking for the only statement that is false.

10 Verbal Reasoning Practice Questions

This section contains 34 texts, and a total of 200 practice questions. These questions are designed to help you develop an awareness of the different techniques and tips mentioned in the previous section and, as such, we have therefore generally included more questions per text than you would anticipate being asked to answer in the exam.

The answers to all questions, together with explanations, can be found from page 344 onwards.

Once you have practised answering all 200 questions, you should be ready to confront the mock exam which features at the back of this book and replicates the actual exam's format (i.e. 11 texts, 4 questions each).

You may want to wait until you have practised all sections in this book before going ahead with the mock exam.

VR 1 Practice — Financial Crisis

TEXT

The 2008 financial crisis was caused by a number of factors which can be difficult for a lay member of the public to understand. At the source of the crisis is the fact that a number of US banks had offered mortgages to so-called "sub-prime" customers (i.e. usually less well-off individuals with a high credit risk) without checking that the customers could actually afford to repay the loans. The bank had then sold the debt to other banks around the world, meaning that almost every bank in the world owned a share of these mortgages, with some owning a bigger share than others. When a large proportion of these "sub-prime" customers failed to repay some of their loans, all exposed banks started experiencing difficulties, having lent money that could not be repaid. This caused a domino effect and a major financial crisis, which included the nationalisation of Northern Rock, the collapse of American investment institutions such as Lehman Brothers, followed by the merger of Merrill Lynch with Bank of America and then the merger of HBOS with Lloyds TSB in the UK. Some commentators have said that bankers' greed was a contributor to the problem.

As if a global crisis wasn't enough, public confidence was also undermined by an alleged pyramid scheme fraud by a prominent American financier. This $50bn alleged fraud consisted of taking money from unsuspecting rich individuals, promising high returns. As new investors paid money into the scheme, the older investors were being paid interest or dividends using the new money, and so on. As it became increasingly difficult to find new money from new investors to pay existing investors and as the old investors started to want their initial investment back, the scheme came apart and the financier had no option but to admit that there was a problem and was arrested. The alleged scam worked on an exclusive basis, i.e. only those who were invited could invest. This created a false sense of security which encouraged very prominent individuals, including bankers, to become victims. Pyramid schemes are non-sustainable models which involve enrolling new members and rewarding the members with money being paid by new members. They clearly exploit the greed and gullibility of those who are easily attracted by high returns. Such schemes are illegal in many countries, including the US and the UK.

PRACTICE QUESTIONS

Q1.1 The HBOS–Lloyds TSB merger could have been avoided if Lehman Brothers had not collapsed.

☐ True ☐ False ☐ Can't tell

Q1.2 The fact that international banks were linked to the American market by owning a share of the sub-prime debt played a key role in the 2008 financial crisis.

☐ True ☐ False ☐ Can't tell

Q1.3 If bankers had not been so greedy, there would have been no financial crisis.

☐ True ☐ False ☐ Can't tell

Q1.4 The 2008 financial crisis has its origin in the US.

☐ True ☐ False ☐ Can't tell

Q1.5 Pyramid schemes do not exist in the UK.

☐ True ☐ False ☐ Can't tell

Q1.6 The alleged fraud was one of the key triggers of the financial crisis.

☐ True ☐ False ☐ Can't tell

Q1.7 The American financier involved in the alleged fraud made a personal gain of $50bn.

☐ True ☐ False ☐ Can't tell

Q1.8 All pyramid schemes will fail eventually.

☐ True ☐ False ☐ Can't tell

VR 2 Practice — Global Warming

TEXT

There is considerable debate about the nature and causes of global warming. A large proportion of politicians believe that global warming is primarily a man-made problem and that each country should make every effort possible to reduce its carbon emissions. As a result, a range of carbon emission reduction measures are being introduced including: encouraging people to use less energy by switching to low-energy light bulbs and switching off unnecessary appliances; and reducing the number of unnecessary car journeys to the bare minimum and encouraging people to switch to public transport. Others believe that the UK is unlikely to make much of a difference since the biggest contributors to carbon emissions are countries such as China, who are refusing to take any remedial action. Others, still, believe that global warming is part of the Earth's natural cycle and, though any action will bring a degree of improvement, such improvement is bound to have little effect overall on the planet.

So, what level of global warming is anticipated for the forthcoming years? Scientists have studied several scenarios which were integrated within climate forecasting models. Assuming that no substantial change takes place, the forecast for the next century includes a rise in the average world temperature of between 1.4 and 5.8 °C and a reduction of the ice cap in the northern hemisphere, whereas in Antarctica (i.e. in the southern hemisphere) the melting of the ice cap would be more than offset by heavier snow falls, with the snow then freezing over the existing layer of ice. Sea levels are expected to increase by between 9 cm and 88 cm. By the end of the 21st century, the average sea level should have risen by between 18 cm and 59 cm. Some scientists predict that the planet's temperature rise caused by humans should continue after the year 2100. The rise in sea level should also continue for millennia after stabilisation of the climate.

Africa is especially vulnerable because of existing pressures on its ecosystems and its low capacity to adapt to change. On all continents, water supply and the threat of flooding in coastal areas will cause problems. On the other hand, areas of the world which are further away from the equator may see an increase in agricultural productivity and colder regions will see their heating needs reduced.

Verbal Reasoning – Practice

PRACTICE QUESTIONS

Q2.1 Switching to low-energy bulbs and encouraging people to use public transport will benefit the combat against global warming.

☐ True ☐ False ☐ Can't tell

Q2.2 Those who believe that global warming is a natural phenomenon also believe that there is no need to take any action.

☐ True ☐ False ☐ Can't tell

Q2.3 China produces the majority of carbon emissions on Earth.

☐ True ☐ False ☐ Can't tell

Q2.4 Global warming is used as an excuse by politicians to reduce the number of cars on the roads.

☐ True ☐ False ☐ Can't tell

Q2.5 In the 21st century, the sea level in Britain is projected to rise by no more than 59 cm.

☐ True ☐ False ☐ Can't tell

Q2.6 The Antarctica ice cap is expected to grow over the 21st century.

☐ True ☐ False ☐ Can't tell

Q2.7 Some countries will experience no negative impact from global warming.

☐ True ☐ False ☐ Can't tell

Q2.8 Over the 21st century, some countries may experience a rise in temperature of over 5.8 °C.

☐ True ☐ False ☐ Can't tell

VR 3 Practice — Free Museum Entry

TEXT

In 2001, the government reintroduced free entry into museums in England, Scotland and Wales, preferring instead to fund museums through governmental subsidies and Heritage Lottery Fund grants. The following year, the number of visitors increased by an average of 70%, with museums such as the V&A registering an increase of 111%.

In addition, a piece of research undertaken by Sara Selwood at City University showed that the museums which saw the biggest increase in visitor figures were also those which had opened new facilities or which had refurbished their facilities in addition to introducing free admission. Some of the increase is due to the same people who previously paid now visiting museums more often and efforts are therefore being made to broaden the appeal of museums to a wider population. As a result of this free-entry policy, some independent museums, who continued charging, have seen a decline in numbers of visitors. The policy is seen as unfair competition. There is also a perception that the subsidies are mostly directed at the already wealthy London museums and do little to encourage museums in the regions.

In 2007, the Department for Culture, Media and Sport (DCMS) announced that the free museum entry policy would be continued at least for another 3 years. Originally, the DCMS had been asked to prepare for a 5% cut in its budget, though the Chancellor, Alistair Darling, later promised that he would increase the department's funding from £1.68 billion in the 2007–08 financial year to £2.21 billion in 2010–11. Many fear though that, in view of the current financial crisis and of the impending Olympic Games, the Arts will be placed on the backburner whilst the government addresses more pressing priorities.

The Conservative Party has developed plans to scrap free entry to museums if it came to power, arguing that allowing museums to set their own entry fees would lead to an improvement in the service they offer. This point of view is likely to anger many members of the public, although perhaps not the 40% of UK residents who, according to a recent poll, seem to be unaware of the existence of the free-entry policy.

Verbal Reasoning – Practice

PRACTICE QUESTIONS

Q3.1 The only impact of the "free-entry" policy has been to encourage people who already went to museums to go more often.

☐ True ☐ False ☐ Can't tell

Q3.2 Some museums have seen an increase in visitor numbers of less than 70%.

☐ True ☐ False ☐ Can't tell

Q3.3 Only the big London museums seem to have benefited from the free-entry policy.

☐ True ☐ False ☐ Can't tell

Q3.4 The increase in visitor numbers is solely due to the free-entry policy.

☐ True ☐ False ☐ Can't tell

Q3.5 Granting free museum entry to the public had never been attempted before.

☐ True ☐ False ☐ Can't tell

Q3.6 The DCMS's budget will increase by £530 million over 3 years.

☐ True ☐ False ☐ Can't tell

Q3.7 The 2012 Olympics will put an end to the free-entry policy.

☐ True ☐ False ☐ Can't tell

Q3.8 A fee-paying entry policy is fairer to small museums.

☐ True ☐ False ☐ Can't tell

VR 4 Practice — EEC, EU, EURO

TEXT

The European Economic Community (EEC) was set up in 1957 by the following countries: Belgium, France, Germany, Italy, Luxembourg and the Netherlands. The UK joined the EEC in 1973. The Maastricht Treaty of 1993 abolished the EEC and replaced it with the European Union (EU). At the time, the EU comprised the same countries as the EEC, but it now includes 27 independent sovereign countries (also known as member states). The main EU institutions are the European Commission, which resides in Brussels (Belgium), and the European Parliament, which sits in Strasbourg (France). The Euro was adopted as the EU's official currency in 1999, though coins and bank notes were not produced until 2002. Fifteen EU countries, collectively known as the Eurozone, have adopted it. In addition, 11 non-EU countries have also adopted the Euro as official currency, including Monaco, the Vatican and Andorra. Sweden and the UK have both declined to join the Euro for the time being.

The UK has adopted a "wait-and-see policy". Arguments in favour of joining the Euro are numerous. By reducing exchange rate uncertainty for UK businesses and tourists, everyone would benefit from lower transaction costs. Adopting the Euro would also encourage greater competition across borders, enabling UK customers to compare prices directly with their neighbours and purchase goods accordingly. On the other hand, adopting the Euro would bring its fair share of problems. For a start, UK interest rates would be set by the European Central Bank in Frankfurt (Germany), which sets interest rates for the whole Eurozone. It has long been argued that the UK economy is more in line with US economy than with European economy and that therefore it needs to keep closer links with US interest rates than European interest rates. In December 2008, the Bank of England was able to reduce UK interest rates drastically in an attempt to boost the UK economy; this would not have been possible had the UK adopted the Euro.

With all this in mind, the most powerful argument against the Euro in the UK is the fact that UK citizens are reluctant to relinquish yet more power to Brussels and to lose their identity in an ever-expanding Europe.

Verbal Reasoning – Practice

PRACTICE QUESTIONS

Q4.1   Monaco is part of the Eurozone.

☐ True   ☐ False   ☐ Can't tell

Q4.2   All original EEC countries are currently in the EU.

☐ True   ☐ False   ☐ Can't tell

Q4.3   All EU institutions are located either in France or in Belgium.

☐ True   ☐ False   ☐ Can't tell

Q4.4   Neither Sweden nor the UK intend to adopt the Euro.

☐ True   ☐ False   ☐ Can't tell

Q4.5   If the UK entered the Eurozone, the Bank of England would lose the power to set interest rates.

☐ True   ☐ False   ☐ Can't tell

Q4.6   The UK would benefit more from adopting the US Dollar as its currency than from adopting the Euro.

☐ True   ☐ False   ☐ Can't tell

Q4.7   Andorra is not an independent sovereign country.

☐ True   ☐ False   ☐ Can't tell

Q4.8   If the UK adopted the Euro as official currency then the Bank of England would cease to exist.

☐ True   ☐ False   ☐ Can't tell

VR 5 Practice — Coq au Vin & Quiche Lorraine

TEXT

"Coq au Vin" is a traditional French dish whose main ingredients are red wine, lardons, onion and occasionally garlic. The word "coq" means "rooster". Traditional recipes use older roosters to produce a richer broth; however, roosters are not easily found and can be tough to eat. Consequently most home cooks use chicken as a substitute. Lardons are frequently used in French cooking and consist of thick slices of pork belly cut in cubes or thick strips. They are often smoked and are a main ingredient for a wide range of dishes including Quiche Lorraine. Although they can be found in some UK supermarkets, lardons are in sparse supply and thick bacon can be used as a substitute. However, bacon is not as fatty as lardons and therefore may taste drier. The original recipe uses the bird's blood, which is added at the end to produce a thick black colour. The fainthearted leave the blood out, though it produces a less rich sauce.

Quiche Lorraine is a dish that dates back to the 16th century, and consisted of an egg, cream and lardon mix on a crust of bread dough. Because of its primarily vegetarian ingredients, it was historically considered a somehow unmanly dish, hence the expression "real men don't eat quiche". There is controversy as to whether cheese formed part of the original dish (although the locals believe it didn't, some food historians do). Today, the Quiche Lorraine is not always served with cheese.

Its name comes from the German "Kuchen", meaning "cake", with "Lorraine" signifying that it comes from the Lorraine region in Eastern France. Lorraine, a region bordering Belgium, Germany and Luxembourg, was first taken by France in 1648, was annexed by the Germans in 1871, and handed back to the French in 1918 following World War I. Its symbol is the Mirabelle plum (a yellow cousin of the greengage), which is often used to make pastries and to make a very refined liqueur.

Verbal Reasoning – Practice

PRACTICE QUESTIONS

Q5.1 Bacon is an essential ingredient of Coq au Vin.

☐ True ☐ False ☐ Can't tell

Q5.2 Bacon can be used as a substitute for lardons in Quiche Lorraine.

☐ True ☐ False ☐ Can't tell

Q5.3 Most home cooks don't follow the traditional Coq au Vin recipe.

☐ True ☐ False ☐ Can't tell

Q5.4 If bacon is used instead of lardons, then garlic should be added to compensate for the dryness.

☐ True ☐ False ☐ Can't tell

Q5.5 Quiche Lorraine is a vegetarian dish.

☐ True ☐ False ☐ Can't tell

Q5.6 Originally, Quiche Lorraine was not a French dish.

☐ True ☐ False ☐ Can't tell

Q5.7 The Lorraine region has remained French since it was handed back by Germany in 1918.

☐ True ☐ False ☐ Can't tell

Q5.8 Mirabelle liqueur is yellow.

☐ True ☐ False ☐ Can't tell

VR 6 Practice — Blu-Ray

TEXT

Blu-Ray – its full name is Blu-Ray Disc (BD) – is the next generation of optical discs developed jointly by a wide range of leading manufacturers, including Dell, Apple, Sony, Philips, Samsung and Sharp. The name of this new technology comes from the fact that it uses a blue-violet laser instead of the red laser currently used by DVD players. Because blue-violet lasers have a shorter wavelength than red lasers, they can be focused with greater precision. This means that data can be packed more tightly onto the disc. Blu-Ray discs can take as much as 25 gigabytes (GB) on each layer. Research carried out by Pioneer has demonstrated that discs can be constructed with up to 20 layers. Hollywood studios have recently announced that they would choose Blu-Ray as their preferred format and would be releasing titles on both normal DVD and BD format for some time. Although the DVD format will eventually disappear, BD players will be able to play DVDs.

The Blu-Ray Disc Association (BRDA) has indicated that British consumers bought over 400,000 BDs in November 2008, an increase of 165% on October 2008 sales. Such an increase could be reasonably explained by three factors: (i) Blu-Ray has won the format war over DVDs and is bound to become more popular; (ii) the release of popular movies such as Batman on Blu-Ray format just before Christmas has boosted sales; and (iii) as Blu-Ray players become cheaper, BDs will sell more. The BRDA is expecting sales of Blu-Ray players to triple over 2009, reaching 2.5 million units Europe-wide. However, there are strong reasons to suspect that such an increase is unrealistic. No Blu-Ray players are manufactured in the UK and, in the context of a falling Pound and a rising Yen, products manufactured in Japan will become more expensive. BDs also remain comparatively expensive against DVDs and, consequently, the average buyer may delay any purchase until better economic times.

Verbal Reasoning – Practice

PRACTICE QUESTIONS

Q6.1 Everyone should replace their DVD players with a Blu-Ray player as soon as possible as DVDs are being phased out.

☐ True ☐ False ☐ Can't tell

Q6.2 Blu-Ray discs are manufactured to store 500GB of data.

☐ True ☐ False ☐ Can't tell

Q6.3 Those who purchase Blu-Ray players can discard their DVD players.

☐ True ☐ False ☐ Can't tell

Q6.4 Blue-violet lasers are safer than red lasers.

☐ True ☐ False ☐ Can't tell

Q6.5 Blu-Ray players would be cheaper if they were manufactured in the UK.

☐ True ☐ False ☐ Can't tell

Q6.6 Sales of Blu-Ray players in the UK are expected to increase over 2009.

☐ True ☐ False ☐ Can't tell

Q6.7 Batman was not released in DVD format.

☐ True ☐ False ☐ Can't tell

Q6.8 Fewer than 200,000 Blu-Ray discs were sold in the UK in October 2008.

☐ True ☐ False ☐ Can't tell

VR 7 Practice — Cyanide & Arsenic

TEXT

Cyanide is a substance commonly found in nature, for example in apple pips, apricot stones and coffee beans. Ingested in small amounts it can cause headaches and cardiac palpitations. Cyanide is sometimes described as having a "bitter almond" smell. However, it can sometimes be odourless. In addition, when it does emit a smell, not all humans have the ability to detect it. Death is likely to occur within 5 minutes if as little as 50 mg is ingested. More substantial amounts would result in instant death. The poison acts by preventing oxygen from reaching the cells, which quickly affects the heart and the brain. As well as being a well-known poison, cyanide has been used by butterfly collectors – who would crush laurel leaves (which contain cyanide) to produce a preservative liquid – as well as in the gold industry where it is commonly used for mining and electroplating.

Arsenic is also colourless but is totally odourless in its normal state. It is a weak acid which is totally soluble in water. When heated in air at atmospheric pressure, it converts directly from solid form to gaseous form. The fumes from the reaction have a similar smell to garlic. Arsenic was used in Victorian times by women, who mixed it with vinegar and chalk and either ingested it or rubbed it into their skin to improve their complexion; the result was a whiter skin which proved that they were not peasants. It has also been abundantly used as a poison, both for humans and also for insects, fungi and bacteria, and is often used to preserve wood. Scientists have often exploited its medicinal virtues; originally used for the treatment of syphilis, it has not been superseded in this role by modern antibiotics. It is, however, currently used for the treatment of some leukaemias, and psoriasis, and new research suggests that it may be better than iodine-124 in locating tumours when doing PET-scan imaging.

PRACTICE QUESTIONS

Q7.1 Most humans would detect cyanide's bitter almond smell when it is present.

☐ True ☐ False ☐ Can't tell

Q7.2 Butterflies caught by collectors were killed using a cyanide-based solution made from laurel leaves.

☐ True ☐ False ☐ Can't tell

Q7.3 Humans should avoid consuming large quantities of apples, apricots and coffee.

☐ True ☐ False ☐ Can't tell

Q7.4 Cyanide is a by-product of gold mining.

☐ True ☐ False ☐ Can't tell

Q7.5 Arsenic does not exist in liquid form.

☐ True ☐ False ☐ Can't tell

Q7.6 Iodine-124 is currently being used to locate tumours.

☐ True ☐ False ☐ Can't tell

Q7.7 Arsenic and cyanide are both toxic to insects.

☐ True ☐ False ☐ Can't tell

Q7.8 Someone who was being poisoned by ingesting water containing arsenic would not be able to detect its presence.

☐ True ☐ False ☐ Can't tell

VR 8 Practice — Chocolate

TEXT

It has often been said that chocolate contains caffeine but this is a myth. In fact, cocoa contains a substance called theobromine, which is a stimulant that is found only in cocoa. Caffeine may be artificially added by chocolate-makers but is not present naturally. Both substances are cardiovascular stimulants. However, fundamentally the effects of theobromine differ widely from those of caffeine. Whilst caffeine is physically addictive, increases emotional stress, stimulates the respiratory system and increases alertness, theobromine is not addictive, is a mild antidepressant, stimulates the muscular system and increases the feeling of well-being. Smoking cigarettes accelerates the dissipation of both substances from the system. As for tea, although it contains more caffeine than coffee, a typical serving contains much less, as tea is normally brewed much weaker.

As well as theobromine, chocolate contains other compounds which are each credited with a range of benefits; for example, recent studies have concluded that chocolate can reduce cholesterol levels through the polyphenols that it naturally contains. Consequently, some manufacturers have sought to fully exploit these newly found health benefits in their advertising and others are going even further by introducing new ingredients into their chocolate products to provide consumers with further benefits. We are now seeing calcium-enriched chocolates which strengthen bones, and can prevent dental caries, osteoporosis and even colon cancer. Soy fibre is being introduced into chocolate to help with cholesterol reduction and phytostanols (saturated phytosterols such as sitostanol and campestanol) are currently being studied as potential cholesterol-lowering compounds for incorporation into chocolate. Soy fibre is derived from the soya bean. Due to its neutral taste and light colour, soy fibre can be incorporated into a variety of high-fibre and reduced-calorie products without affecting traditional quality. A particularly new area of development is the addition of mood-enhancing plants or compounds such as ginseng, ginko or even royal jelly. This has led to the introduction of a wide range of chocolates which claim to improve brain activity, enhance memory or even have an aphrodisiac effect.

Verbal Reasoning – Practice

PRACTICE QUESTIONS

Q8.1 Drinking tea may lead to increased emotional stress.

☐ True   ☐ False   ☐ Can't tell

Q8.2 Smoking compensates for the effects of caffeine and theobromine.

☐ True   ☐ False   ☐ Can't tell

Q8.3 Chocolate is not addictive.

☐ True   ☐ False   ☐ Can't tell

Q8.4 Chocolate can only contain caffeine if coffee is mixed with it.

☐ True   ☐ False   ☐ Can't tell

Q8.5 Phytostanols are substances occurring naturally in plants.

☐ True   ☐ False   ☐ Can't tell

Q8.6 Soy fibre contains phytostanols.

☐ True   ☐ False   ☐ Can't tell

Q8.7 The risks of developing osteoporosis can be reduced by eating calcium-enriched foods.

☐ True   ☐ False   ☐ Can't tell

Q8.8 Some of the advertised health benefits of enhanced chocolate are unproven.

☐ True   ☐ False   ☐ Can't tell

VR 9 Practice — Pregnancy Food

TEXT

Pregnant women should be aware of the consequence of eating cheese during pregnancy. Cheese constitutes an important source of calcium and protein to pregnant women; however, some varieties of cheese may encourage the growth of bacteria which could harm an unborn child. Women avoiding high-risk cheese are very unlikely to be affected by such bacteria such as listeria. Hard cheeses such as Cheddar, Edam, Gruyère, feta and Parmesan, and soft and processed cheeses such as Boursin, goat cheese without a white rind, mozzarella and ricotta are safe to eat in pregnancy because listeria is present in such small numbers that the risk is considered extremely small. Mould-ripened soft cheeses such as Brie and Camembert, blue-veined cheeses such as Roquefort and Stilton, and soft unpasteurised cheeses must be avoided. All yoghurts, crème fraiche and sour cream are safe to eat, whether they are natural, flavoured or biologically active.

Fish is a good meal choice during pregnancy as it contains omega-3 fatty acids that help baby's brain development. However, the expectant mother should avoid some varieties such as shark and swordfish, which contain high levels of methyl-mercury, a substance which may affect baby's nervous system. These fish live longer and are therefore accumulating more mercury in their flesh than other fish. Be aware too that most types of fish contain traces of mercury, so a pregnant woman may want to limit her weekly consumption of safer varieties too. It is recommended that no more than 350 g of lower-mercury fish such as salmon, shrimp or canned light tuna be consumed in a week (which is equivalent to approximately two meals). Of those 350 g, only half should come from canned "white" albacore tuna, which tends to contain more mercury than light tuna (which is a mix of different low-mercury tuna species). Women who have any doubt about mercury levels or the provenance of the fish should limit their fish consumption to 175g per week.

Verbal Reasoning – Practice

PRACTICE QUESTIONS

Q9.1 Pregnant women should avoid goat cheese with a white rind.

☐ True ☐ False ☐ Can't tell

Q9.2 A pregnant woman eating no other cheese than Cheddar cannot get listeria infection.

☐ True ☐ False ☐ Can't tell

Q9.3 Pregnant women should steer clear of cheese.

☐ True ☐ False ☐ Can't tell

Q9.4 A sandwich made only from ham and Gruyère between two slices of bread is safe for a pregnant woman to eat.

☐ True ☐ False ☐ Can't tell

Q9.5 It would normally be considered safe for a pregnant woman to eat 150 g of a fish pie made exclusively of the following ingredients: salmon, white albacore tuna, shrimp, crème fraiche, Cheddar, Parmesan.

☐ True ☐ False ☐ Can't tell

Q9.6 White tuna is the species of tuna with the longest life expectancy.

☐ True ☐ False ☐ Can't tell

Q9.7 Once ingested by a fish, methyl-mercury tends to stay in its body for some time.

☐ True ☐ False ☐ Can't tell

Q9.8 Assuming all other factors equal, a young fish from one species will contain less mercury than an older fish from the same species.

☐ True ☐ False ☐ Can't tell

VR 10 Practice — The Grass is Greener

TEXT – LETTER DATED 5 JANUARY

Dear Sir

I am writing regarding the parking ticket which I found on my car this morning and would like to explain why I believe it should be cancelled. On 16 December, I parked my car legally within the white markings on Green Avenue, a small street parallel to the street in which I live. This is a road where anyone is free to park for free all year round. This morning, as I was setting out for work, I found my car on a nearby piece of grass, with a parking ticket for £120, stating that I was being fined because my car was illegally parked on the grass. This is NOT where I had left it.

I gather from a notice that I found on a lamp post near where I originally parked the car that the road has been resurfaced recently. The notice was dated 17 December and announced that parking would be suspended between 19 December and 24 December, both dates included, to allow resurfacing work to take place during that time. It was confirmed to me by the Council that the resurfacing work did indeed take place at some stage between those two dates. Because I was away from the country between 18 December and 2 January, I was not able to move my car from its normal parking space and I know from having talked to neighbours that the workers moved the car before starting the resurfacing work. Since I was not responsible for moving the car, I don't see why I should have to pay for it!

I feel that this parking fine is unfair because the notice given to remove my car was posted after I had parked it there and did not give me enough time to remove the car. It is also unfair of you to expect that, around Christmas time, people would be around to read the notice in the first place.

I therefore hope that you will cancel the ticket and look forward to hearing from you soon with the good news.

Best regards
John Rover

PRACTICE QUESTIONS

Q10.1 The car's owner was fined for being in breach of the parking suspension.

☐ True ☐ False ☐ Can't tell

Q10.2 The car remained parked on the grass for at least a week.

☐ True ☐ False ☐ Can't tell

Q10.3 John Rover lives in a street where parking is normally free.

☐ True ☐ False ☐ Can't tell

Q10.4 The resurfacing work lasted 5 days.

☐ True ☐ False ☐ Can't tell

Q10.5 John Rover did not use his car on 17 December.

☐ True ☐ False ☐ Can't tell

Q10.6 Although dated 17 December, the parking suspension notice was not placed on the lamp post before 18 December.

☐ True ☐ False ☐ Can't tell

Q10.7 The parking ticket was placed on the car on or before 24 December.

☐ True ☐ False ☐ Can't tell

Q10.8 Legally, councils are only required to give two days' notice for parking suspensions.

☐ True ☐ False ☐ Can't tell

VR 11 Practice — The Bard

TEXT

After three years of meticulous research, X-rays and infrared imaging, experts have finally lifted all doubts: the only known portrait of William Shakespeare painted whilst he was alive has been found! The painting was unveiled on Monday in London by Professor Stanley Wells, president of the Foundation Shakespeare Birthplace, an association which manages the museum in Stratford-upon-Avon, where the poet was born.

The painting was made in 1610, several years before the death of the great English poet and writer. It is part of a collection owned for centuries by the family of Alex Cobbe, a restorer of objects of art, who inherited it. The painting was very well appreciated within his family but no one had made the link with the poet until Alex saw a portrait of Shakespeare with an uncanny similarity to his own painting at the National Portrait Gallery in London. This was a painting from the Folger Shakespeare Library in Washington, which had, for a long time, been deemed to have been painted whilst Shakespeare was still alive, before analyses made 70 years ago concluded that the paint dated from the 19th century.

Realising that he was the owner of the original version, which had been copied, he contacted Professor Stanley Wells, who was at first dubious because the oldest known paintings and busts of Shakespeare had, until then, all been done just after his death in 1616.

Professor Rupert Featherstone of the University of Cambridge looked at the pigments used whilst experts from the University of Hamburg dated the oak plank on which the portrait was painted. Their conclusions were positive: the painting was made when Shakespeare was still alive. Another favourable point: the painting was found by the Cobbes with another portrait which represented the Count of Southampton, one of Shakespeare's main financial sponsors.

Verbal Reasoning – Practice

PRACTICE QUESTIONS

Q11.1 The Cobbes' painting was made approximately six years before Shakespeare's death.

☐ True ☐ False ☐ Can't tell

Q11.2 The Cobbes' painting was the only portrait of Shakespeare ever painted during his lifetime.

☐ True ☐ False ☐ Can't tell

Q11.3 The Folger Shakespeare Library copy of the painting was painted 70 years ago.

☐ True ☐ False ☐ Can't tell

Q11.4 Shakespeare was born in a museum.

☐ True ☐ False ☐ Can't tell

Q11.5 The portrait was painted on wood rather than on a canvas.

☐ True ☐ False ☐ Can't tell

Q11.6 The Count of Southampton met Shakespeare during his lifetime.

☐ True ☐ False ☐ Can't tell

Q11.7 The Folger Shakespeare Library copy of the painting was made over three centuries after the original portrait was painted.

☐ True ☐ False ☐ Can't tell

Q11.8 Alex Cobbe restored the original Shakespeare portrait inherited by his family.

☐ True ☐ False ☐ Can't tell

VR 12 Practice — Delay Compensation Package

TEXT

Euro MPs have recently adopted a new law compensating bus, coach and boat passengers for delays and cancellations.

Maritime transport companies will have the obligation to "provide information to their passengers as well as compensation if their journey is disrupted or interrupted", the Parliament explains. Compensation will vary between 25% of the price of the ticket for delays between one and two hours and 50% if the delay exceeds two hours. Compensation is 100% of the ticket price if the company does not provide suitable alternative means of transport or information on alternative means of transport.

For buses and coaches, companies will also need to provide a substitute or information about substitute modes of transport. If required, they will also need to pay half the ticket price.

New EU legislation had already been adopted in 2005 for plane delays, with passengers denied boarding because of overbooking, or delays caused by other airline hiccups, receiving compensation of 250 Euros for short-haul flights, rising to 600 Euros for long-haul flights. If a flight is cancelled, airlines have to give passengers meals, refreshments and overnight accommodation (including a transfer to the hotel) free of charge or find them alternative transport to their final destination. Passengers are also entitled to complimentary refreshments on board the aircraft if they are delayed beyond a specified number of hours, which depends on the distance they are due to fly. Those who are most affected are the budget airlines, as the compensation sums represent a huge proportion of their average fares.

PRACTICE QUESTIONS

Q12.1 A delay of one hour on the bus will give rise to compensation of 25% of the price of the ticket.

☐ True   ☐ False   ☐ Can't tell

Q12.2 Compensation in the airline industry is not related to the cost of the ticket.

☐ True   ☐ False   ☐ Can't tell

Q12.3 Compensation for airline delays cannot exceed 600 Euros.

☐ True   ☐ False   ☐ Can't tell

Q12.4 The introduction of the new compensation rules will lead to an increase in ticket prices.

☐ True   ☐ False   ☐ Can't tell

Q12.5 It is possible for airline delay compensation to be higher than the price paid for the ticket.

☐ True   ☐ False   ☐ Can't tell

Q12.6 It is possible for ferry delay compensation to be higher than the price paid for the ticket.

☐ True   ☐ False   ☐ Can't tell

Q12.7 Boat companies are legally obliged to organise an alternative mode of transport for their passengers.

☐ True   ☐ False   ☐ Can't tell

Q12.8 All airline passengers who are entitled to the 600-Euro compensation package for long-haul flights are also entitled to complimentary refreshments on board the aircraft.

☐ True   ☐ False   ☐ Can't tell

VR 13 Practice: Saving Neil Armstrong's Spacesuit

TEXT

A fundraising campaign was launched a few days ago to preserve the spacesuit worn by Neil Armstrong when he became the first astronaut to walk on the Moon.

The US National Air and Space Museum is trying to raise $500,000 to safeguard the spacesuit and build a climate-controlled display case.

The spacesuit curator at the Air and Space Museum in Washington said:

"In most of the 46 years since the spacesuit was used, we've owned it at the Smithsonian Air and Space Museum; it was transferred to us by NASA after they finished testing it. It was on display until 2006, at which point we decided to take it off display and place it in our state-of-the-art facility, which is at cool temperature and low humidity, just to preserve it and figure out a way in which we can further display it, in readiness for the 50th anniversary of Neil Armstrong's first step on the Moon.

"The suit is a very complex machine made of many different materials, about 12 different types of fabric combined together in one. Now, to preserve and conserve each textile individually would be very easy, but we would have to take the suit apart and we are not prepared to do that. We have to conserve it all as one thing. We want to use what are now state-of-the art conservation techniques of imaging and photography so we are able to map the suit entirely, get a very close-up look at it, and provide virtual visitors on the internet with a 360-degree experience. We will also develop a special display support, which will allow air to circulate around the suit. We are also going to buy a special display case, which will provide the climate that I discussed earlier and will enable us to display the suit on time for that 50th anniversary in 2019."

Verbal Reasoning – Practice

PRACTICE QUESTIONS

Q13.1 In what year was this piece of text most likely written?

    A. 2005.
    B. 2008.
    C. 2012.
    D. 2015.

Q13.2 Which one of the following statements is the author most likely to agree with?

    A. All fabrics used to make the spacesuit require low temperature and low humidity to be preserved.

    B. All fabrics used to make the spacesuit require air circulation to be preserved

    C. Visitors to the museum will be able to see the spacesuit for themselves, albeit through a glass wall.

    D. Visitors to the museum will only be able to see the spacesuit via interactive computer screens.

Q13.3 Until 2006, the suit was on display but not in a special atmosphere.

    ☐ True   ☐ False   ☐ Can't tell

Q13.4 The $500,000 that the museum is trying to raise will cover the full cost of the climate-controlled display care and of the photography/imaging work.

    ☐ True   ☐ False   ☐ Can't tell

VR 14 Practice — Sleepover

TEXT

Everyone knows that sleeping too little is bad; it makes you feel tired and irritable; and it can contribute to obesity, high blood pressure, diabetes and heart disease. But now, those who sleep too much also have cause for concern: research carried out over the last 10 years appears to show that adults who usually sleep less than 6 hours or more than 8 are at risk of dying earlier than those who sleep between 6 and 8 hours.

An analysis of the results of 16 different studies by Professor Cappuccio shows that 12% more of the short sleepers (i.e. those who sleep less than 6 hours per night) had died when they were followed up, compared to the medium sleepers (i.e. those who sleep 6-8 hours per night). However, 30% more of the long sleepers had died compared to the medium sleepers. That increase in mortality risk is roughly equivalent to the risk of drinking several units of alcohol a day, though less than the mortality risk that comes from smoking.

Professor Cappuccio was aware that some of those who sleep too long might be depressed or might be using sleeping pills. He made allowances for this and found that the link was still there. His own theory is that people who sleep over 8 hours may have an underlying health problem that is not yet showing other symptoms.

But not everyone agrees. Professor Youngstedt of Arizona State University carried out a study with 14 young adults, asking them to spend 2 extra hours in bed every night for 3 weeks. The participants complained of soreness and back pain. They also suffered from "increases in depressed mood" and also "increases in inflammation", specifically higher levels of a protein called IL-6 in the blood, connected with inflammation.

Anyone studying sleep has to contend with a range of difficulties. You have to take with a pinch of salt the number of hours people say they sleep each night. Apparently we have a tendency to overestimate how long we have been asleep. And when it comes to quality of sleep, all experts agree that it is even harder to measure than how long you sleep.

Verbal Reasoning – Practice

PRACTICE QUESTIONS

Q14.1 What conclusion can be drawn from Professor Cappuccio's research?

　　　A. People who sleep more than 8 hours would be less likely to die if they made efforts to sleep less than 6 hours.

　　　B. Depression can stop you from sleeping enough hours.

　　　C. Taking sleeping pills increases your mortality risk.

　　　D. Sleeping more than 8 hours may be the first sign of a terminal illness.

Q14.2 What conclusion can be drawn from Professor Youngstedt's research?

　　　A. People who sleep 8 hours tend to be more depressed than those who sleep only 6 hours.

　　　B. Spending 2 hours more in bed than you normally do may increase your risk of depression.

　　　C. IL-6 can cause depression.

　　　D. Sleeping more than 8 hours may be the first sign of a terminal illness.

Q14.3 Which assumption is Professor Cappuccio making?

　　　A. The average person sleeps 7 hours a day.

　　　B. People with depression have higher mortality than those who are not depressed.

　　　C. Smoking is less dangerous than drinking.

　　　D. People with underlying health problems tend to oversleep rather than undersleep.

VR 15 Practice — Earth 2.0

TEXT

A haul of planets from NASA's Kepler telescope includes a world sharing many characteristics with Earth. Officially named Kepler-452b, this new world orbits at a very similar distance from its star as the Earth, though its radius is 60% larger than the Earth's. Astronomers tend to get excited about such worlds because they might be small and cool enough to host liquid water on their surface and might therefore be hospitable to life. NASA's science chief called the new world "Earth 2.0".

Kepler-452b joins other so-called exoplanets, such as Kepler-186f, that are similar in many ways to Earth. However, determining which is most Earth-like depends on the properties one considers. Kepler-186f, announced in 2014, is smaller than the new planet, but orbits a red dwarf star that is significantly cooler than our own. However, Kepler-452b orbits a parent star which belongs to the same class as the Sun; it is just 4% more massive and 10% brighter. The mass of Kepler-452b cannot yet be measured and so astronomers have to rely on models to estimate a range of possible masses, with the most likely being five times that of the Earth.

The new world is included in a haul of 500 new possible planets sighted by the Kepler space telescope around distant stars. Twelve of the new candidates are less than twice Earth's diameter, orbiting in the so-called habitable zone around their star. The zone refers to a range of distances at which the energy radiated by the star would permit water to exist as a liquid on the planet's surface if certain conditions are met. Around 20% of Sun-like stars, of which there are countless, have an Earth-sized planet in their habitable zone.

While similar in size and brightness to the Sun, Kepler-452b's host star is 1.5 billion years older than ours. Scientists therefore believe it could point to a possible future for the Earth. It is not known if Kepler-452b is a rocky planet or a small gas planet but, based on its small radius, Kepler-452b has a reasonable chance, between 49% and 62%, of being rocky. If it is a rocky planet, it may be subject to a runaway greenhouse effect similar to that seen on Venus; the increasing energy from its ageing sun might be heating the surface and evaporating any oceans. It could be experiencing now what the Earth will undergo more than a billion years from now.

PRACTICE QUESTIONS

Q15.1 Which of the following statements is definitely false?

    A. Kepler-452b has a diameter 60% larger than the diameter of the Earth.
    B. The radius of a planet can be used as an indicator of how rocky it is likely to be.
    C. Earth 2.0 is smaller than Kepler-186f.
    D. Venus experienced a runaway greenhouse effect.

Q15.2 Which of the following statements can reasonably be concluded from the passage?

    A. The Earth's oceans will eventually disappear.
    B. The Sun has a remaining lifespan of over 1.5 billion years.
    C. All planets orbiting within the habitable zone of their sun contain liquid water.
    D. The Sun is getting bigger and brighter as it gets older.

Q15.3 Which of the following statements is the author most likely to agree with?

    A. Exoplanets are rocky.
    B. Exoplanets revolve around a star similar to the Earth's Sun.
    C. Exoplanets contain liquid water on their surface.
    D. Exoplanets are common in the universe.

Q15.4 There is no liquid water on Venus.

    ☐ True   ☐ False   ☐ Can't tell

VR 16 Practice — Dyeing To Bake

TEXT

Liquid Dye is made out of synthetic colourings with a water base, usually found in little plastic squeezy bottles. Being water-based, it is the least intense and weakest of all food colourings, meaning you will need to use more of it to achieve a brighter or deeper colour. If you use a significant amount, the extra liquid has the potential to thin and throw off a recipe. It is thus most suited to recipes requiring lighter colours.

Liquid Gel Dye is a synthetic colouring with a water, glycerine and/or corn syrup base, which is available in small dropper bottles that contain a thick gel-like liquid. It is harder to find than liquid dye and, because of its thick texture, it can be harder to incorporate into thick or stiff dough. However the colour in liquid gel dye is more concentrated than traditional liquid food colourings, so you need less, which is important in recipes where you want to minimise the amount of liquid added (such as in sweets or icing recipes). Since you need less, there is less of a chance the colouring will adversely flavour the food too.

Gel Paste Dye is a synthetic colouring with a water, glycerine and/or corn syrup base, usually found in small pots or jars. It is an even more concentrated form of liquid gel dye and is therefore thicker; you only need a small amount, so it can be slightly less messy than using dropper bottles. Gel paste dye is very effective in dyeing a large amount of mix (like cake mix) and produces dark, saturated colours. It is easy to add too much colouring, which cannot be undone. Online reviews by users suggest that red dyes "produce a weird metallic taste".

Powdered Dye is a synthetic colouring with no water, glycerine or corn syrup, found in jars. Since there is no liquid in powdered dyes, it's great in recipes where any added liquid can lead to a disaster, like in crystal sugar, chocolate, macaroons or meringues. Powdered dye won't dry out like other food dyes and has an extremely long shelf life – great for producing really dark shades of colour.

Verbal Reasoning – Practice

PRACTICE QUESTIONS

Q16.1 With regard to liquid dyes, which of the following conclusions is the author most likely to <u>disagree</u> with?

    A. Using large quantities of liquid dyes will not affect taste.
    B. Liquid dyes are good to achieve pastel tones.
    C. It is not advisable to make macaroons with liquid dye.
    D. When using liquid dyes to obtain a bright colour, it is best to reduce the amount of water/milk used in the recipe by an equivalent amount.

Q16.2 An amateur baker has a stock of each of the four types of dye, but the labels setting out the ingredients are missing. He wishes to bake a bright red cake with a stiff mix for someone who is allergic to glycerine. Which is the most suitable dye to use?

    A. Liquid dye.
    B. Liquid gel dye.
    C. Gel paste dye.
    D. Powdered dye.

Q16.3 Which conclusion can be drawn from the passage?

    A. Gel paste dye dries out more quickly than liquid dye.
    B. Red gel paste dye is not a natural product.
    C. Non-red gel paste dye does not taste metallic.
    D. Powdered dye does not affect taste.

Q16.4 Which conclusion can be drawn from the passage?

    A. One cannot use two types of dye in the same cake mix.
    B. Gel paste dye is hard to incorporate into stiff dough.
    C. Powdered dye is not water soluble.
    D. Gel paste dye is more expensive than liquid gel dye.

Q16.5 Someone with a corn allergy cannot use liquid gel or gel paste dyes.

    ☐ True   ☐ False   ☐ Can't tell

VR 17 Practice — A Battle Of Wills

TEXT

A woman cut out of her mother's will was awarded a £200,000 inheritance in what could prove a landmark ruling. She will now be able to buy her housing association property. Ms Jackson went to court after her mother left her entire £600,000 estate to a range of animal and other charities when she died in 2006. The Court of Appeal ruled that she should receive a third of the estate, in a ruling which could significantly weaken people's right to leave money to those they want to inherit it, it is thought.

Ms Jackson had disappeared at the age of 16 with her boyfriend; her mother never forgave her and refused to leave her a single penny of her estate, which was instead left to charities such as the Wildlife Fund and the RSPB. Ms Jackson, who was an only child born two months after her father died, had previously won the right to an inheritance of £50,000 after a district judge concluded that she had been "unreasonably" excluded by her mother. That ruling was subsequently reversed by the Appeal Court, who ruled that she was entitled to a share of the money. Justifying the decision, Lady Justice Arden said that Ms Jackson's mother had been "unreasonable, capricious and harsh".

Experts say the ruling means you can still disinherit your children but you'll have to explain why and what connects you to those you do leave money to. That'll make it easier for adult "disinherited" children to challenge wills and claim greater sums by way of reasonable provision.

In previous cases:
- Animal charities won an appeal to inherit property worth £350,000 despite claims it had been a verbal "deathbed gift" to the homeowner's nephew.
- A builder who cleaned an elderly man's gutters for free was left £500,000 when the pensioner died but faced a court battle with the family to keep the money. The court awarded him the full amount.
- Last year, a 98-year-old woman left £300,000 to a window cleaner instead of her "favourite nephew", who challenged the will in the High Court and won the case.

Verbal Reasoning – Practice

PRACTICE QUESTIONS

Q17.1 How much did Ms Jackson receive in total?

   A. £200,000.
   B. £250,000.
   C. A third of £650,000 (£600,000 + £50,000).
   D. The value of her housing association property.

Q17.2 The value of Ms Jackson's housing association property is:

   A. Less than £200,000.
   B. £200,000.
   C. More than £200,000.
   D. Unknown.

Q17.3 If this case acts as a precedent, what is the most likely conclusion that could be drawn from the passage?

   A. People will have to leave all their money to their children.
   B. Charities will no longer be able to be included in wills.
   C. Wills will be valid as long as the children inherit something.
   D. Wills will only be valid if the sum of money left to the children represents a reasonable percentage of the value of the estate.

Q17.4 Which of the following cannot be reasonably concluded from the passage?

   A. Courts do not always rule in favour of the relatives.
   B. The charities involved in Ms Jackson's case received £400,000.
   C. Ms Jackson's mother was not mentally competent enough to draw up a reasonable will.
   D. Charity donations through wills will decrease.

Q17.5 Following the judgement, at least one third of a deceased person's estate should go to the children.

☐ True   ☐ False   ☐ Can't tell

VR 18 Practice — Fat Chance

TEXT

Supermarket shelves are full of oils of various provenances. But do you know which ones are best to cook with? Obvious, isn't it?! Vegetable fats are good and animal fats are bad. Well, you may need to think again. There are three main types of fat: monounsaturated, polyunsaturated and saturated. When fats and oils are exposed to temperatures close to 180 °C, they undergo an oxidation process, which leads to the formation of aldehydes and lipid peroxides. The same happens at room temperature, albeit far more slowly, leading to lipids going rancid. It so happens that consuming aldehydes, even at small doses, is linked to an increase in the risk of heart disease and cancer.

Corn oil and sunflower oil are rich in polyunsaturates and therefore generate substantial levels of aldehydes when heated, at a level 20 times higher than recommended by the World Health Organization (WHO).

Butter, goose fat, olive oil and cold-pressed rapeseed oil produce far fewer aldehydes because they are richer in monounsaturated and saturated fatty acids, which makes them more stable when heated. In fact, saturated fats hardly undergo this oxidation reaction at all. When it comes to cooking, it doesn't matter whether the olive oil is extra virgin or not; the antioxidant levels present in the extra-virgin products are insufficient to protect us against heat-induced oxidation.

We have known for a while that saturated fat may, after all, not be so bad. Previously scientists had examined the links between eating saturated fat, such as butter, and heart disease. Despite looking at the results of nearly 80 studies involving more than half a million people, they were unable to find convincing evidence that eating saturated fats leads to greater risk of heart disease. One prominent cardiologist was quoted as saying: "Saturated fat makes you less hungry. There is certainly a strong argument that an over-reliance in public health on saturated fat as the main dietary villain for cardiovascular disease has distracted from the risks posed by other nutrients, such as carbohydrates (e.g. bread, potatoes, pasta), which people started to consume in larger quantities to compensate for a lower intake in saturated fats. A high consumption of carbohydrates is associated with changes linked to diabetes and heart disease."

PRACTICE QUESTIONS

Q18.1 Which of these statements can be concluded from the passage?

    A. Aldehydes form at a temperature of 180 °C.
    B. Rancid oil does not contain aldehydes.
    C. Heated saturated fats contain high levels of aldehydes.
    D. Aldehydes tend to be generated from polyunsaturated fats.

Q18.2 Which one of the following oils would the author most likely conclude is not good for use in a cold salad dressing?

    A. Sunflower oil.
    B. Extra-virgin olive oil.
    C. Rapeseed oil.
    D. None of the above.

Q18.3 Which of these statements cannot be concluded from the passage?

    A. Butter is healthier when heated up than when cold.
    B. Hot butter is healthier than hot sunflower oil.
    C. Cold butter is healthy to eat in small quantities.
    D. Eating butter makes you less likely to eat other potentially unhealthy foods.

Q18.4 Which of these statements is the author most likely to agree with?

    A. Potatoes fried in goose fat cannot cause heart disease.
    B. The public was misled about the dangers of saturated fats.
    C. Pasta with extra-virgin olive oil is healthier than pasta alone.
    D. At room temperature, olive oil goes rancid more quickly than sunflower oil.

Q18.5 Which of the following options best ranks the three types of fat in increasing level of oxidation when heated?

    A. Polyunsaturated < Monounsaturated < Saturated.
    B. Saturated < Monounsaturated < Polyunsaturated.
    C. Monounsaturated < Polyunsaturated < Saturated.
    D. Saturated < Polyunsaturated < Monounsaturated.

VR 19 Practice: Snooping

TEXT

Some of the most popular messaging services in the world, such as WhatsApp, Skype or Apple's iMessage, could soon be banned by the British government because the encryption methods they use are not accessible by the security services.

Concerns were earlier expressed by both the UK and the US governments, alleging that such services could make it easier for terrorists to communicate without the fear of seeing their communications intercepted. The Prime Minister said: "In our country, do we want to allow a means of communication between people which, even in extremis, with a signed warrant from the Home Secretary personally, we cannot read?" His answer was no.

The Prime Minister hinted that he wanted corporations such as Facebook, Apple or Microsoft to stop using such applications completely or provide a backdoor to their encryption.

But take a look at Apple's privacy policy and you will see what the problem is: "Apple has no way to decrypt iMessage and FaceTime data when it's in transit between devices. So unlike some other companies' messaging services, Apple doesn't scan your communications, and we wouldn't be able to comply with a wiretap even if we wanted to."

Some of the CEOs of the companies targeted have expressed concerns that tampering with encryption would only help criminals and would threaten the security of consumers who rely on it for services such as online banking.

What is also clear is that advanced encryption is an important part of the security offered by such applications and it is hard to see how those American companies could offer a different product in the UK from what they offer everywhere else in the world.

PRACTICE QUESTIONS

Q19.1 Assuming all the information contained in the passage is correct, which of the following assertions can be concluded from the text?

    A. Messages can sometimes be too securely encrypted to be read by the person receiving them.

    B. The UK version of iMessage could become less secure than the version of iMessage sold in many other countries.

    C. Only messages originating from the UK or the US have a highly secure level of encryption.

    D. No warrant is required to intercept Skype communications.

Q19.2 Which of the following can be concluded from the passage?

    A. Should Apple decide to continue providing iMessage, it may have no choice but to break the law.

    B. If Apple scanned communications, it could decipher encrypted communications in transit.

    C. Communications made via Skype are monitored.

    D. A warrant signed by the Home Secretary is essential to intercept communications.

Q19.3 According to the passage, the biggest risk is that:

    A. Customers may receive undecipherable messages.
    B. Terrorists may intercept customers' personal messages.
    C. Terrorists may communicate without being caught.
    D. The state is unable to monitor terrorists' bank accounts.

Q19.4 Which of the following is the author most likely to conclude from the passage?

    A. A ban on messaging services would be unenforceable.

    B. Skype and iMessage use the same type of encryption.

    C. The government's preferred option is to obtain a backdoor into the encryption.

    D. If the UK government imposed that it should be granted backdoor access, the software companies may no longer wish to make their systems available in the UK.

VR 20 Practice: Breaking The Sound Barrier

TEXT

Travelling at 4.5 times the speed of sound on a commercial airliner is something that we may all live to experience. Two companies of the Airbus group, Astrium and EADS, have registered a patent with the US Patent Office for a project called "Ultra-rapid air vehicle and method of aerial locomotion". The future plane, if it sees the light of day, would be much faster than Concorde (which flew the distance between London and New York in 3 hours and was retired in 2003). It would link London to New York in 1 hour (as opposed to seven to eight currently) and Paris to Los Angeles in three hours. This project was unveiled in a YouTube video by Deepak Gupta, founder of the India-based intellectual property drafting service Patent Yogi and a man with a passion for aeroplanes who, according to the newspaper *Les Echos*, "spends all his time on YouTube trying to find licences and patents which have been deposited".

Equipped with a single triangular wing, the plane would carry 20 passengers for distances of about 5,500 miles (Concorde could carry up to 120 passengers). A rocket engine would propel the plane on a near-vertical ascent to an altitude of 20 miles. Two stratojets would then catapult the plane at supersonic speed on a horizontal trajectory. The aircraft would then cruise on the edge of space, high above conventional aircrafts, before slowing down and entering normal air traffic close to its destination.

The patent filed recognises the issue of supersonic aircrafts making sonic booms as they break the sound barrier. This boom is seen as one of the main reasons Concorde was not a commercial success, with noise complaints leading to it being banned from operating at high speed over land by many countries, negating the main attraction of travelling on the jet. Details are limited on how the supersonic bang would be reduced, but the height at which the new aircraft would fly and the "narrow" angle of the supersonic shock wave coming off its nose would help reduce it because it has a longer distance to dissipate before it reaches the ground.

If you're eager to give it a try, don't get too excited yet. Airbus files for hundreds of patents a year, many of them weird. Last summer, it filed a patent for bicycle-style seats on planes that would make it possible to cram more passengers in the same amount of space. And last autumn, it patented an aircraft cabin shaped like a giant flying saucer.

PRACTICE QUESTIONS

Q20.1 Which of the following statements can be deduced about Deepak Gupta from the passage?

    A. He is a patents and trademarks lawyer/attorney.
    B. He is a plane spotter.
    C. Airbus is one of his clients.
    D. None of the above.

Q20.2 Which of the following statements can be deduced from the text?

    A. The new plane is not at risk of crashing with normal planes.
    B. Normal aircrafts fly at an altitude below 20 miles.
    C. The new plane is unlikely to ever be built.
    D. The new plane could also fly like a normal plane if needed.

Q20.3 If we assume that any plane reaching its destination takes one hour to refuel and be prepared before its next flight, which of the following statements holds true for a London-to-New-York route?

    A. Concorde could carry more passengers in 24 hours than the new plane.
    B. Concorde could carry fewer passengers in 24 hours than the new plane.
    C. Both planes could carry the same number of passengers in 24 hours.
    D. It is not possible to calculate which plane could carry more passengers in 24 hours.

Q20.4 Which of the following is the author most likely to conclude from the passage?

    A. Concorde could only fly to countries bordering an ocean.
    B. The London-to-New-York Concorde line was not profitable.
    C. The new plane could potentially fly to any destination without risking a ban for excess noise.
    D. Airbus will eventually increase the new plane's capacity by introducing bicycle-style seats.

VR 21 Practice — Radioactive Waste

TEXT

Scientists are thinking hard about what the world will look like in 100,000 years' time and how to best protect our radioactive waste. Many think that it should be buried in the ground.

Waste will obviously not just be dumped underground in its raw state. It will be coated with glass, and various other materials, placed in steel and copper canisters, and inserted in concrete tunnels. Clay is effective for geological disposal because it does not allow water or anything leaking from a canister to flow through it. Clay also flexes, helping to dampen shockwaves from earthquakes and protecting the canisters from damage. Rocks such as granite are brittle and crack when they are stressed; and although water cannot travel through granite, it can flow along its cracks. In these rocks, a facility would be located where there were very few cracks and waste canisters would be entirely surrounded by a thick layer of clay called bentonite, which swells when in contact with water. This seals any gaps between the waste and the rock and also cushions the canisters from earthquakes. Incidentally, bentonite is also used to purify wine, cider, beer and vinegar by removing excess protein and to make cat litter. It has laxative properties, acts as a shield against poison ivy, is used as a desiccant (due to its absorption properties) for products at risk from moisture degradation and is being studied for use in battlefield wound dressings.

That's all very well, but how can we make sure that those who live here in 100,000 years' time understand what we did? Whether we write things on paper (which is highly degradable) or on computers (which version of Microsoft Windows will we be on by then!?), keeping information accessible and available for that long is a hard task. Some proposed to mark each sealed disposal site with monoliths inscribed in the six official UN languages, e.g. English, but will people be able to decipher them then? If we can't understand the significance of 5,000-year-old pyramids, how will someone who discovers a radioactive concrete sarcophagus in 50,000 years' time make sense of it and know how to handle its danger? The Scandinavians have tried to come up with landscapes which "make you feel this is a bad and inhospitable place", a bit like in the Edvard Munch painting *The Scream*. But whatever solution is right, it will only need to be implemented when the sites are sealed, in just over a century.

PRACTICE QUESTIONS

Q21.1 Out of those four materials, which one will be furthest away from the radioactive waste?

    A. Glass.
    B. Clay.
    C. Granite.
    D. Copper.

Q21.2 Which of the following is the author most likely to agree with?

    A. Munch's *The Scream* depicts a nuclear apocalypse.
    B. No element remains radioactive for over 100,000 years.
    C. Kitchen sinks can be made out of granite.
    D. The canisters are designed to last over 100,000 years.

Q21.3 Which of these options is the least likely use for bentonite?

    A. Sealing the floor of landfills to prevent underground water contamination.
    B. Keeping boxes containing moisture-sensitive objects dry.
    C. Anti-diarrhoea treatment.
    D. Increasing water retention in soils to increase agricultural yields.

Q21.4 Which of the following is the author most likely to agree is <u>not</u> an intended purpose for bentonite in the context of nuclear waste disposal?

    A. Protect the canisters during earthquakes.
    B. Protect the canisters from damage by external substances.
    C. Stop the granite from cracking during earthquakes.
    D. Contain any material leaking from the canisters.

Q21.5 Which of the following is the author most likely to disagree with in relation to warning future generations?

    A. Books and computers are not a viable solution.
    B. In 100,000 years, no one will speak English.
    C. In 100,000 years, humanity will have self-destructed.
    D. We still have much to learn about the pyramids.

VR 22 Practice — Frankenburger

TEXT

He didn't succumb to Google's appetising offer. Biochemist Patrick Brown, founder of the start-up company Impossible Foods, rejected a proposal for a Google buy-out to the tune of 200 to 300 million dollars to acquire his innovation: vegetal (i.e. plant-based) meat.

It is actually Google who had first initiated research in that field in 2013, when it financed a Dutch scientist who went on to create an artificial burger from beef stem cells. A total of 20,000 muscle fibres are needed so that the whole thing looks like a burger, to which are added salt, breadcrumbs and egg powder as well as beetroot juice and saffron. Without those last two ingredients the burger would look grey, far from the real colour of meat. In contrast, Patrick Brown has invented a vegetal burger, which is made from a secret recipe containing not a single traditional ingredient. Only a small clue is given on the company's website: "We have looked at all animal products at molecular level and have selected the proteins and nutrients which are specific to plant seeds in order to recreate the wonderfully complex experience of eating meat."

Taste-wise, the Google burger (often called Frankenburger by the media) was tested in London by volunteers who felt it had an intense taste close to real meat but lacked fat and therefore tasted a little dry. No official tasting of the vegetal burger has yet taken place, though a journalist from the New-York-based *Wall Street Journal* who tried it said it was amazing and "had the appearance, the taste and cooks on the grill like a real burger"; all that without the taste of blood, states the article.

As for the cost, Google spent 250,000 Euros developing their burger and in 2015 it was estimated that it would cost only 10 Euros to make one, which opens the door to possible retail. Impossible Foods has not revealed the price of its innovation but hopes to manufacture its burger by the end of 2015, with a retail price of 20 Dollars (18 Euros) to remain competitive in the burger market.

According to Patrick Brown, people are prepared to stop consuming meat if there are "new choices on offer which are more delicious and satisfying". As to whether vegetarians will try the Frankenburger, the jury is out, given that some will struggle with the fact that it still contains animal stem cells, even if they are donated voluntarily by the animal.

Verbal Reasoning – Practice

PRACTICE QUESTIONS

Q22.1 Which of the following can be concluded from the passage with regard to the two types of burgers (Impossible Foods (IF) and Google), based on 2015 data and assuming both companies intend to make a profit?

  A. Google burgers will have a lower retail price than IF burgers
  B. Google burgers cost less to manufacture than IF burgers.
  C. Google has manufactured 25,000 burgers so far.
  D. The IF burger will retail at less than 1.8 times the price of the Google burger.

Q22.2 With which of the following statements are the readers of the passage most likely to disagree?

  A. The Google burger does not require animal slaughter.
  B. Pure vegetarians are likely to prefer the IF burger to the Google burger on ethical grounds.
  C. The Google burger is not vegetarian.
  D. The IF burger may be more appealing to New York customers than London customers.

Q22.3 Patrick Brown is a vegetarian.

  ☐ True ☐ False ☐ Can't tell

Q22.4 Beetroot juice and saffron modify the colour but not the taste.

  ☐ True ☐ False ☐ Can't tell

Q22.5 Adding fat to the Google burger would enhance its taste and texture.

  ☐ True ☐ False ☐ Can't tell

Q22.6 Without added colourant, the Google burger looks grey because it lacks blood.

  ☐ True ☐ False ☐ Can't tell

VR 23 Practice — Microwaves

TEXT

Microwaves are the best known and the most useful waves. Amongst their use, you will of course find the microwave oven, but also Wi-Fi, mobile phones and GPS. Their wavelength ranges from 1 millimetre (300 GHz frequency) to 1 metre (0.3 GHz), frequency and wavelength being inversely proportionate. Beyond that, as frequency decreases, you will find FM radio waves and then long waves.

Microwave ovens and Wi-Fi work at the same frequency of 2.4 GHz (12.5 cm wavelength); the difference lies in the nature of the wave produced. The oven behaves like a cavity that creates a stationary wave, exciting the water molecules present in the food and causing a rise in temperature. Wi-Fi, however, only sends impulses containing bundles of information. Mobile phones work on the same principle but with frequencies of 0.8 GHz, 1.8 GHz and 2.6 GHz.

There is an urban legend that a microwave oven can help calculate the speed of light. This is not entirely stupid. We know that the velocity of a wave is calculated as the product of its frequency and its wavelength. Place on a plate some chocolate, marshmallows or grated cheese and switch the microwave oven on. Quickly some melted zones and non-melted zones will appear as a result of the non-homogeneous heating taking place inside (and that is why the plate inside the microwave usually turns, thus resolving the issue). The microwaves inside the oven are like guitar strings. They vibrate but they are forced to be stationary at their two fixation points (i.e. the walls). Between the two, one observes areas of large amplitude (i.e. where the intensity is maximal) and areas where the strings seem stationary (i.e. where the intensity is nil). In the areas of high amplitude, chocolate and cheese melt. The distance between two melting zones is a good indicator of half of the wavelength. Multiplying the wavelength by the frequency should therefore give us the speed of light. Easy!

Not quite, warns Professor J.M. Courty. Though he agrees that the principle is correct, he states that waves found in an oven are more complex than a guitar string because of the irregularities in the oven walls, the presence of a fan, electrical resistance and other factors. The hot spots are not evenly spread, making it impossible to calculate the wavelength.

PRACTICE QUESTIONS

Q23.1 Which of these statements can be concluded from the text?

A. Microwaves are safe for humans.
B. You can cook food with a Wi-Fi device.
C. Microwaves travel at the speed of light.
D. Microwaves can escape from a microwave oven.

Q23.2 Which of these statements can be concluded from the text?

A. FM waves have a shorter wavelength than mobile phone signals.
B. Mobile phones emit continuous waves.
C. FM waves have a higher frequency than long waves.
D. Microwave ovens emit waves with a shorter wavelength than mobile phones.

Q23.3 Which of the following statements would the author be less likely to agree with?

A. If a microwave oven's melting zones were equally spread, they would be 6.25 cm apart.
B. Microwave ovens are suitable for melting cheese.
C. Microwave ovens with non-rotating plates are less effective.
D. The distance between melting zones is the same across all microwave ovens.

Q23.4 Which of the following statements would the author most likely disagree with?

A. All microwave ovens use waves at the same frequency.
B. To calculate the speed of light using a microwave oven, one would need to use an oven without a rotating plate.
C. Microwave ovens with rotating plates use rotating waves and not waves with two fixation points.
D. Stirring food in the middle of the microwaving process would make the food heat up more homogeneously.

| VR 24 Practice | American Queen |

TEXT

Steamboats (aptly named!) have been through a few cycles since John Fitch first operated a primitive one on the Delaware River in 1787. Originally steamboats were not the opulent creatures we picture today. They were cargo vessels, stripped down for maximum speed, since quick delivery, especially for livestock and produce, was vital. People were an afterthought. Then railways came along, making steamboats an also-ran in the cargo-moving race. Increasingly, steamboats catered for passengers, with on-board entertainment and such. Fares varied, just like on ocean-going ships of the day (and you could also work on-board in exchange for passage).

The new owners of *American Queen* (capacity 420 passengers) have returned to the traditional steamboating audience: a crowd with a lot of grey hair and no interest in the parasailing and snorkelling you find offered on Caribbean cruises. The nightly song and dance shows are generally introduced with the phrase "Remember when". The *American Queen* barely pays lip service to the idea of on-board exercise, with only a small gym. Most activities are of the sit-and-listen variety, e.g. talks about steamboat history, piano bar and eating. Food on-board is served in a large dining room. The service in the dining room is a little rocky since the staff is green and therefore more or less learning on the job. But the food is better than food on a boat has the right to be. Even though my ticket cost £1,872, the dessert on the second night convinced me that I hadn't nearly paid enough. Anyone who doesn't feel stuffed with what is being served in the dining room can eat at the River Grill on a rear deck, and at the front of the boat a little snack bar sells hot dogs, snacks and cappuccinos.

Along the journey, we come across various towns filled with historic mansions crying out to be toured. Various cotton, sugar and tobacco plantations can also be visited on the way. There is a riverboat casino in Natchez and a string of land-based gaming parlours in Vicksburg.

At each stop, the cruise line sets up a free hop-on/hop-off bus circuit to take guests to nearby attractions, some of which grant free admission to passengers from the boat. But for an additional fee – £36 was typical – the more adventurous can take a variety of premium tours.

Verbal Reasoning – Practice

PRACTICE QUESTIONS

Q24.1 Which of these statements about steamboats cannot be deduced from the passage?

    A. They were originally designed to carry animals and goods.
    B. Some passengers could travel without paying any money.
    C. They used to carry cotton, sugar and tobacco.
    D. They were not powered by steam.

Q24.2 Which of these statements cannot be deduced about the *American Queen* from the passage?

    A. Cruises are mostly attended by older people.
    B. There are few opportunities to exercise on-board.
    C. There is more than one food outlet on-board.
    D. There is a casino on-board.

Q24.3 Which of these statements is the author most likely to agree with?

    A. Food on-board is good value for the price of the cruise.
    B. Food portions served in the dining room are too small.
    C. Some of the dining room waiters can get sick when sailing.
    D. Passengers of the *American Queen* often tend to go on Caribbean cruises too.

Q24.4 The writer enjoyed his dessert on the second night.

    ☐ True   ☐ False   ☐ Can't tell

Q24.5 All premium tours incur an additional fee.

    ☐ True   ☐ False   ☐ Can't tell

Q24.6 Vicksburg and Natchez are towns on the Delaware River.

    ☐ True   ☐ False   ☐ Can't tell

Q24.7 John Fitch was the inventor of steamboats.

    ☐ True   ☐ False   ☐ Can't tell

Q24.8 Ocean-going ships used to charge fixed fees.

    ☐ True   ☐ False   ☐ Can't tell

VR 25 Practice — Forest Fire

TEXT

The scientists could barely believe their eyes. More than 20,000 hectares of forest were charred but, in the middle of the devastation, a group of cypresses was still standing tall and green. When a fire swept through an experimental plot in Andilla, in the Spanish province of Valencia in 2012, it gave researchers a perfect opportunity. The plot was part of a European-Union-financed project set up to test the resistance of over 50 varieties of Mediterranean cypress to a pathogenic fungus. After the 2012 fire, it also provided anecdotal evidence of the peculiar resilience of the species in the face of fire. Indeed, all the common oaks, holm oaks, pines and juniper had completely burnt but only 1.3% of the cypresses had ignited. The Valencia fire led to a three-year study to find the reasons behind the resilience of the species and discover if it could provide buffer zones to hinder or prevent the rapid spread of wildfires.

In the past, this species was not studied in-depth or only a few parameters were measured. Furthermore, using different techniques, the results of flammability tests in vegetation can be different or even contradictory. A crucial difference of the new tests is that they were performed not only on dead dry samples but also on live fine twigs with leaves taken from different crown heights, which revealed one of the key traits of the species: its high-water content. Tests revealed that the Mediterranean cypress, because of the particular structure of its leaves, is able to maintain a high-water content even in situations of extreme heat and drought, and this is a very favourable starting point concerning fire risk. The litter on the forest floor, made up of small fragments of leaves, also forms an intricate and compact layer and is slow to decompose. The thick and dense litter layer acts as a 'sponge' and retains water, and the space for air circulation is reduced.

According to scientists, the species has a great plasticity in terms of soil, climate and altitude. It can grow in all soils, even degraded ones, apart from those that are water-logged, and it thrives from sea level to altitudes of more than 2,000 metres. The species has been introduced in Latin America and could grow without problems in the temperate climate of California, Chile or Argentina.

PRACTICE QUESTIONS

Q25.1 Which of the following would best protect a house from fires?

- A. Building its walls with Mediterranean cypress wood.
- B. Encircling the house with rows of Mediterranean cypress.
- C. Encircling the house with a mix of cypresses and oaks.
- D. Planting juniper bushes all around the house.

Q25.2 Which of the following is least likely to contribute to fires?

- A. Large dead leaves on the forest floor.
- B. Fast-decomposing leaves.
- C. Compact forest floors.
- D. High winds.

Q25.3 Which of the following statements about the fire resistance of Mediterranean cypresses cannot be deduced from the text?

- A. It requires live cypresses.
- B. It was discovered by chance.
- C. It is only effective if the cypresses are planted in groups.
- D. It was proven through a European-Union-funded study.

Q25.4 Which of the following is not a suitable planting ground for Mediterranean cypresses?

- A. In drought-prone areas.
- B. In marshes.
- C. At high altitude.
- D. Near common oaks.

Q25.5 Which of the following statements can be deduced from the text?

- A. The presence of fungus on cypresses slows fire.
- B. Previous tests had only been performed with dead material.
- C. Oak leaves decompose fast.
- D. Before 2012, the flammability resistance of cypresses was well known but never studied.

VR 26 Practice — I am a Berliner

TEXT

"Rent brake" – that is the name of a controversial law introduced in Germany to cap the level of rents charged by landlords in order to slow down undesirable price rises. Until the fall of the Berlin wall (1989), which separated communist East Berlin from the capitalist West during the cold war, the area near the central station was known as the *death strip*. Today it's a property hotspot and it is hard to believe that a place where people could have been shot simply for standing there is now a place where people can eat ice cream and canal boats drift by, filled with contented-looking middle-aged Germans drinking huge beers. Now, the area's gruesome past is a sexy selling point for estate agents trying to drum up business: crumbling concrete watchtowers dwarfed by gleaming glass-fronted apartment buildings.

A few years ago, anyone with a decent permanent job would have easily found a flat in central Berlin. But with a growth of 50,000 people per year, a city once renowned for the bohemian lifestyle that comes with cheap housing was seeing rent rises of 10% per year. Consequently the government introduced a cap on rents, whereby landlords cannot charge more than 10% above a local average set by the authorities. The move is seen by most Berliners, half of whom rent, as a breakthrough, and it appears to be working since, in the month following the introduction of the law, rents fell by 3%. In some areas, such cap is necessary, as in Munich where people are not able to pay those prices. There, you have the Paris or London effect, where no one lives in the city centre, bar the very rich.

But the law may well backfire. Small investors will be hit the hardest because the legal level set by the authorities is below market value and often much less than the mortgage that an individual buy-to-let investor may have taken on. Instead of renting out their flats, owners may simply sell them, thus causing a shortage in rental properties and thus an increase in rents. This would not help those looking to rent a property. And when potential tenants mention to a landlord that the rent they are asking for is 20% above the legal limit, they may suddenly be told that the flat is no longer available. This is because, although rents are capped, tenants can waive their new right and accept a higher rent. Coupled with low supply, this could spell disaster and, by the looks of it, it won't be long before it happens.

PRACTICE QUESTIONS

Q26.1 Which of the following statements is the author most likely to agree with?

    A. The "rent brake" law was first tested in London and Paris.
    B. Before Berlin, the "rent brake" law was tested in Munich.
    C. The new law might help repopulate city centres.
    D. In Munich, rents are high but property prices are affordable.

Q26.2 Which of the following statements can be deduced from the passage?

    A. The average rent in Berlin is 3% below the cap.
    B. In time, all landlords will charge rent below the cap.
    C. Landlords can charge rents up to 10% higher than the cap.
    D. A landlord can charge rent over the cap if the tenant agrees

Q26.3 Which of the following statements is the author most likely to disagree with?

    A. The landlords who charge rent above the cap are those with high mortgage repayments.
    B. The law would be made more effective by removing the waiver clause.
    C. Landlords with mortgages may incur losses.
    D. The fall in rent levels may be short-lived.

Q26.4 Which of the following statements about Berlin cannot be deduced from the passage?

    A. There is a river or canal near the central station.
    B. Berlin has the same demography as Munich.
    C. There are still remnants of the East/West split era in Berlin.
    D. Berlin used to be affordable for the standard German.

VR 27 Practice — Part-Time

TEXT
In the US, the employment statistics do a good job concealing the true nature of the workforce. The unemployment rate has dropped dramatically since the recession ended, largely because millions of Americans are now no longer considered part of the workforce. This is an easy way to boost the employment rate without actually creating new jobs. Another growing trend is that of part-time work. Part-time work and low wages go hand in hand. Part-time workers usually are not afforded the same benefits or pay conditions as those working full-time. They are also brought on with a just-in-time attitude and are treated as such when no longer needed.

Companies looking to cut benefits and offer little commitment to future workers will opt to go the part-time route. It is embedded in the nature of low wage labour. This is one major reason companies have been able to boost profits while filtering profits to the top: slash wages, cut benefits and squeeze productivity out of workers. It is a good model at the top and simply does not foster a middle class. Why would anyone struggling with part-time work want to commit to buying a home? Long-term purchases are pushed off into the future. The US is still having a tough time getting back to full-time employment even after the current recovery. However, the percentage of the workforce now working part-time is near record highs.

In Japan, companies generally expect their employees to put in long hours of overtime. However, women, who also have household chores to do and children to take care of, find it hard to work at the same pace as men who, traditionally, are not sharing the burden of such responsibilities. Many of them inevitably opt for part-time jobs, which enables them to combine work and domestic duties. At present, 25% of all female salaried workers are part-timers and the number is on the rise. Part-time work places women at a disadvantage. Part-time workers' wages are considerably lower than those of full-time employees for the same amount of time worked, and part-time work tends to involve menial labour and often seasonal work. Additionally, because salary and promotion in Japanese companies are often based on seniority, it is extremely difficult for women either re-entering the labour force or switching from part-time to full-time work to climb the ladder.

PRACTICE QUESTIONS

Q27.1 Which of the following statements is the author most likely to agree is the reason for the fall in unemployment in the US?

  A. New jobs have been created.
  B. Full-time employees have been forced to work part-time.
  C. People previously classified as unemployed have been re-classified as "employed".
  D. People previously classified as unemployed have been re-classified as not relevant for statistical purposes.

Q27.2 Which of the following statements is the author most likely to disagree with in relation to part-time workers in both the US and Japan?

  A. They are not highly regarded by employers.
  B. They tend to earn less per hour than full-time workers.
  C. They tend to be recruited to address short-term needs.
  D. The majority are women.

Q27.3 Which of the following statements is the author most likely to agree with in regard to Japan?

  A. Age-related pay is common in companies.
  B. Three-quarters of part-time workers are men.
  C. Few men take on a share of household chores.
  D. Part-time workers rarely get paid for their overtime hours.

Q27.4 Which of the following can be deduced from the passage?

  A. In the US, there are more part-timers than full-timers.
  B. Few US part-timers are likely to buy a house.
  C. There are no accurate employment records in Japan.
  D. Most Japanese women whose children have left home tend to mostly work full-time.

VR 28 Practice — Antibiotics

TEXT

Bacteria have a talent for learning new ways to survive, thus rendering some of the best drugs ineffective. And so, in the same way that we would buy a new car after having written off the previous one, when a drug has stopped fulfilling its role, we just move on to another one. Apply that model to antibiotics and you soon have a situation where none of the drugs available work anymore, so-called "antibiotics apocalypse". One way in which we, as a society, have responded to this problem since the 1980s has been to intensify research to find new classes of antibiotics. But, to use the driving analogy, isn't it time that we took driving lessons instead of simply changing car every time we crash one? We, indeed, need to learn to use antibiotics more responsibly.

Some healthcare systems are making substantial progress and the UK is at the front of that. However, taking a global view, we are way away from resolving the issue. In the UK alone, despite good awareness of the dangers of overusing antibiotics, approximately 10 million out of the 40 million antibiotic prescriptions given each year are deemed inappropriate. Patients have been criticised for an 'addiction' to the drugs and doctors are being reproached to be a 'soft touch' by being too keen to prescribe them, or rapidly wilting under patient demand. Consequently, patients are taking antibiotics for conditions for which they would never work, such as viral infections (colds, sore throats) or conditions which would resolve themselves without any treatment. And, as a result, we risk seeing multi-drug-resistant infections, which may cause death, like in the old days.

In many countries, unlike in the UK where a prescription from a doctor is required, antibiotics are simply available over the counter without the need for a prescription or seeing any kind of health professional. And there is also another problem in the misuse of antibiotics in livestock and fish farms, which all serves to exacerbate the problem along the food chain as and when people consume them unknowingly.

There are promising new drugs potentially coming out. Indeed a US research group has found a new method of growing bacteria, which has yielded 25 potential new antibiotics. But we are not out of the woods yet until we can grow up and become more responsible!

Verbal Reasoning – Practice

PRACTICE QUESTIONS

Q28.1 Which of the following is not a cause of antibiotic overuse?

  A. Doctors giving in to patients' insistent requests.
  B. Self-medication by patients.
  C. Lack of research into new antibiotics.
  D. Lack of patient understanding of the purpose of antibiotics.

Q28.2 Which of the following is not a consequence of antibiotic overuse?

  A. Patients with a cold may spend longer recovering from it.
  B. There is a constant need to develop new antibiotics.
  C. Some patients may die.
  D. It is possible for people who have never used antibiotics to treat an illness to become resistant to them.

Q28.3 Which policy would the author most likely agree could best resolve the problem of antibiotic overuse in the UK?

  A. Stepping up research efforts into new antibiotics.
  B. Criminalising inappropriate prescriptions by doctors.
  C. Making antibiotics available over the counter.
  D. Running an awareness campaign amongst the population.

Q28.4 Which statement is the author most likely to agree with?

  A. Antibiotics are addictive.
  B. Antibiotics can be deadly, even at normal dose.
  C. Antibiotics should not be taken whilst driving.
  D. Antibiotics do not kill viruses.

Q28.5 Which of the following statements is the author most likely to agree with?

  A. If left untreated, colds simply resolve themselves.
  B. A quarter of doctors wrongly prescribe antibiotics.
  C. Doctors need to be firmer with demanding patients.
  D. Most doctors prescribe antibiotics inappropriately because they are unable to reach the correct diagnosis.

Q28.6 Some doctors prescribe antibiotics, knowing they will not work.

  ☐ True   ☐ False   ☐ Can't tell

VR 29 Practice: Eighty Hours

TEXT

US medical residencies (i.e. medical training posts) traditionally require lengthy hours. The public and the medical education establishment recognise that such long hours are counter-productive since sleep deprivation increases the rate of medical errors and may affect learning. However, the phenomenon persists in order to create a higher entry barrier and reduce costs for medical facilities. To counter some of the risks, the Accreditation Council for Graduate Medical Education (ACGME) – a trade association that accredits residency/training programmes – capped the number of weekly work hours. These standards came into effect in 2003:

- An 80-hour weekly limit, averaged over 4 weeks.
- A 24-hour limit on continuous duty with up to 6 additional hours for continuity of care and education.
- At least 10 hours of rest period between each shift.
- In-house night shifts not more than once in 3 nights, averaged over 4 weeks.
- One day in 7 free from patient care and educational obligations.
- No new patient to be accepted after 24 hours of continuous duty.

Whilst these limits are voluntary, adherence has been mandated for accreditation.

A study of over 8 million hospital admissions of Medicare beneficiaries published in 2007 comparing mortality rate before and after implementation of the new standards showed no difference in mortality. However, it is largely felt that actual duty hours (as opposed to reported duty hours) have not changed substantially. One issue is that statutes do not provide whistle-blower protection to residents who report work hour violations. Secondly, the penalty for work hour violation is loss of accreditation, which would adversely affect the medical resident since he/she would not be able to become board certified in his/her field of medicine.

Research from Europe and the United States on non-standard work hours and sleep deprivation found that night-shift workers are subject to higher risks of gastrointestinal disorders, cardiovascular disease, breast cancer, miscarriage, pre-term birth and low birth weight of their newborns.

PRACTICE QUESTIONS

Q29.1 Which statement is the author most likely to disagree with?

　　A. Some doctors work over the limit.

　　B. Many doctors report a lower number of hours than they actually work.

　　C. Residents caught working over the limits risk losing their accreditation.

　　D. Amnesty is granted to doctors who speak up.

Q29.2 Which of the following is the author most likely to disagree with in relation to the ACGME standards?

　　A. It is possible for a doctor to work over 80 hours in a week.
　　B. Doctors can be on shift for up to 30 continuous hours.
　　C. A doctor cannot work more than 3 nights in any week.
　　D. A doctor finishing work at 8pm must not start his next shift before 6am the next day.

Q29.3 Which of the following is the most likely reason for the limited impact of the ACGME standards on mortality rates?

　　A. Doctors did not work over 80 hours/week before anyway.
　　B. Residents are not usually adhering to the regulations.
　　C. The mortality rate calculations are flawed.
　　D. The regulations are not mandatory.

Q29.4 Which of the following statements is the author most likely to agree with?

　　A. Making fewer doctors work longer hours is more expensive than making more doctors work fewer hours.

　　B. Non-trainees also have to adhere to the regulations.

　　C. Long hours act as a deterrent to future medical applicants.

　　D. The regulations risk decreasing the standard of training.

Q29.5 Doctors working long hours are at higher risk of cardiovascular disease.

　　☐ True　　　　☐ False　　　　☐ Can't tell

VR 30 Practice — Science Funding

TEXT

Whenever a medical charity awards money to a university, that money often only covers the direct cost of a research project and not the overheads (e.g. electricity, rent, lab maintenance). Since 2008, that gap has been funded by the state-funded Charity Research Support Fund (CRSF). Typically the additional money provided by the fund adds an extra 25% to the charitable grant. But, since 2010, austerity has meant that the state's additional funding was frozen, despite the fact that charitable grants have grown in size. Consequently, in 2015, UK medical charities are finding that universities are increasingly rejecting research grants because they cannot make up for the relative drop in government financial support.

Typically a university will always accept funding from the larger organisations but the challenge is whether they will accept funding from the smaller charities. That, in turn, will impact on the range of diseases that are being researched.

The head of the Association of Medical Research Charities (AMRC) stated: "I understand that this may be a consequence of the tough financial environment or could simply be a 'blip'. However, some members of the association have already been spending their research fund overseas. This trend has not necessarily increased in the past five years. But, if universities' money declines further then we will look abroad."

The head of policy of one of the Association's major members, the Wellcome Trust, said that the Wellcome Trust "wouldn't fund the full economic costs of research in universities" and that it was "important to us that it's a partnership with government", a view shared by nearly all members of the association.

Research organisations such as the Institute of Cancer Research (ICR) and the University of Oxford are encountering growing difficulties taking charitable funding. A researcher at the ICR said that the shortfall was currently covered by fundraising and royalties but that this impaired any ability to invest for the future and buy new buildings and state-of-the-art equipment. At Oxford, the biggest university recipient of charity research funding in the UK, more medical science divisions have started to run a deficit, largely due to a relative reduction in the CRSF.

PRACTICE QUESTIONS

Q30.1 What is the main cause of grants being rejected by universities?

A. Government funding has been withdrawn.
B. There is a lack of medical researchers.
C. Charities struggle to raise funds from the general public.
D. Government funding has not increased in line with charity funding.

Q30.2 Which of the following is the author most likely to disagree with?

A. Some research centres are finding other ways to make up the funding shortfall.
B. Charities are increasingly redirecting their funds abroad.
C. Some research centres are running at a loss.
D. The Wellcome Trust is refusing to increase funding to compensate for a relative drop in government funding.

Q30.3 Which of the following statements is the author most likely to agree with?

A. Smaller charities are often given preference by research centres over larger charities.
B. Smaller charities often deal with different diseases than larger charities.
C. Smaller charities are less likely to send their funds abroad than larger charities.
D. Smaller charities tend to be more effective fundraisers than larger charities.

Q30.4 Which of the following is the author most likely to disagree with?

A. Charities are threatening to redirect their funds abroad.
B. Universities will consider not taking charitable grants because they cannot afford to cover the related overheads.
C. The funding gap issue is affecting mostly the smaller research centres.
D. Lack of funding may make research centres stagnate instead of developing.

VR 31 Practice — Children's Books

TEXT

The Education Secretary has recently called for a return to English literature classics. One has to wonder whether they are actually still relevant. Look at the list of today's most read children's books and you will see that today's youngsters are growing up in a very different literary landscape to their parents; The Famous Five and the Chronicles of Narnia have given place to the likes of Jeff Kinney's *Diary of a Wimpy Kid*, the complete and ever-growing works of David Walliams, and Liz Pichon's *Tom Gates* series. Only the prolific Roald Dahl remains sandwiched between the bookends by these newer arrivals at the top of the literary pops. And when it comes to the 19th century classics, many children have simply never heard of them.

Millions of children are readers because of *Diary of a Wimpy Kid*; Jeff Kinney's work is perfect for turning reluctant readers on to books. With 50% words and 50% cartoons, the books are 100% hilarious and children agree; the text does not look so scary and it therefore appeals to the more hesitant or reluctant readers. There is also no doubt that the popularity has more to do with the content rather than just the aesthetics. The children in these books are often in great peril and the adults tend to be either non-existent, evil or weak in comparison to the young protagonists. And to be honest, you only have to look at Dahl's work to see that there is nothing new here in taste or in style.

All that being said, it turns out that a major publisher has recently reissued a series of 20 classics of children's literature: an indication that they have an enduring appeal, even if that is mostly because the parents are buying them on their children's behalf. A spokesperson for the publisher said: "Books such as *Treasure Island* or *The Wizard of Oz*, respectively by Stevenson and Baum, have been firm favourites across many generations, and by giving them striking new jackets we will ensure that they remain popular for many years to come."

Some of the more challenging classics such as those written by Dickens or Jules Verne are often used in their abridged editions, which try to maintain the richness of the language and contain graphics. However, many such books remain sitting lonely on school library shelves, waiting for someone to borrow them, because they are often not made available in electronic formats.

Verbal Reasoning – Practice

PRACTICE QUESTIONS

Q31.1 Which of the following is not labelled as a writer of classics?

    A. Roald Dahl.
    B. Jules Verne.
    C. Liz Pichon.
    D. Charles Dickens.

Q31.2 What of the following statements on Roald Dahl is correct?

    A. His books are no longer popular.
    B. He is considered a classic 19th century author.
    C. The style of his books is similar to that of newer books.
    D. He wrote *Treasure Island*.

Q31.3 Which of the following is not a reason for the success of new children's books over classics?

    A. They tend to be illustrated.
    B. They are available in formats other than paper.
    C. Parents prefer their children to read modern stories.
    D. Children's characters play a more active role.

Q31.4 Which of the following statements about classics can be deduced from the passage?

    A. Children like them so much that publishers are reprinting them in their original format.
    B. Complex words and phrases put children off reading them, even in their abridged versions.
    C. Some classics are too hard for children to read in their original versions.
    D. They are mostly bought by libraries.

Q31.5 *Treasure Island* and *The Wizard of Oz* are 19th century classics.

    ☐ True   ☐ False   ☐ Can't tell

VR 32 Practice — Dismaland

TEXT

Dismaland, the "bemusement park" set up by Banksy, is closing its doors today at the end of its intended run. Billed by the artist himself as a pop-up "family attraction unsuitable for children", it had room for 4,500 paying customers every day in the course of its five-week run, largely supported by countless social media postings around the world. People were not just queuing up at the doors, they lined the beaches! And each day, those at the back of the queue never made it to the front despite seamless organisation. This compares to a mere 3,500 people per day who visited the V&A's exhibition on fashion designer Alexander McQueen this year and 3,907 who visited the Tate's most popular exhibition in its history on Henri Matisse. It is worth noting though that David Hockney's exhibition at the Royal Academy in 2012 attracted 7,512 visitors a day.

Visit Somerset described the event as "a global phenomenon of major importance" with some observers pointing out that Banksy had definitely put Weston-super-Mare on the map. "Only the elusive Bristolian could have pulled off such an expensive and logistically difficult challenge," an official said.

From a tourism perspective, many Dismaland visitors said that they had never been to the town before and that they would be likely to return. And the major benefit was that every B&B and hotel bed was full throughout September. Tourist chiefs estimated it had brought £20m to the town.

One of the reasons for the success of the temporary park is that Banksy has a unique approach, always trying to convey a message (often political or social) through his art. Indeed many artists who visited the exhibition felt empowered to make their own art more political, more message driven. Banksy art, being easily accessible, is popular with people who don't generally like the sort of conceptualism inflicted onto them by the art establishment. So does that mean that we will be seeing Banksy's bemusement park in many other places around the country? Most likely not. One of the reasons why Banksy chose Weston-super-Mare is that he has a personal connection to the town. This is what gave the exhibition poignancy.

The Local Gazette, 27 September

PRACTICE QUESTIONS

Q32.1 Which of the following can be deduced from the passage?

A. More people visited the Hockney exhibition than the Banksy bemusement park across their respective runs.
B. The Banksy bemusement park reached full visitor capacity across the five-week run.
C. Beaches had to close to make space for queuing.
D. The queuing system for Dismaland was disorganised.

Q32.2 Which of the following can be deduced from the passage?

A. The exhibition was reserved solely for locals.
B. Children were banned from visiting the exhibition.
C. Hotels in the area are not normally full in September.
D. The exhibition opened its doors early September.

Q32.3 Which of the following can be deduced from the passage?

A. Some tourists visited the attraction more than once.
B. Banksy was born in Weston-super-Mare.
C. Banksy has a connection with Bristol.
D. McQueen was alive at the time of the exhibition of his work.

Q32.4 With which of the following statements cannot be deduced from the passage?

A. Banksy's exhibition is influencing other artists.
B. Banksy's art is often found outdoors.
C. Banksy's art is easy to understand.
D. Banksy's art often contains a message.

Q32.5 Which of the following statements is the author most likely to agree with?

A. Following closure, the exhibition will tour the UK.
B. The exhibition was a one-off.
C. Any further exhibition will take place in a larger venue.
D. Bristol has been chosen as the venue for the next exhibition.

VR 33 Practice — Indian Rugby

TEXT

Walking round the streets of Kolkata (formerly known as Calcutta), I showed passers-by a rugby ball and asked them whether they could name the sport. One teenager came up with "Hockey?" whilst another teenager guessed "Basketball?" A 13-year-old thought it might be handball whilst a 14-year-old just had no clue. One middle-aged man simply said: "Sorry, no idea, this is not a game we play here." And yet, ironically, those of you who are familiar with Rugby Union will know that one of the famous trophies is the Calcutta Cup, the annual game played between England and Scotland which has its origins here in the 1870s.

When I talked to him, the president of the Indian Rugby Football Board felt that such lack of understanding is making it difficult for the sport to attract the money it needs to raise awareness of the game and encourage promising players; sponsors can be found but it is hard work and they do not stay more than a year or two. Another issue is that the country only counts two clubs: Mumbai and Kolkata, both of which are member-only establishments (set up way back under British rule). And though both clubs (which host all tournaments) are welcoming, their oak-panelled clubhouses and trophy cabinets carry an air of elitism. Shaking off that stuffy image and showing more international rugby on Indian TV would help revitalise the image of the sport and would encourage more sponsors to come forward and would help popularise the game.

Like football, hockey and badminton (in decreasing order of popularity) have already done, rugby could learn from the success of cricket's Indian premier league, creating a made-for-television format tournament with Bollywood owners, music and razzmatazz that attracts international players by making it financially viable, thus ensuring that cricket remains the most popular sport in India. Not that the sport is totally devoid of backers. Birla Tyres sponsors an annual Kolkata tournament, though the sums involved remain pitiful. Its chief executive said: "On the face of it, there is no business reason to sponsor rugby; it's a closed circle of people who really watch or play the sport. We didn't just want to be yet another sponsor of cricket. The Rugby World Cup gets watched in India – perhaps not as widely as football or cricket, but still; rugby will have a revival and our participation means that, as the sport revives, our association with it will mean an increased visibility for us."

PRACTICE QUESTIONS

Q33.1 Which of the following can be deduced from the passage?

A. The Calcutta Cup is part of the Six Nations Tournament.
B. The Calcutta Cup match is played in Kolkata.
C. There is at least one England v. Scotland match each year.
D. Rugby was invented in the 1870s.

Q33.2 Which of the following is the author most likely to agree with?

A. No rugby is shown on Indian television.
B. Rugby is not popular because the Indian team is not strong enough to participate in international tournaments.
C. Rugby is not popular because its tournaments lack a show business element.
D. Rugby is not popular because it is considered a dangerous game for adults only.

Q33.3 Which of the following is the author most likely to disagree with?

A. Rugby is seen as an old-fashioned and elitist sport.
B. Rugby is less popular than badminton.
C. Football is less popular than cricket.
D. Hockey is more popular than football.

Q33.4 Which of the following is the author most likely to agree with?

A. Rugby needs to attract a different kind of sponsor.
B. Increasing the appeal of rugby would attract more sponsors
C. Birla Tyres is currently the only sponsor of rugby in India.
D. International cricketers want to play for India because they like the spectacle surrounding the game.

Q33.5 Which of the following is the author most likely to agree with in respect of the role to be played by TV stations?

A. They should recruit international players as commentators.
B. They should broadcast more international rugby games.
C. They should start broadcasting the Rugby World Cup.
D. They should find wealthier advertisers.

VR 34 Practice

Plastic Bags

TEXT

A 5p tax on plastic bags was recently introduced in England. The price hike affects only retailers with 250 or more employees and, unlike schemes in other parts of the UK, paper bags are exempt from a charge. Evidence from countries such as Wales, Ireland and Scotland shows that charging 5p per plastic bag used in a shop reduces plastic bag consumption by between 60% and 90%. However, does it really matter that much? Plastic bags can take 1,000 years to degrade and can harm seabirds and other animals who may ingest them. However, they only represent 0.1% of all litter. On beaches they account for only 2% of all pieces of litter. So basically introducing a 5p tax will have a big effect on a tiny problem.

Reusable bags are a current trend but they are not much better for the environment. For example, a cotton bag would need to be used 131 times compared with a regular plastic bag before they become better in terms of global warming. And if you consider that 40% of plastic bags would be reused as bin liners, this goes up to 173 times. Most people are unlikely to reuse a bag that many times and, in any case, cotton bags need to be washed, which also has an environmental cost in terms of the water and detergent it uses – not counting the risk of harbouring bacteria caused by storing them in car boots: a great breeding ground! In America, this has pushed shops to create zones where reusable bags are allowed and zones where they are banned; this had the effect of increasing sales of goods in areas where they were allowed and decreasing sales of goods in areas where they were banned, with an impact on employment.

And what of the argument that plastic bags clog up landfill? In San Francisco, following introduction of a plastic bag tax, people started using more paper bags, causing an even bigger landfill problem. In Austin, Texas, people started throwing away more heavy-duty plastic reusable bags. Not including the environmental cost of washing those reusable bags. All this led some experts to conclude that such policy is basically a totemic policy. You can be seen to be doing something and it sounds dramatic, but it won't have much impact on society. It is worth noting also that since the 5p tax is not passed on by the retailers to the government, it may only benefit the profits of those retailers. The 5p charge may also push people to shop online more as retailers will deliver to your door without using bags, whilst also reducing the number of car journeys made.

PRACTICE QUESTIONS

Q34.1 Which of the following can be deduced from the passage?

    A. Plastic bags do not actually harm wildlife.
    B. The policy is not the same in different parts of the UK.
    C. Cotton bags take less time to degrade than plastic bags.
    D. Plastic bags degrade faster in landfill than on beaches.

Q34.2 Which of the following can be deduced from the passage?

    A. The money raised by the government through the tax will be used to promote environmental schemes.
    B. 5p is not a high enough amount to make people switch away from plastic bags.
    C. Retailers will feel compelled to donate the money to charity.
    D. This policy may increase the sale of bin liners.

Q34.3 Which of the following is the author most likely to agree with?

    A. Reusable bags play an important role in reducing landfill waste.
    B. Reusable bags are more environmentally friendly than standard plastic bags.
    C. Reusable plastic bags do not need to be washed.
    D. Online shopping is more environmentally friendly than physical shopping.

Q34.4 Which of the following is the author most likely to agree with?

    A. Cotton bags are a potential infection risk to shops.
    B. Reusable plastic bags are more hygienic than cotton bags.
    C. It is nearly impossible to clean cotton bags.
    D. Placing goods directly in the car boot is a hygienic solution.

11 Verbal Reasoning Answers to Practice Questions

VR 1 – Financial Crisis

Q1.1 – CAN'T TELL. All we know is that the merger followed the collapse of Lehman Brothers. Although there might have been a link, the text does not suggest any.

Q1.2 – TRUE. The text clearly states that American banks sold the sub-prime debt to banks around the world and that it was the failure to repay those sub-prime debts which started the collapse.

Q1.3 – CAN'T TELL. It is commonly accepted that bankers' greed played a key role in the onset of the financial crisis; however, for the purpose of the exam, you must stick to what the text is saying. The text states that "some commentators have said that bankers' greed was a contributor to the problem". It does not specify the extent of the role played by greed, or imply whether the financial crisis could have been avoided if greed had not been present. We simply know that it contributed.

Q1.4 – TRUE. The second sentence of the text explicitly states that the source of the crisis is linked to US banks. Again, there might have been other reasons elsewhere, but you must stick to what the text says and not use any additional knowledge or preconceptions you may have.

Q1.5 – CAN'T TELL. At the very end, the text says that pyramid schemes are illegal in the UK, which is not the same as saying that they do not exist. The text contains no information to suggest that any pyramid schemes actually operate in the UK. It is highly likely that several are in existence, and you may well be aware of some of them; however, you must ensure that you do not use any external knowledge to answer the question. Based on what we are given, we cannot say whether pyramid schemes exist in the UK.

Q1.6 – FALSE. There are several elements in the text which point towards a "False" answer. First, the beginning of the second paragraph implies that the alleged fraud was in addition to the financial crisis. Second, the second

Verbal Reasoning – Practice

paragraph clearly indicates that the alleged fraud affected rich individuals, whereas the first paragraph is clear in saying that the financial crisis had its roots in the "less well-off" population. Although it is possible that the alleged fraud contributed to some extent to the financial crisis, the text does not allow us to say that it was a key trigger.

Q1.7 – CAN'T TELL. The text talks about a $50bn fraud. We do not know whether this was the total amount of money invested by those who participated in the scheme or whether this was the amount of money that the financier made. In addition, we are told that this is an "alleged" fraud, which places further ambiguity on the statement.

Q1.8 – TRUE. The text clearly states that pyramid schemes are unsustainable.

VR 2 – Global Warming

Q2.1 – TRUE. The text suggests that there are different schools of thought on the topic of global warming; however those who criticise these measures argue that they will have little effect, not that they will have no effect at all. It is possible that such effect is very minimal (it is impossible from the text to determine how much of an effect this is likely to have), but this is enough to answer "True" to this question.

Q2.2 – CAN'T TELL. The text merely states that they believe it will have little effect. This is not the same as saying that there is no need to take action. So we can't say.

Q2.3 – CAN'T TELL. The text says that China is one of the biggest contributors. There is no suggestion that it is the biggest contributor of carbon emissions.

Q2.4 – CAN'T TELL. Nothing in the text suggests that global warming is used as an excuse to reduce the number of cars (which does not mean that it isn't the case).

Q2.5 – CAN'T TELL. The text states that the average sea level will rise by between 18 and 59 cm. Since this is the average sea level, this means that some sea levels are expected to rise by less than 18 cm and others by more than 59 cm. In fact, the previous sentence says that individual sea levels could rise by anything between 9 cm and 88 cm. This may or may not include Britain; nothing in the text points one way or another.

Q2.6 – TRUE. The text states "a reduction of the ice cap in the northern hemisphere, whereas in Antarctica (i.e. in the southern hemisphere) the melting of the ice cap would be more than offset by heavier snow falls, with the snow then freezing over the existing layer of ice".

The use of the word "whereas" opposes two statements, with the events in Antarctica being opposed to the events in the northern hemisphere. Since the northern hemisphere ice cap is reducing, this implies that the Antarctica ice cap is not (though this does not necessarily mean that it is actually increasing; it could simply be remaining stable). However, the phrase "more than offset" indicates that snow will be falling at a higher rate than the ice is melting, which points towards an actual increase of the ice cap.

Q2.7 – CAN'T TELL. The text does mention at the end that some areas of the world may see some benefits but there is nothing about these countries not experiencing any negative impacts. This lack of information means that we cannot conclude decisively.

Q2.8 – TRUE. We are told that the average world temperature will rise by between 1.4 and 5.8 °C. So, it is possible that the average rise will be 5.8 °C. This then means that some countries will see rises below 5.8 °C and some countries will see rises above 5.8 °C. The use of the word "may" in the assertion makes it a true statement according to the text. If the assertion had been "some countries will experience a rise of temperature of over 5.8 °C", then we could not have concluded either way since we cannot know for sure what the average rise will be and therefore whether any countries will actually experience such a high rise.

VR 3 – Free Museum Entry

Q3.1 – FALSE. The text states that some of the increase is due to the same people visiting museums more often. This suggests there are other reasons.

Q3.2 – TRUE. On average the increase was 70%. Since we know that at least one museum had an increase of 111% then there has to be others with less than 70% increase in visitors.

Verbal Reasoning – Practice

Q3.3 – FALSE. The text states that the subsidies are mostly directed towards London museums. The use of the term "mostly" implies that others have benefited too, though perhaps not to the same extent. It is therefore incorrect that <u>only</u> London museums have benefited.

Q3.4 – CAN'T TELL. The question uses the word "solely". It could only be true if the text clearly showed that there could be no other explanation for the increased visitor numbers than the introduction of the new policy. The text states that the number of visitors increased the following year but does not say why. It also suggests a link with the fact that some museums have refurbished their facilities, so this may have accounted for some of the increase. For statement Q3.4 to be false, we would need proof that there was at least another factor which contributed to the increased visitor numbers. We know that there is a possible link with the refurbishment and new facilities of some museums but we don't know whether this actually had an impact. We therefore cannot conclude either way.

This is a typical case of a question where you have to leave your common sense on the side and solely concentrate on what the text is telling you. To most people, it is obvious that the new policy cannot be the sole contributor to the increased visitor numbers and that, consequently, the statement in Q3.4 is actually false. However, the text is inconclusive in that regard. It only suggests that there may be a link with some other factors.

Q3.5 – FALSE. The first sentence says that "In 2001, the government <u>reintroduced</u> free entry into museums …", which means that it had been done before.

Q3.6 – CAN'T TELL. The figure of £2.21 billion – £1.68 billion = £0.53 billion = £530 million over 3 years is correct. However, all we know is that this is what the Chancellor promised. We cannot say if this <u>will</u> actually happen.

Q3.7 – CAN'T TELL. We know that the free-entry policy will be extended by at least 3 years. The text therefore leaves open the possibility that it may be extended by more. The last sentence indicates that the Arts may suffer from the current financial crisis and the Olympic Games, but there is no indication that this will affect the free-entry policy. There is no indication either that it will not be affected; therefore we cannot conclude either way.

Q3.8 – CAN'T TELL. What the second paragraph tells us is that independent museums have seen a decline since the introduction of free entry.

Therefore a fee-paying policy would be fairer to independent museums because it would place them on an even footing. We are being asked to determine whether a fee-paying entry policy would be fairer to smaller museums. This would be true if the text showed that the independent museums are also the smaller ones. Unfortunately, the text does not allow us to determine this; therefore we cannot conclude either way.

VR 4 – EEC, EU, EURO

Q4.1 – FALSE. The Eurozone is defined as the 15 countries from the EU who have adopted the Euro. The text says that, in addition, 11 non-EU countries have adopted the Euro including Monaco. Therefore Monaco, although it uses the Euro, is not in the officially-defined Eurozone.

Q4.2 – CAN'T TELL. Although, if you know your history, you will know that this statement is true, we cannot conclude it from the text. The text tells us that in 1993, the statement was true. For the statement to be true currently, we would need confirmation that none of the original countries have left the EU since 1993. The text does not say anything on the matter. It only states that there are now 27 countries but does not list them. Remember to base your conclusions on the text only and not on your general knowledge.

Q4.3 – FALSE. The first paragraph does state that the main EU institutions are in Belgium and France. However, there are other institutions which reside somewhere else; in fact the text states that the European Central Bank is in Germany. The statement that all institutions are based in Belgium or in France is therefore false.

Q4.4 – FALSE. We know that both countries have declined to join the Euro, but that is not an indication of future intention. The first sentence of the second paragraph says that the UK has adopted a wait-and-see policy, which means that it remains open. Therefore the fact that neither country intends to adopt the Euro is incorrect.

Q4.5 – TRUE. The second paragraph states clearly that interest rates would be set by the European Central Bank in Frankfurt. It also later states that if the UK had joined the Euro, the Bank of England would not have been able to reduce interest rates drastically to boost the UK economy.

Q4.6 – CAN'T TELL. The only mention of the US is in a statement which says that "It has long been argued that the UK economy is more in line with

Verbal Reasoning – Practice

US economy than with European economy and that therefore it needs to keep closer links with US interest rates than European interest rates." There is nothing in the text which suggests that, if two countries have economies which are aligned, they would benefit overall by having a common currency (since the text presents both pros and cons). This is all speculative and nothing in the text allows us to draw such a definitive conclusion.

Q4.7 – CAN'T TELL. The text says that the EU includes 27 independent sovereign countries, but this does not mean that there are not any other independent sovereign countries outside the EU. The fact that Andorra is a non-EU country (which the text states) does not mean that it is not an independent sovereign country. In the absence of any further information, we cannot conclude either way.

Q4.8 – CAN'T TELL. What the text says is that, should the UK adopt the Euro, UK interest rates would be set by the European Central Bank in Frankfurt. There is no mention of the Bank of England disappearing (it may be needed to fulfil other roles). However, since there is no mention of the Bank of England remaining either, we cannot conclude either way.

VR 5 – Coq au Vin & Quiche Lorraine

Q5.1 – FALSE. The list of main ingredients in the first sentence does not contain bacon. Bacon may be used as a substitute for lardons and therefore cannot be labelled "essential".

Q5.2 – TRUE. The first paragraph is clear in suggesting that thick bacon can be used as a substitute for lardons.

Q5.3 – TRUE. The traditional recipe uses rooster. The first paragraph states that most home cooks use chicken as a substitute. Therefore, it follows that most home cooks don't follow the traditional recipe.

Q5.4 – CAN'T TELL. The text says that using bacon makes the dish drier. The text also says that occasionally garlic is used. What we don't know is what the effect of garlic is. Although there does not seem to be much logic behind the statement, we cannot actually say whether there is a link between the two.

Q5.5 – FALSE. We are told that Quiche Lorraine is made with lardons. The first paragraph clearly states that lardons are made of pork, so Quiche Lorraine contains meat.

Q5.6 – TRUE. Quiche Lorraine comes from the Lorraine region, which, the text states, was first taken by France in 1648 (i.e. the 17th century). The first sentence of the second paragraph says that the dish dates back to the 16th century, i.e. before it became French.

Q5.7 – CAN'T TELL. The text does not state what happened to the Lorraine region after 1918 and does not state anywhere that it has remained French since then (Note: in fact it briefly became German again during WWII, but this is not information which can be found in the text). Therefore we cannot conclude either way.

Q5.8 – CAN'T TELL. The Mirabelle fruit is yellow, but there is no indication of the colour of the liqueur.

VR 6 – Blu-Ray

Q6.1 – FALSE. If the industry wanted people to switch to BD players as soon as possible then they would only release new titles in BD format (since BD readers can also read DVDs). The fact that titles will still be released in DVD format for some time means that there is no rush to switch to BD.

Q6.2 – CAN'T TELL. We know that each disc layer can take 25 GB and we know that Pioneer has "demonstrated that Blu-Ray discs can be constructed with up to 20 layers. Therefore, 20 x 25 = 500GB is the total possible capacity of a Blu-Ray disc; however, we can't tell whether they are or will be actually manufactured at maximum capacity. We simply know that it is possible to achieve this level.

Q6.3 – TRUE. Those who purchase BD players will also be able to play DVDs on them. Therefore DVD players will become redundant and can therefore be discarded.

Q6.4 – CAN'T TELL. The text does not deal with the safety aspect of the two types of lasers. Therefore we simply cannot answer the question.

Q6.5 – CAN'T TELL. What the text actually says is that because Blu-Ray players are manufactured abroad, the fluctuations in exchange rates will make them more expensive than what they cost at present, i.e. we are comparing the cost to a UK consumer of a foreign product before and after currency fluctuation. There is nothing to indicate whether manufacturing the product in the UK would be cheaper. For example, if we assume that the current cost of a Blu-Ray player is £1,000, then exchange rate pressures may increase this cost to £1,200, say. But this may still be cheap in comparison to what it would cost to manufacture the product in the UK (which could be £2,000 say).

Q6.6 – CAN'T TELL. We know that sales of Blu-Ray readers are expected to triple over 2009, but this figure is Europe-wide. We are not told of expectations over the UK. All we know about the UK is that the sales of Blu-Ray discs have increased (which does not necessarily mean that the sales of players has increased and, in any case, a past increase in sales does not necessarily translate into a future increase in sales). So, although there may be good reasons to believe that the statement is true, we cannot conclude for certain on the basis of the text. In fact, the final sentence suggests that economic uncertainty and adverse exchange rates could go against Blu-Ray in the short term.

Q6.7 – CAN'T TELL. We are told that Batman was released in Blu-Ray format but nothing indicates that it wasn't released in DVD format as well. Therefore we cannot tell either way.

Q6.8 – TRUE. The sale of 400,000 discs in November 2008 represents an increase of 165% on October 2008 figures. Therefore the number of discs sold in October would be calculated as 400,000 / 2.65, which is below 200,000.

VR7 – Cyanide & Arsenic

Q7.1 – CAN'T TELL. We know that some humans cannot detect its smell; however, we don't know the percentage of humans who can. Therefore we cannot say whether "most humans" (i.e. over 50%) would detect the smell when present.

Q7.2 – CAN'T TELL. The text says the cyanide in the crushed leaves was used to make a preservative liquid. However, we don't know how the butterflies were killed.

Q7.3 – CAN'T TELL. We are not told how much fruit a human being would need to eat to suffer harmful effects and whether anyone could realistically eat all of these in a reasonable amount of time for the cyanide concentration to be harmful. There is certainly nothing in the text which suggests that eating too much of the cyanide-containing fruit could be detrimental to humans. We therefore simply cannot conclude whether the statement is true or false from the information given.

Q7.4 – CAN'T TELL. The text only says that cyanide is used in mining. We can't conclude whether cyanide is a by-product of mining or not.

Q7.5 – CAN'T TELL. We are told that arsenic converts directly from solid to gaseous form when heated in air at atmospheric pressure. Nothing indicates that a liquid form is not possible under different conditions.

Q7.6 – CAN'T TELL. We are told that arsenic is better than iodine-124 to locate tumours; however, we don't know whether iodine-124 is what is being used currently.

Q7.7 – CAN'T TELL. We are told explicitly that arsenic is a poison to insects, so the answer now depends on whether cyanide is toxic to insects or not. Although we know from the text that cyanide is toxic to humans and that it is also being used in a preservative liquid for butterflies; we cannot conclude that it is toxic to insects.

Q7.8 – CAN'T TELL. Several elements point towards this statement being true including the following: (i) arsenic is totally soluble in water; (ii) arsenic is colourless; and (iii) arsenic is odourless in its normal state. However, the text does not say anything about taste.

VR8 – Chocolate

Q8.1 – TRUE. From the text, we know that tea contains caffeine and that caffeine increases emotional stress. Therefore we can conclude that drinking tea (and the caffeine within it) may lead to increased emotional stress. If the statement had said that "drinking tea always leads to increased emotional stress" then the answer would have been "Can't tell". Indeed the text tells us that it is caffeine (and not tea) which leads to increased emotional stress. It could well be that there are other substances in tea which coun-

Verbal Reasoning – Practice

teract the effects of caffeine. We simply don't know. What makes this statement true is the presence of the word "may" within it, which simply indicates that it is possible, rather than definite.

Q8.2 – CAN'T TELL. The text says that smoking cigarettes accelerates the dissipation of both substances from the system. This is not the same as compensating for the effects. Nothing in the text mentions the impact of cigarette smoking on the effect of caffeine.

Q8.3 – CAN'T TELL. From the text, we know that theobromine is not addictive, but that does not mean that chocolate isn't.

Q8.4 – FALSE. The text tells us that chocolate does not contain caffeine naturally and that any caffeine found in chocolate has been added artificially. However, this could be achieved by other means than by adding coffee (for example, the text tells us that there is caffeine in tea).

Q8.5 – CAN'T TELL. The name "phytostanols" contains the root "phyton" which, in Greek, does mean "plant" and the context does suggest that phytostanols may be a natural substance; however, the text itself (remember: all that matters is what we can conclude from the text itself) does not give enough information to enable us to conclude that this is the case.

Q8.6 – CAN'T TELL. Soy fibre and phytostanols are both discussed within the text, one as a cholesterol-lowering tool and the other one simply as being under investigation. There is nothing to suggest whether soy fibre contains phytostanols.

Q8.7 – TRUE. The text states that calcium-enriched chocolates can prevent osteoporosis. This suggests that it is either the calcium, the chocolate or both which prevent osteoporosis. However, the context here is a discussion on how different types of new ingredients can bring different health benefits, so clearly we are being told that it is the calcium enrichment which is making a difference and we can generalise the statement.

Q8.8 – CAN'T TELL. The text presents some benefits as proven (e.g. soy fibre lowering cholesterol, calcium enrichment strengthening bones, preventing dental caries, etc.) but also says that some of the benefits are just claims made by manufacturers (e.g. improving brain activity, enhancing memory, aphrodisiac). The use of the word "claim" suggests that the author may have a cynical view of such claims; however it does not mean that they are unproven (indeed, it could simply be due to the author's ignorance of such proofs). The only thing that we know is not proven is the cholesterol-reducing effect of phytostanols, but, as far as we know from the text, no manufacturer has made such a claim.

VR9 – Pregnancy Food

Q9.1 – CAN'T TELL. We know that goat cheese without a white rind is safe. However, we don't know if the presence of a white rind makes it unsafe.

Q9.2 – FALSE. The text states that Cheddar is safe to eat, but then goes on to explain that this is because the level of bacteria is so low that the risk is extremely small. In addition, the final sentence of the first paragraph states that women avoiding high-risk cheese are very unlikely to be affected by listeria. Although the risk is very small, it still exists and it is therefore incorrect to state that a woman eating Cheddar only cannot get listeria infection. If the wording of the statement were "is unlikely to get listeria infection", the statement would be true.

Q9.3 – FALSE. The recommendations are that many cheeses are actually, on the whole, safe for pregnant women. The first paragraph also states that cheese can be beneficial to pregnant women. The text actually encourages pregnant women to eat cheese, though remaining careful about which they should eat. Nowhere does it state that women should steer clear of cheese, even if it reminds the reader that every cheese has its risk.

Q9.4 – CAN'T TELL. We know that Gruyère is safe, but we don't know whether ham and bread are safe.

Q9.5 – TRUE. The whole meal weighs 150 g so, although we don't know exactly how much fish it contains, we know it will be under the 175 g which constitutes the absolute safe limit for women who have doubts. All the ingredients described are either safe cheeses or low-mercury fish and we know there are no other ingredients ("made exclusively of the following ingredients") so the pie is safe to eat in this quantity.

Q9.6 – CAN'T TELL. All we know from the text is that (i) longer living fish tend to have greater mercury levels; and that (ii) canned white tuna contains more mercury than light tuna, which is a mix of low-mercury tuna species. We know nothing about other species of tuna (which are not being canned) and therefore cannot conclude either way.

Verbal Reasoning – Practice

Q9.7 – TRUE. This is the principle which underlines the whole of the second paragraph. We are being told that fish which live longer are accumulating more mercury (hence why they may be unsafe). The word "accumulating" is an explicit answer to the question.

Q9.8 – TRUE. We know from the text that mercury builds up in the body with age. Therefore it makes sense for a young fish to have less mercury than an older fish of the same species. However, there is always a risk that external conditions such as living in a mercury-polluted river or sea could make this assumption wrong. But since the question says that we must assume that all other factors are equal then we can confidently conclude that the assertion is true.

VR10 – The Grass is Greener

Q10.1 – FALSE. The parking suspension applies to the bay in the street in which he normally parks. Because John Rover left his car in that bay before the resurfacing took place, the car was moved onto a piece of grass and he was fined for parking on the grass (as the ticket says) and not for remaining parked in the bay after the suspension took effect (although he was also guilty of that latter offence, this is not what he was fined for).

Q10.2 – TRUE. We know that the letter was dated 5 January, on which date he discovered the car parked on the grass, together with the ticket. We also know that the car was moved before the resurfacing commenced (from the neighbour's testimony) and that the resurfacing work took place between 19 and 24 December. This means that the car was moved before 24 December. So the car was on the grass at least between 24 December and 5 January, which is over a week.

Q10.3 – CAN'T TELL. All we know is that parking is normally free on Green Avenue, which is parallel to the street in which he lives. We don't know whether parking is free in his own street.

Q10.4 – CAN'T TELL. We know that parking was suspended between 19 December and 24 December (i.e. 6 days) and that, during that time, the road was resurfaced. We don't know whether the resurfacing took place during the entire period or not.

Q10.5 – CAN'T TELL. We know that he used his car on 16 December, since he said he parked it in Green Avenue on that day, and that he left the country on 18 December. There is nothing in the text which enables us to conclude that he did not use his car on 17 December.

Q10.6 – CAN'T TELL. All we know is that he did not see the notice on 17 December. We cannot conclude it wasn't there (though it is possible).

Q10.7 – CAN'T TELL. The parking ticket was placed on the car because the car was parked on the grass. The car would have been moved onto the grass between the time the notice was put up and the time the work started. So this could be at any time between 17 December and 24 December. However, we don't know when the ticket was placed on the car. This could have been at any time before 5 January when John Rover found it on his car.

Q10.8 – CAN'T TELL. The text does not deal with the legal aspect. All we know is that the notice was signed two days before the day of the suspension. Whether this was legal or not cannot be concluded from the text as it stands.

VR11 – The Bard

Q11.1 – TRUE. We are told that the painting was made in 1610, several years before his death. Later on, we are told he died in 1616. Since we ignore in which month he died or the painting was made, we can conclude that the use of the word "approximately" makes the sentence true.

Q11.2 – CAN'T TELL. We know that it was painted during his lifetime and that all other known pieces were done afterwards. But we cannot conclude definitively that there are no other paintings which were also done during his lifetime. Some may well be hidden in other places. This is reiterated in the first paragraph which states that it is the "only *known* portrait".

Q11.3 – FALSE. It was found to be a fake 70 years ago but it was painted in the 19th century, therefore over 100 years ago.

Q11.4 – CAN'T TELL. Although this seems absurd, we can't actually conclude either way from the text. The text says: "Foundation Shakespeare Birthplace, an association which manages the museum in Stratford-upon-Avon, where the poet was born." What this really says is that Shakespeare

Verbal Reasoning – Practice

was born in Stratford-upon-Avon rather than in the museum, but, since we don't actually know where exactly he was born in that town, we can't conclude that he wasn't born in a museum.

Q11.5 – TRUE. The text states that the portrait was painted on an oak plank.

Q11.6 – CAN'T TELL. We know that he lived at the same time as he was financing him, but nothing in the text links the two men as having met. We only know their two portraits were found in the same place.

Q11.7 – FALSE. The painting was made in 1610. The copy dates from the 19th century, i.e. between 1800 and 1899, which makes it between 190 and 289 years later i.e. under three centuries.

Q11.8 – CAN'T TELL. We know that he owns the painting and is a restorer, but we don't know whether he actually restored the portrait.

VR12 – Delay Compensation Package

Q12.1 – CAN'T TELL. The text is actually ambiguous on this matter. Intuitively one would think that buses and coaches would follow the same rules as boats, but the text only mentions the need to pay half of the ticket price "if required" without mentioning anything about how such requirement is assessed or whether the 25% also applies for smaller delays.

Q12.2 – TRUE. The amounts are fixed and therefore are not linked to ticket prices.

Q12.3 – FALSE. As well as the potential maximum of 600 Euros, the text also mentions having to provide complimentary refreshments on board the aircraft if the delay is beyond a specified number of hours. This will add to the costs.

Q12.4 – CAN'T TELL. Although this is a possibility, there is nothing in the text that remotely addresses this issue.

Q12.5 – TRUE. Since the compensation amount is fixed at an arbitrary level, it is of course possible that an airline with cheap tickets could pay more in compensation than the price paid for the ticket. This is a fact that is emphasised in the last sentence of the text.

Q12.6 – FALSE. There is no mention in the text of any reason why compensation should go over 100%. In fact, we know that it would normally be 50% and would only increase to 100% if no information was provided.

Q12.7 – FALSE. Companies only have an obligation to provide information. We can get this from two places: the first sentence of the second paragraph states this explicitly; also, the compensation of 100% is only payable if companies fail to provide alternative means of transport or information on alternative modes of transport. There is therefore no need for them to actually organise it.

Q12.8 – CAN'T TELL. The 600 Euros are payable for delays but we don't know how many hours of delay are needed. We also know that there are complimentary refreshments on board the aircraft for those who have been delayed beyond a specified number of hours, though the text says nothing about what those hours are. Therefore we have no means of assessing whether there is an exact match between the two numbers of hours required to trigger each part of the compensation package.

VR13 – Saving Neil Armstrong's Spacesuit

Q13.1 – D: 2015. The 50th anniversary of Neil Armstrong's first step on the Moon is in 2019. Therefore the event took place in 1969. The quote from the curator mentions that those first steps were 46 years previously. Therefore the year is 1969 + 46 = 2015.

Q13.2 – C: Visitors to the museum will be able to see the spacesuit for themselves, albeit through a glass wall. The text mentions that the suit was being displayed up until 2006 and that the museum is now seeking a new display case. This still leaves open the possibility that the display case may only be for remote viewing; however, the word "further" in the phrase "to preserve it and figure out a way in which we can further display it" points to the fact that it will be displayed in a similar fashion as before. Within the context of the whole sentence, it implies that the intention is to display it as it had previously been, albeit within a more controlled environment. Looking at the other options:

- **A: All fabrics used to make the spacesuit require low temperature and low humidity to be preserved.** The text states that conserving each textile individually would be very easy but that it would require taking the suit apart. That implies that different fabrics require different

Verbal Reasoning – Practice

conditions. From the text, we can't conclude whether all fabrics require low temperature and low humidity. Indeed it is perfectly possible that one fabric actually requires high humidity and that the low humidity is just a compromise to preserve at least the 11 other fabrics which require it. It is also very plausible that some fabrics don't actually require any specific conditions and would be quite happy at normal room temperature. The problem with the statement is the word "all".

- **B: All fabrics used to make the spacesuit require air circulation to be preserved.** In a similar argument to Option A, it is possible that some fabrics would be happy with no air circulation. The use of the word "all" in the statement means that we cannot reasonably infer that this is correct.

- **D: Visitors to the museum will only be able to see the spacesuit via interactive computer screens.** If Option C is correct then Option D is not. At a stretch, it may be possible to infer from the text that the spacesuit is not for public display other than through interactive screens, i.e. visitors to the museum would actually see an interactive image of the spacesuit in the same way that internet users would. However, on top of the reasons outlined above to justify Option C, one also wonders why they would bother placing the suit in a display case as opposed to, say, some locked vault with a camera in it. The use of a display cabinet implies that it is designed to be seen physically.

Q13.3 – CAN'T TELL. We are told that in 2006 the suit was taken off display and placed in "our state-of-the-art facility, which is at cool temperature and low humidity, just to preserve it and figure out a way in which we can further display it". From this we can deduce that it wasn't previously stored in a state-of-the-art facility with low humidity and temperature, but not that it was simply left without any kind of special atmosphere.

Q13.4 – CAN'T TELL. We know that the museum is trying to raise the $500,000 for that purpose; however, this is the amount it is trying to raise. It is perfectly possible that the project will cost more but that some of the money has already been raised either internally (i.e. the museum will invest some of its own funds) or externally (i.e. from benefactors). All we can conclude is that the $500,000 in question is the shortfall in funding, but not necessarily the full cost.

VR14 – Sleepover

Q14.1 – D: Sleeping more than 8 hours may be the first sign of a terminal illness. Professor Cappuccio suggests that the increased mortality of those who sleep over 8 hours is partially due to the fact that some people might be more depressed, take sleeping pills or have an underlying health problem. Therefore it would be correct to conclude that sleeping over 8 hours may be the first sign of a terminal illness. Note that the statement contains the word "may", which indicates that this would not necessarily be systematically the case, i.e. it is not saying that everyone who sleeps long hours has a terminal illness, but simply that sleeping long hours might be a cause for concern. If the statement did not contain the word "may" but was more definite, it would be incorrect. Looking at the other options:

- **A: People who sleep more than 8 hours would be less likely to die if they made efforts to sleep less than 6 hours.** Nothing in the part of the text relating to Professor Cappuccio's work points to the fact that it is the duration of sleep which causes the higher mortality. Instead of showing a cause, it simply establishes a link, i.e. there are other factors coming into play, such as depression. Professor Cappuccio's contention is that people are the victims of certain illnesses which increase their mortality risk and, independently, cause them to sleep longer; nothing more. Therefore, forcing oneself to sleep fewer hours would not necessarily decrease the mortality risk.

- **B: Depression can stop you from sleeping enough hours.** Whilst in reality depression can, in some cases, reduce one's hours of sleep, there is nothing in the text related to Professor Cappuccio which links depression to short sleeping times. He only links depression to longer sleeping times.

- **C: Taking sleeping pills increases your mortality risk.** Whilst this may be the case for some individuals, there is nothing in the text which suggests it. What would be more likely to increase mortality would be the depression or the stress that is causing those people to take the sleeping pills, and not the sleeping pills themselves.

This question really highlights the danger of confusing association (i.e. X and Y co-existing in a situation) and causation (X causing Y). The fact that two facts occur simultaneously indicates that they may be linked but does

Verbal Reasoning – Practice

not necessarily indicate that one is the cause of the other. Indeed, Y might cause X, or some other factor, Z, might cause both X and Y.

Q14.2 – B: Spending 2 hours more in bed than you normally do may increase your risk of depression. The Youngstedt study made the participants spend 2 hours more in bed than their normal amount. The results confirm that participants experienced "increases in depressed moods". Looking at the other options:

- **A: People who sleep 8 hours tend to be more depressed than those who sleep only 6 hours.** The study does not compare a group of people who sleep 6 hours with another group who sleep 8 hours. It looks at changes within each individual. Also it looks at people who spend two hours more in bed than usual and does not mention any number with regard to what their normal sleep hours might be. It is very possible that all participants normally sleep 8 hours and that they were asked to sleep for 10 hours.

- **C: IL-6 can cause depression.** The text mentions only a connection with inflammation, not depression. Even so, this would be association and not causation.

- **D: Sleeping more than 8 hours may be the first sign of a terminal illness.** The text does not mention anything about 8 hours or terminal illnesses, only depression.

Q14.3 – B: People with depression have higher mortality than those who are not depressed. Professor Cappuccio attributes the higher mortality to the fact that some participants who oversleep may be depressed. This can only be true if he makes the assumption that depression would lead to death somehow (suicide, self-neglect, etc.). Looking at the other options:

- **A: The average person sleeps 7 hours a day.** He is only looking at different groups who sleep different hours. The results imply that the normal range is 6-8 hours but this in no way assumes that the average person sleeps for 7 hours per night.

- **C: Smoking is less dangerous than drinking.** If anything, we may be able to construe from the text that smoking is more dangerous than drinking, although the text is very vague with regard to the amounts involved. In any case, that would be a conclusion rather than an assumption.

- **D: People with underlying health problems tend to oversleep rather than undersleep.** Professor Cappuccio offers as an explanation for the higher mortality amongst oversleepers that some may have underlying health problems. The text does not say anything about his possible explanations for the higher-than-normal mortality amongst undersleepers. It is possible that health factors may also have an impact on their mortality. As such we cannot conclude that he made that assumption.

VR15 – Earth 2.0

Q15.1 – C: Earth 2.0 is smaller than Kepler-186f. The text states that "Kepler-186f is smaller than the new planet" (i.e. Kepler-452b/Earth 2.0). Looking at the other options:

- **A: Kepler-452b has a diameter 60% larger than the diameter of the Earth.** If its radius is 60% larger than Earth's radius, then so is its diameter (2 x radius).

- **B: The radius of planet can be used as an indicator of how rocky it is likely to be.** The sentence "based on its small radius, Kepler-452b has a reasonable chance, between 49% and 62%, of being rocky" indicates that the radius is an indicator of how rocky it might be.

- **D: Venus experienced a runaway greenhouse effect.** This is made clear in the sentence "it may be subject to a runaway greenhouse effect similar to that seen on Venus".

Q15.2 – A: The Earth's oceans will eventually disappear. In the final paragraph, the text describes how an increase in energy from an ageing sun will lead to evaporation of any oceans, making it clear also that this is a process that the Earth will undergo in a billion years' time. Looking at the other options:

- **B: The Sun has a remaining lifespan of at least 1.5 billion years.** The "1.5 billion years" referred to in the text is the difference in age between the two suns. It has nothing to do with longevity.

Verbal Reasoning – Practice

- **C: All planets orbiting within the habitable zone of their sun contain liquid water.** All we know from the text is that the habitable zone is a zone where the levels of energy would make it possible to have liquid water "if certain conditions are met". Therefore we cannot conclude that all planets within that zone would contain liquid water.

- **D: The Sun is getting bigger and brighter as it gets older.** We know that the increasing energy from the ageing star around which Kepler-452b orbits may be evaporating the oceans and we are told that the same will happen to Earth later. So what we can surmise from that is that it is anticipated that the Sun will give out higher levels of energy; but the text is not conclusive as to whether this will involve the Sun getting bigger and brighter.

Q15.3 – D: Exoplanets are common in the universe. Though the term "exoplanet" is not precisely defined in the text, it provides sufficient background to help us conclude that an exoplanet is a planet that is similar to the Earth (see beginning of paragraph 2). We are told at the end of the penultimate paragraph that "around 20% of Sun-like stars, of which there are countless, have an Earth-sized planet in their habitable zone". That would suggest that there exist a large number of planets of similar size to the Earth, which would qualify as exoplanets. This would make exoplanets common. Looking at the other options:

- **A: Exoplanets are rocky.** We know that Kepler-452b is an exoplanet but that it has a probability of being rocky of 49% to 62%, therefore we can't assert confidently that exoplanets are rocky (as this implies that they should all be). In fact, the text suggests that rockiness is linked to the radius.

- **B: Exoplanets revolve around a star similar to the Earth's Sun.** This is not the case for Kepler-186f which, we are told, "orbits a red dwarf star that is significantly cooler than our own".

- **C: Exoplanets contain liquid water on their surface.** All we know from the text is that exoplanets would need to orbit within the habitable zone in order to have the potential to have surface water. It does not follow that all planets within the habitable zone will contain surface water. The habitable zone only makes it possible.

Q15.4 – CAN'T TELL. We know from the text that Venus experienced a runaway greenhouse effect, i.e. increased energy from the Sun caused oceans to evaporate. So the statement could be true; however, it is not clear whether that process is completed or in progress. Therefore we cannot say conclusively that there is no liquid water remaining on Venus.

VR16 – Dyeing To Bake

Q16.1 – A: Using large quantities of liquid dyes will not affect taste. Though the paragraph dealing with liquid dye does not state directly that using large quantities of liquid dye will not affect taste, the paragraph on liquid gel dye explains that, because liquid gel dyes are more concentrated, you need to use a smaller amount, with less of a chance that the colouring will adversely flavour the food. Therefore using large quantities of liquid dye is likely to affect the taste. Looking at the other options:

- **B: Liquid dyes are good to achieve pastel tones.** The text states that liquid dyes are most suited to recipes requiring lighter colours. That would include pastel colours.

- **C: It is not advisable to make macaroons with liquid dye.** The paragraph on powdered dye suggests that, when making macaroons, adding any liquid can lead to a disaster. Therefore it would indeed not be advisable to use liquid dyes when making macaroons.

- **D: When using liquid dyes to obtain a bright colour, it is best to reduce the amount of water/milk used in the recipe by an equivalent amount.** Bright colours can only be achieved by using large amounts of liquid dye. One can therefore conclude that problems would be avoided by reducing the quantities of milk/water accordingly.

Q16.2 – D: Powdered dye. If the cake is for somebody who is allergic to glycerine then this rules out liquid gel and gel paste dyes, both of which potentially contain that ingredient (we can't be sure since the label is missing, hence the risk cannot be taken). Using liquid dye would require large quantities, which would thin the mix. Hence using powdered dye would be the most suitable option.

Q16.3 – B: Red gel paste dye is not a natural product. The first line of the gel paste dye paragraph states that this type of dye is synthetic; therefore, red or not, it is not natural. Looking at the other options:

Verbal Reasoning – Practice

- **A: Gel paste dye dries out more quickly than liquid dye.** All we know is that powdered dye will not dry out like the other types of dye; but nothing in the text gives any indication about the relative drying times of the other dyes.

- **C: Non-red gel paste dye does not taste metallic.** The text only refers to red gel paste dye as having been found to taste metallic by some users. The absence of comments about other colours does not in any way mean that they do not taste metallic as well.

- **D: Powdered dye does not affect taste.** The text does not address the link between powdered dye and taste. Therefore we cannot infer anything.

Q16.4 – B: Gel paste dye is hard to incorporate into stiff dough. We are told that liquid gel dye has a thick texture which makes it harder to incorporate into stiff dough. We are also told that gel paste dye is thicker than liquid gel dye; hence we can conclude that it will be even harder to incorporate into stiff dough. Looking at the other options:

- **A: One cannot use two types of dye in the same cake mix.** Nothing in the text suggests that they cannot be mixed.

- **C: Powdered dye is not water soluble.** Nothing in the text suggests it is not water soluble. Particularly the fact that it is not water-based cannot be interpreted as such.

- **D: Gel paste dye is more expensive than liquid gel dye.** All we know from the text is that gel paste dye is more concentrated than liquid gel dye. That may impact on price but we are not told how.

Q16.5 – FALSE. We are told that liquid gel and gel paste dyes have a water, glycerine and/or corn syrup base. The "and/or" indicates that corn syrup may or may not be present and suggests that some brands do not contain corn syrup (if corn syrup was always included then the use of "and/or" would make no sense). Therefore those allergic to corn could use both types of dyes and would simply need to select the variants that do not include corn syrup.

VR17 – A Battle Of Wills

Q17.1 – A: £200,000. She had originally been awarded £50,000 but the decision was overturned and the amount increased to £200,000. The total amount ever available was £600,000 therefore Option C (a third of 650,000) is incorrect. Option D (the value of her housing association property) is also incorrect. All we know from the text is that she will use the money to buy her property; there is nothing in the text that links the amount received to the value of the property.

Q17.2 – D: Unknown. All we know from the text is that she will be able to buy the property using the money (£200,000) received. We don't know its price. It is possible the property is worth less than £200,000; it may also be worth more (and she will simply use the £200,000 as part payment).

Q17.3 – D: Wills will only be valid if the sum of money left to the children represents a reasonable percentage of the value of the estate. Ms Jackson was offered £50,000, a decision which was overturned by the Court of Appeal, who ruled that she should be entitled to a "share of the money". This suggests therefore that the original £50,000 awarded was not calculated as a share (i.e. a percentage in this case) of the money, but as a fixed sum which would appear reasonable. Hence Option D is a more likely conclusion than Option C ("Wills will be valid as long as the children inherit something").

With regard to Options A and B, since Ms Jackson was only granted a third of the money, the remaining two thirds went to the charities to which the money had originally been granted. Therefore there is no ground to conclude that people will need to leave all their money to their children or that charities would be excluded from wills.

Q17.4 – C: Ms Jackson's mother was not mentally competent enough to draw up a reasonable will. All we know is that the decision by the mother to cut out her daughter was deemed unreasonable (most likely because it was driven by revenge). There is nothing to suggest that the mother was mentally incompetent. Looking at the other options:

- **A: Courts do not always rule in favour of the relatives.** The case of the builder who cleaned the gutters proves it.

Verbal Reasoning – Practice

- **B: The charities involved in Ms Jackson's case received £400,000.** The case was brought by the daughter to reclaim some of the £600,000 for herself, when the full amount was originally granted to the charities. She managed to reclaim £200,000; this means that the charities are then left with the remainder, i.e. £400,000.

- **D: Charity donations through wills will decrease.** The case will likely lead to more wills being contested by relatives on grounds of unreasonableness. This will in turn lead to lower amounts being granted to charities, in favour of relatives.

Q17.5 – CAN'T TELL. In truth we do not know how the money has been apportioned and, particularly, whether the judges considered that one third was an appropriate amount for a child to receive in absolute (in which case there would be a problem if there were more than 3 children) or whether it was reasonable for someone to give two thirds of their fortune to non-relatives, in which case the relatives would need to share one third between them. The text merely implies that children will have a better chance of winning their case if they feel they have been hard done by and want to contest a will on grounds of unreasonableness.

VR18 – Fat Chance

Q18.1 – D: Aldehydes tend to be generated from polyunsaturated fats. The second paragraph states that corn oil and sunflower oil are rich in polyunsaturates and therefore generate substantial levels of aldehydes. This shows that polyunsaturates produce aldehydes. However, in order to conclude that aldehydes tend to be generated from polyunsaturates we also need to show that nothing else generates substantial amounts of aldehydes. We get the answer from the third paragraph, which states that monounsaturated and saturated fats produce far less aldehydes. Therefore we can conclude that aldehydes tend to be generated from polyunsaturates.

Note that it is very possible that another type of fat not described in the text may also produce aldehydes; however, the question is asking what the author is most likely to conclude as opposed to which sentence can be definitely concluded from the text. This is where this format of question differs from the "true/false/can't tell" format. Looking at the other options:

- **A: Aldehydes form at a temperature of 180 °C.** We can actually conclude from the text that this is false because, though it does state that an oxidation process producing aldehydes takes place around 180 °C, it also states that this could equally happen at room temperature if the oil is left around for a long period of time. Therefore aldehydes can also form at much lower temperatures.

- **B: Rancid oil does not contain aldehydes.** Paragraph 1 is clear about the fact that the oxidation process leading to the formation of aldehydes can also happen at room temperature, leading to the lipids going rancid. Therefore we can logically conclude that rancid oil does contain aldehydes.

- **C: Heated saturated fats contain high levels of aldehydes.** The text states that saturated fats hardly undergo the oxidation reaction; therefore we can reasonably conclude that heated saturated fats would in fact contain very low levels of aldehydes.

Q18.2 – D: None of the above. From the text, we can only conclude that there is an issue when the oils are heated (in which case one would want to avoid sunflower oil). There is nothing in the text to indicate that any of the oils mentioned would be detrimental at cold temperatures. Based on the text there is therefore no reason to suspect that any of the three oils mentioned would be bad for use in a cold salad dressing.

Q18.3 – A: Butter is healthier when heated up than when cold. This assertion does not really make much sense. In light of the text, all we can reasonably conclude from the text is that butter is not likely to be more dangerous when hot than when cold, but it is far from saying that it would actually be healthier when heated up. Looking at the other options:

- **B: Hot butter is healthier than hot sunflower oil.** We know from the text that hot butter does not produce many aldehydes whereas sunflower oil does. So the assertion would be a logical conclusion, at least as far as heart disease is concerned.

- **C: Cold butter is healthy to eat in small quantities.** The last paragraph actually relates to saturated fats in general, and not just those which are heated up. We know from paragraph 3 that butter contains saturated fats and we also know from the last paragraph that eating saturated fats can cut hunger and stop other foods such as carbohydrates from being eaten. So it is reasonable to conclude that small quantities of butter can be healthy to eat.

Verbal Reasoning – Practice

- **D: Eating butter makes you less likely to eat other potentially unhealthy foods.** This is dealt with in the last paragraph.

Q18.4 – B: The public was misled about the dangers of saturated fats. It is explained in the last paragraph that saturated fats were unfairly vilified at the expense of the message on other issues such as overconsumption of carbohydrates. Looking at the other options:

- **A: Potatoes fried in goose fat cannot cause heart disease.** The text suggests that goose fat poses a minimal danger; however, it does link carbohydrate consumption (potatoes are carbohydrates, we are told) to heart disease and therefore we can conclude that this sentence is actually incorrect.

- **C: Pasta with extra-virgin olive oil is healthier than pasta alone.** This could only be concluded if the text explained how the addition of olive oil could produce a health benefit. All we know about olive oil is that it is stable when heated, not that it neutralises the harmful impact of carbohydrates on the risk of diabetes or heart disease.

- **D: At room temperature, olive oil goes rancid more quickly than sunflower oil.** We know that olive oil is more stable when going through the oxidation process (which also causes oil to go rancid when left at room temperature), whereas sunflower oil tends to oxidise more substantially. Based on the text, there is no reason to suspect that at room temperature the process would be the total opposite (i.e. olive oil going rancid faster than sunflower oil).

Q18.5 – B: Saturated < Monounsaturated < Polyunsaturated. We know from paragraph 3 that oils rich in monounsaturated and saturated fatty acids are stable and produce far fewer aldehydes than polyunsaturated fats. Therefore both will feature at the bottom of the scale and polyunsaturated fats will be at the top (as they oxidise the most).

We are also told that saturated fats hardly undergo any oxidation at all, which implies that the aldehydes produced by fats such as butter or olive oil come mostly from the monounsaturates. Hence saturated fats are at the bottom of the scale when it comes to oxidation, followed by monounsaturated fats.

VR19 – Snooping

Q19.1 – B: The UK version of iMessage could become less secure than the version of iMessage sold in many other countries. The government wishes to gain a backdoor access to the encryption, which may make the system less secure (see the penultimate paragraph). It means that the UK version could be less secure than the versions sold in countries that have not passed such law. Looking at the other options:

- **A: Messages can sometimes be too securely encrypted to be read by the person receiving them.** The only entities mentioned within the text as not being able to read the encrypted material are the government and Apple, not the users.

- **C: Only messages originating from the UK or the US have a highly secure level of encryption.** There is nothing in the text explicitly mentioning the situation in other countries. In fact, the last paragraph suggests strongly that every country in the world uses the same highly secure versions of messaging systems.

- **D: No warrant is required to intercept Skype communications.** The only paragraph referring to warrants is the second paragraph, which suggests that the Prime Minister is concerned that, even with a high-profile warrant, the government would not be able to access the information. It does not suggest in any way that no warrant is required to intercept Skype communications.

Q19.2 – A: Should Apple decide to continue providing iMessage, it may have no choice but to break the law. If a law is passed which imposes that the government be given access to intercept communications, then Apple would not be able to comply because it "has no way to decrypt [information] whilst it's in transit between devices", adding later that it "wouldn't be able to comply with a wiretap even if [they] wanted to". As such, the only way to avoid breaking the law would be to stop providing the iMessage service. Looking at the other options:

- **B: If Apple scanned communications, it could decipher encrypted communications in transit.** This contradicts the text (see explanation for Option A).

Verbal Reasoning – Practice

- **C: Communications via Skype are monitored.** In fact the text suggests the opposite since Skype is listed as one of the messaging systems that the government wants to gain access to. It is possible that Skype communications are monitored by the company that owns the software but nothing in the text suggests it.

- **D: A warrant signed by the Home Secretary is essential to intercept communications.** The only paragraph mentioning the Home Secretary is the second, within a quote by the Prime Minister. The purpose of the quote is to highlight the fact that, even with a warrant signed by the highest authority in the UK, monitoring is not currently possible because of the encryption levels. It does not suggest that warrants have to be signed by the Home Secretary.

Q19.3 – C: Terrorists may communicate without being caught. The passage concerns the monitoring of communications through interception whilst in transit. It states explicitly in the second paragraph that both the UK and US government fear that the existing messaging systems currently enable terrorists to communicate freely without fearing interception. Looking at the other options:

- **A: Customers may receive undecipherable messages.** The text only talks about communication in transit, not when received. In any case, it does not mention anything that would affect the functionality of the messaging systems from the user's point of view but only the fact that governments may be granted backdoor access.

- **B: Terrorists may intercept customers' personal messages.** That is in fact possible but that is not presented as a risk within the text. The text is clearly about stopping terrorists communicating.

- **D: The state is unable to monitor terrorists' bank accounts.** The issue is to do with messages in transit and not someone's financial records sitting on a bank server. The only mention of bank accounts refers to the fact that a weakened level of encryption may make it easier for criminals to access bank accounts online. It does not relate to or hint at the fact that the state cannot monitor terrorists' bank accounts.

Q19.4 – D: If the UK government imposed that it should be granted backdoor access, the software companies might no longer wish to make their systems available in the UK. The final paragraph states that it is hard to see how different products could be offered in the UK and in the rest of the world. From that we can conclude that either they will simply no longer make the product available in the UK at all or that the products made available in the rest of the world may be made less secure to match the products retailed in the UK. However, at the beginning of the same paragraph, we are told that advanced encryption is an important part of the security offered by such applications, hinting that they may not compromise on security. We can therefore deduce that it would be sensible for the author to conclude that the products may be withdrawn from the UK market. But to be sure this is the most likely conclusion, we also need to look at the other options:

- **A: A ban on messaging services would be unenforceable.** Nothing in the text suggests that a ban would be unenforceable. It may be true but we cannot deduce it from anything in the text.

- **B: Skype and iMessage use the same type of encryption.** All we know from the text is that they both use very secure encryption methods, which does not mean that they are the same.

- **C: The government's preferred option is to obtain a backdoor into the encryption.** From the text, we can see that the government is concerned with stopping terrorists communicating amongst themselves, not necessarily with snooping on them. Since the ban is presented on an equal footing with the backdoor entry (see third paragraph) then we cannot conclude that it would favour a backdoor into the encryption.

VR20 – Breaking The Sound Barrier

Q20.1 – D: None of the above. Looking at the other options:

- **A: He is a patents and trademarks lawyer/attorney.** We only know that he founded an intellectual property drafting service called Patent Yogi, but the text does not mention or suggest he is an attorney.

- **B: He is a plane spotter.** We only know that he has a passion for planes but nothing suggests he engages in plane spotting. In fact the

Verbal Reasoning – Practice

text suggests he spends most of his time on his computer engaging in patent-spotting.

- **C: Airbus is one of his clients.** Nothing suggests he works with Airbus.

Q20.2 – B: Normal aircrafts fly at an altitude below 20 miles. The text says that the new plane will ascend to an altitude of 20 miles before being catapulted horizontally, cruising at the edge of space high above conventional aircrafts. Therefore it can be deduced that conventional aircrafts fly below an altitude of 20 miles. Looking at the other options:

- **A: The new plane is not at risk of crashing with normal planes.** Though it is correct that it will fly way above conventional aircrafts, it will need to enter normal air traffic close to its destination (see end of the second paragraph). As such, the risk of crashing with normal planes is real.

- **C: The new plane is unlikely to ever be built.** The text does refer to the fact Airbus filed strange patents before and hints at the fact that the project may not see the light of day or that it is a long way off. However, it does not go as far as saying or implying that it is unlikely that the new plane will ever be built, but merely that it is possible it may not.

- **D: The new plane could also fly like a normal plane if needed.** Nothing in the text suggests this is the case.

Q20.3 – A: Concorde could carry more passengers in 24 hours than the new plane. The new plane could do 12 trips in 24 hours (each flight would last one hour, followed by a one-hour maintenance period. Total: 2 hours), thus carrying 12 x 20 = 240 passengers in total, which is twice the number that Concorde could carry at any one time.

Concorde took 3 hours to make the London-to-New York trip, to which we must add one hour of maintenance, so 4 hours in total. Therefore it could make 6 trips in 24 hours. Since each trip could contain 120 passengers, this would equate to 720 passengers in total.

Note that for this question you don't actually need to make all the calculations. All you need to ascertain is that Concorde can actually make more than 2 trips per day.

Q20.4 – C: The new plane could potentially fly to any destination without risking a ban for excess noise. We know that the problem with Concorde was that some countries had banned it from flying over their territory because of the supersonic boom. We also know that the supersonic boom is unlikely to be heard with the new plane. This lifts any restrictions due to excess noise. Looking at the other options:

- **A: Concorde could only fly to countries bordering an ocean.** All we know from the text is that many countries banned it from flying over their territory. That does not mean that they all banned it and, as such, we cannot conclude that it had to fly to a country bordering an ocean.

- **B: The London-to-New-York Concorde line was not profitable.** The text only mentions commercial success rather than profitability. But even if we take one to mean the other, in the text it is linked to the fact that Concorde was banned by many countries because of excess noise. It does not relate to any routes that it was actually flying.

- **D: Airbus will eventually increase the new plane's capacity by introducing bicycle-style seats.** The mention of bicycle-style seats is indeed raised in relation to increased capacity, and so this could potentially end up being true. However, the author labels those seats as a weird idea, and so he/she would be unlikely to conclude that they would be a viable option to increase capacity for the new plane. Option C is a more likely conclusion.

VR21 – Radioactive Waste

Q21.1 – C: Granite. We are told that the waste will be coated with glass, inserted into steel and copper canisters, which would then be surrounded by a layer of clay and buried in granite.

Q21.2 – C: Kitchen sinks can be made out of granite. The text mentions that water cannot travel through granite (unless it is cracked) so there is no reason why kitchen sinks could not be made from granite. Looking at the other options:

- **A: Edvard Munch's *The Scream* depicts a nuclear apocalypse.** The text only mentions that the Scandinavians took inspiration from the type of landscape depicted in the painting. We are not informed of what the painting actually represents, and nothing hints at it.

Verbal Reasoning – Practice

- **B: No element remains radioactive for over 100,000 years.** Anyone with any knowledge of physics and chemistry will know that this is incorrect, but one must use only the text to draw a conclusion. If this statement were true, then no one would have to worry about people living in 100,000 years' time needing to be informed about the dangers of nuclear waste. In fact, the whole premise of the text is that waste could remain radioactive for that long.

- **D: The canisters are designed to last 100,000 years.** There are two reasons why this statement is not a conclusion one can draw easily from the text. First, the text does not suggest that the canisters themselves are built in any material which could last that long. Second, the majority of the text talks about how to minimise the consequences of a possible leak, thus hinting the canisters may well not last that long. All we can conclude is that the whole set-up is designed to ensure that we are protected against the waste for 100,000 years, but not that the canisters themselves are designed for that purpose. Had there been no other suitable option, Option D would have been a possible candidate, but Option C is more definite.

Q21.3 – C: Anti-diarrhoea treatment. We are told that bentonite has laxative properties and so this is the last thing you would want to take if you had diarrhoea! Looking at the other options:

- **A: Sealing the floor of landfills to prevent underground water contamination.** This is a possible use because we know that bentonite swells and makes a barrier when in contact with water. It would therefore stop elements from seeping into the ground much as it stops nuclear waste from escaping once leaked from the canisters.

- **B: Keeping boxes containing moisture-sensitive objects dry.** We are told it is a desiccant due to its absorption properties. Therefore it would be suitable to keep a box's contents dry.

- **D: Increasing moisture retention in soil to increase agricultural yield.** Placing a layer of bentonite underground would stop water from flowing away and downwards.

Q21.4 – C: Stop the granite from cracking during earthquakes. The granite is located on the outside of the whole protection system and therefore is not protected by the clay. Instead, we are told that the clay is there

375

to stop water infiltration and seal the gap between the rock and the canisters. The text also states that clay would not allow anything leaking from a canister to flow through it. This therefore makes Option D (contain any material leaking from the canisters) true and Option B (protect the canisters from damage from external substances) a conclusion someone could likely draw even though it is not explicit in the text. Option A is also true because the text states that the clay would flex, helping to dampen shock waves from earthquakes.

Q21.5 – C: In 100,000 years, humanity will have self-destructed. There is nothing in the text which hints at self-destruction for anyone to draw that conclusion. In fact the whole premise of the text is that people will be around in 100,000 years and that we need to protect and inform them. Therefore this is a claim that the author is likely to disagree with. Looking at the other options:

- **A: Books and computers are not a viable solution.** The text strongly suggests that both media are ephemeral in different ways and the fact that everyone is busy trying to find a more durable solution means that books and computers are not a long-term option.

- **B: In 100,000 years no one will speak English.** There are several factors which would help the author conclude that. First he mentions the fact we can't understand the secrets of the pyramids, which are just 5,000 years old. Second, he questions whether people will be able to decipher any of the six official UN languages, which includes English.

- **D: We still have much to learn about the pyramids.** The text is quite clear about that.

VR22 – Frankenburger

Q22.1 – D: The IF burger will retail at less than 1.8 times the price of a Google burger. We know that the planned retail price for the IF Burger is 18 Euros. The manufacturing price for a Google burger is estimated at 10 Euros and therefore its retail price will be higher if the company is to make a profit. The ratio of 18 over an amount greater than 10 will be lower than 1.8. Looking at the other options:

- **A: Google burgers have a lower retail price than IF burgers.** All we know from the text is that the Google manufacturing cost is lower than

Verbal Reasoning – Practice

the IF retail price. There is nothing in the text that hints as to what the Google retail price would be. This in fact could be set at any level, provided it is above 10 Euros so that they can make a profit.

- **B: Google burgers cost less to manufacture than IF burgers.** There is nothing in the text that enables us to deduce the level of the IF manufacturing cost. All we know is that they will be lower than 18 Euros so that the company can make a profit.

- **C: Google has manufactured 25,000 burgers so far.** If you have chosen this option then you have probably considered that a spend of 250,000 Euros for a burger costing 10 Euros would mean they have made 25,000 burgers. However, the development cost would include all the research and technology costs and is in no way linked to the manufacturing cost of a single burger.

Q22.2 – D: The IF burger may be more appealing to New York customers than London customers. All we know is that a London audience somewhat liked the Google burger and that one New York journalist found the IF burger amazing. Nothing suggests which would do better in either location. Looking at the other options:

- **A: The Google burger does not require animal slaughter.** The text says that the "meat" is made from stem cells. Those of you who are the most clued up on stem cells may guess that those can be collected without actually killing the animal BUT this would be the wrong way to reach that conclusion since you are not supposed to use any external knowledge to answer questions. Instead, the clue is given in the last paragraph where it is stated that "it still contains animal stem cells, even if they are donated voluntarily by the animal". Obviously this does not mean that the animal actually gave its consent but, in that context, it does imply that the animal is not killed to provide those stem cells.

- **B: Pure vegetarians are likely to prefer the IF burger to the Google burger on ethical grounds.** We know that the IF burger is made from seeds and is therefore pure vegetarian, whereas the Google burger is made of products derived from meat. The last paragraph indicates that this would put off some vegetarians, even though no animal is hurt.

- **C: The Google burger is not vegetarian.** The burger is made of muscle fibres grown from stem cells. It is still meat, albeit obtained in a more humane way.

Q22.3 – CAN'T TELL. All we know is that Patrick Brown invented a vegetal burger. We know nothing about his dietary preferences.

Q22.4 – CAN'T TELL. The text explicitly states that both beetroot juice and saffron need to be added to stop the burger looking grey. This is not to say that it does not add anything to the taste as well. The text is silent on the matter.

Q22.5 – TRUE. The text states that London volunteers felt it tasted a little dry because it lacked fat.

Q22.6 – CAN'T TELL. We know from the text that without colourant (albeit natural, e.g. beetroot juice and saffron), the burger looks grey. But the text does not address the reason for the lack of colour.

VR23 – Microwaves

Q23.1 – C: Microwaves travel at the speed of light. The text tells us that velocity of a wave = frequency x wavelength. It also tells us that, for microwaves, multiplying wavelength by frequency should give us the speed of light. Therefore we can conclude that the velocity of a microwave is the speed of light. The text then contains a number of objections, but these are more to do with the design of microwave ovens than microwaves themselves. Looking at the other options:

- **A: Microwaves are safe for humans.** All we can conclude from the text is that they are in common use in products used by humans but not that they are safe.

- **B: You can cook food with a Wi-Fi device.** The second paragraph explains that, though the two work on the same wavelength, the oven's stationary waves are the key to cooking food, whereas the Wi-Fi system only sends impulses. This suggests that one can't cook food with Wi-Fi, though this cannot be definitely concluded. As such, the answer is probably false, or at best a "can't tell". Either way, it cannot be concluded that it is true.

- **D: Microwaves can escape from a microwave oven.** There is no such suggestion in the text.

Verbal Reasoning – Practice

Q23.2 – C: FM waves have a higher frequency than long waves. The last line of the first paragraph suggests that FM radio waves have a higher frequency than long waves. Looking at the other options:

- **A: FM waves have a lower wavelength than mobile phone signals.** The text confirms in the first paragraph what you should already know i.e. that as wavelength increases, frequency decreases. The last sentence indicates that FM radio waves have a lower frequency (and therefore a higher wavelength) than microwaves (mobile phone signals are microwaves as the first sentence suggests).

- **B: Mobile phones emit continuous waves.** This is not discussed in the text. All we know is that microwaves can be stationary (e.g. microwave oven) or sent in impulses (e.g. Wi-Fi).

- **D: Microwave ovens emit waves with a shorter wavelength than mobile phones.** The text states that microwave ovens operate at a frequency of 2.4 GHz. Mobiles phones operate at 0.8 GHz, 1.8 GHz or 2.6 GHz. Therefore it may be true to say that microwave ovens have a higher frequency (and therefore a shorter wavelength) than many mobile phones (i.e. those with frequency 0.8 or 1.8) but not all, since some mobile phones have a frequency greater than 2.4 GHz.

Q23.3 – D: The distance between melting zones is the same across all microwave ovens. The text in fact suggests that the melting zones within the same microwave oven may not be at the same distance (see last paragraph) as this will be influenced by the fan, electrical interference, irregularities in the wall, etc. Therefore, there will also be inconsistencies from one oven to another. This statement is therefore false. Looking at the other options:

- **A: If a microwave oven's melting zones were equally spread, they would be 6.25 cm apart.** The penultimate paragraph tells us that the distance between two melting zones is half the wavelength. Since the wavelength for a microwave oven is 12.5 cm (second paragraph) then the distance between two melting zones is 6.25 cm. The statement is therefore definitely true.

- **B: Microwave ovens are suitable for melting cheese.** The text does suggest that microwave ovens can be used for melting cheese. And although this is conditional on having a rotating plate to avoid non-uniform melting, this statement is, on the whole, true.

- **C: Microwave ovens with non-rotating plates are less effective.** The text clearly explains that more homogeneity is achieved with the help of a rotating plate.

Q23.4 – C: Microwave ovens with rotating plates use rotating waves and not waves with two fixation points. The text clearly states that microwave ovens work with waves resembling guitar strings in that they are fixed at both ends. The use of rotating plates is to ensure that different parts of the food are exposed to the hot spots. Looking at the other options:

- **A: All microwave ovens use waves at the same frequency.** It is clearly stated that the frequency for microwave ovens is 2.4 GHz.

- **B: To calculate the speed of light using a microwave oven, one would need to use an oven without a rotating plate.** The whole calculation rests on the ability to measure the distance between the hot spots. Using rotating plates would make the food move and would make identification of the hotspots impossible.

- **D: Stirring food in the middle of the microwaving process would make the food heat up more homogeneously.** Microwaves heat the food heterogeneously. The use of a rotating plate helps expose various other parts of the food to the hot spots. Stirring the food would help reduce temperature differences between the various parts of the food by making different parts of the food exposed to the hot spots when the food is placed back into the microwave and making sure that parts of the food which may never reach a hot spot have a chance to do so. (Note: stirring would also make the temperature more uniform by mixing hot and cold areas of the food, though this point is more contentious because it is something we can only surmise; it cannot be easily deduced from the text.)

VR24 – American Queen

Q24.1 – C: They used to carry cotton, sugar and tobacco. All we know is that steamboat cruises include visits to cotton, sugar and tobacco plantations, which we presume are bordering the river and may therefore well have been carried by those boats. Nothing indicates those were the actual goods carried by steamboats. Looking at the other options:

- **A: They were originally designed to carry animals and goods.** The first paragraph describes how the boats were designed to transport livestock and produce.

- **B: Some passengers could travel without paying any money.** The end of the first paragraph states that you could work on-board in exchange for passage. This implies that work was in lieu of money.

- **D: They were powered by steam.** The words "aptly named" in the first sentence means that the name reflects the reality. Therefore steamboats were powered by steam.

Q24.2 – D: There is a casino on-board. The only casinos mentioned in the text are those in Natchez and in Vicksburg. There is no hint of a casino on-board the *American Queen*. Looking at the other options:

- **A: Cruises are mostly attended by older people.** There are several clues to this. This is a "crowd with a lot of grey hair"; although younger people can have grey hair of course, this use of "a lot of" points to an older crowd. Then the text talks about a fairly sedentary lifestyle and contrasts it with the more sporty activities of the Caribbean cruises. Finally the passage talking about "song and dance" and the use of the phrase "remember when" also point to an older audience.

- **B: There are few opportunities to exercise on-board.** The text mentions that the boat "barely pays lip service to the idea of on-board exercise, with only a small gym".

- **C: There is more than one food outlet on-board.** The text mentions the large dining room, the River Grill and the snack bar.

Q24.3 – A: Food on board is good value for the price of the cruise. The sentence "The food served is better than food on a boat has the right to be" means that the food is exceeding the expectation of the food one would expect to see on a boat. Looking at the other options:

- **B: Food portions served in the dining room are too small.** If anything, the text hints to portions being generous: "Anyone who doesn't feel stuffed with what is being served in the dining room..."

- **C: Some of the dining room waiters can get sick when sailing.** Nothing in the text points to anyone getting sick on board. For the sake of clarity, the word "rocky" in the text refers to substandard service and the word "green" refers to the waiters being young or new. They have nothing to do with boat movement and sickness.

- **D: Passengers of the *American Queen* often tend to go on Caribbean cruises too.** There is no suggestion in the text that this is the case. In fact the text suggests they may attract crowds with different interests.

Q24.4 – TRUE. "Even though my ticket cost £1,872, the dessert on the second night convinced me that I hadn't nearly paid enough." This suggests that the price of the cruise was cheap for the quality of the food served (epitomised by that dessert). The writer is suggesting he would have paid more for that level of quality.

Q24.5 – TRUE. The last sentence clearly indicates that an additional fee is payable for premium tours. The fact that the £36 is a "typical" amount only indicates that most fees would be around that amount, not that some would be free of charge.

Q24.6 – CAN'T TELL. The only mention of the Delaware River is on the second line as the home of the first steamboat. We are not actually told about the river on which the *American Queen* operates and therefore on which Vicksburg and Natchez are located.

Q24.7 – CAN'T TELL. We are told only that John Fitch was the first to operate a steamboat, not that he was the inventor. We therefore cannot conclude either way.

Q24.8 – FALSE. The last sentence of the first paragraph is clear: "Fares [on steamboats] varied, just like on ocean-going ships..." Therefore fares on ocean-going ships were variable, not fixed.

Verbal Reasoning – Practice

VR25 – Forest Fire

Q25.1 – B: Encircling the house with rows of Mediterranean cypress. The text explains that cypresses tend not to burn whereas other trees such as oaks and juniper tend to burn completely. Therefore the best protection would be achieved with Mediterranean cypresses. Building the walls out of cypress (Option A) would obviously offer some protection but not as much as having a protective hedge that would stop the fire from reaching the house in the first place. Any option involving other trees such as oak (Option C) and juniper (Option D) would not offer any protection.

Q25.2 – C: Compact forest floors. The text explains the fact that the cypress has a high-water content but also that the debris it produces is small, decomposes slowly and therefore forms a compact floor which acts like a sponge and reduces air circulation. Therefore out of the four options on offer, compact forest floors (Option C) would be least likely to contribute to fires (they actually hold fires back).

Q25.3 – D: It was proven through a European-Union-funded study. The only reference to a European-Union-funded project is in reference to the plot of land that burnt in Valencia. The fire highlighted the fact that cypresses didn't burn that easily, which then led to a proper study. We do not actually know from the text whether that study was funded by the European Union. Looking at the other options:

- **A: It requires live cypresses.** The text actually points out that the new study did not just look at dead dry samples but also at live fine twigs, which is how it was identified that the fire resistance of the cypress was linked to a high-water content. Therefore fire resistance would only be achieved with live cypresses.

- **B: It was discovered by chance.** The first paragraph clearly indicates that the fire wasn't planned and that, without that fire, the difference in fire resistance amongst the various trees would have remained unknown ("The scientists could barely believe their eyes" and "the 2012 fire…provided anecdotal evidence").

- **C: It is only effective if the cypresses are planted in groups.** The key to fire resistance is the compact floor and the high-water content of the leaves. A single tree, isolated trees, or the presence of other trees would undermine the ability to obtain a compact floor and would allow a fire to bypass the barrier.

Q25.4 – B: In marshes. The last paragraph explains that the tree would not grow in water-logged areas, thus excluding marshes. Paragraph 2 explains that the cypress's ability to retain water in droughts and extreme heat (making Option A true), the final paragraph says that it can thrive at high altitudes (Option C) and the fact that it survived living near common oaks in Andilla (paragraph 1) makes Option D suitable (note that its proximity to common oaks may undermine the cypress's ability to act as a fire shield but this is not to say that it cannot be planted near them).

Q25.5 – B: Previous tests had only been performed with dead material. This comes from the sentence: "A crucial difference of the new tests is that they were performed not only on dead dry samples but also on live fine twigs" in paragraph 2. Looking at the other options:

- **A: The presence of fungus on cypresses slows fire.** The text only talks about fungus as the topic for the original piece of research, but not as a fire-retardant.

- **C: Oak leaves decompose fast.** We don't know if the issue with oak leaves is because they decompose fast or because they contain less water.

- **D: Before 2012, the flammability resistance of cypresses was well known but never studied.** The findings that followed the 2012 fire came as a surprise to the scientists and therefore we can deduce that the resistance of cypresses was not known.

VR26 – I am a Berliner

Q26.1 – C: The new law might help repopulate city centres. The author mentions that the law is necessary because in some areas such as Munich (following in the footsteps of Paris and London), high rents led to no one living in city centres. Lower rents would therefore encourage people to move back to city centres. However, paragraph 3 argues that the law may not have the desired effect, hence we can only conclude that the new law *might* help repopulate city centres.

Verbal Reasoning – Practice

The law was not tested in Paris, London or Munich (Options A and B); those cities are merely quoted as examples of city centre desertion. Also, the text does not mention anything about property prices in Munich (Option D); it merely talks about high rents.

Q26.2 – D: A landlord can charge rent over the cap if the tenant agrees. This is addressed in the penultimate sentence of the text: "tenants can waive their new right and accept a higher rent." Looking at the other options:

- **A: The average rent in Berlin is 3% below the cap.** The text mentions that rents fell by 3% in the month following the introduction of the law. But since we know nothing about rent levels pre-implementation we cannot conclude anything. For example, if all rents were 3% above the cap prior to the introduction of the cap, then the average new level would be exactly at the cap.

- **B: In time, all landlords will charge rent below the cap.** Since there is nothing forcing landlords to charge under the cap (as tenants can waive their rights) and that there is anecdotal evidence that tenants who refuse a higher rent are not taken on, we can in fact surmise that some landlords will simply force tenants to opt out and therefore will charge rent above the cap (unless the opt-out clause is removed, but nothing in the text suggests that).

- **C: Landlords can charge rents up to 10% higher than the cap.** The text states that the cap is set at 10% above a local average set by the authorities. There is no mention of anything being limited to 10% above the cap. In fact, once the cap is set, landlords can charge what they want if the tenant waives his rights.

Q26.3 – A: The landlords who charge rent above the cap are those with high mortgage repayments. Landlords with high mortgage repayments may well decide to charge over the cap in order to cover their repayments (though in fact the text suggests that they are likely to sell the property). However, the problem with this sentence is that it implies that they are the only ones who would charge higher rents. That cannot actually be deduced from the text. Looking at the other options:

- **B: The law would be made more effective by removing the waiver clause.** In essence, the cap is not effective because landlords can still charge what they want. If all landlords decided to charge rents higher than the cap then tenants would have no choice but to pay the higher levels of rents and the law would be pretty much pointless. Thus removing the waiver clause and imposing the cap would ensure lower rents.

- **C: Landlords with mortgages may incur losses.** Landlords with mortgages are singled out in the text as the new law may result in income from rent becoming lower than mortgage repayments (i.e. causing a loss), which would force them to sell.

- **D: The fall in rent levels may be short-lived.** Though this is not specifically stated in the text, it is discussed that the issues faced by landlords with mortgages will likely lead to rent increases, and that some landlords have already decided to charge over the cap. The final sentence of the text (and the use of the word "may") helps conclude that the statement is a reasonable conclusion to reach.

Q26.4 – B: Berlin has the same demography as Munich. Other than the fact that rents have gone up in both cities, the text offers little comparison between the two. As such, we cannot deduce that they have the same demography.

We know there is a river or canal (Option A) because the text talks about canal boats. We know there are remnants of the East/West split era (Option C) because the text mentions the crumbling watchtowers, and we know that Berlin used to be affordable (Option D) because the text talks about the fact it had cheap housing.

VR27 – Part-Time

Q27.1 – D: People previously classified as unemployed have been reclassified as not relevant for statistical purposes. The text states that "the unemployment rate has fallen largely because millions of Americans are now no longer considered part of the workforce."

Options A and C are not suitable because they imply that people have been given jobs whereas the text states they are no longer part of the workforce. Option B would be a valid reason if the release of work by forcing people to be part-time had then caused unemployed people to take up part-time jobs. But this is not mentioned in the text anywhere and, in any case, that would

Verbal Reasoning – Practice

also mean that unemployed people had become employed and not that they were "no longer part of the workforce".

Q27.2 – D: The majority are women. There is nothing about women and part-time work in the part of the text dealing with the US. With regard to Japan, all we know from the text is that 25% of salaried women work part-time. There is nothing in the text about the proportion of women amongst the part-time working population. Looking at the other options:

- **A: They are not highly regarded by their employers.** The last sentence of the first paragraph indicates that part-timers are treated as a disposable resource in the US. As for Japan, the whole paragraph suggests that they are paid less and get more menial work.

- **B: They tend to earn less per hour than full-time employees.** The text raises this for both the US ("not afforded the same...pay conditions") and Japan ("Part-time workers' wages are considerably lower than those of full-time employees").

- **C: They tend to be recruited to address short-term needs.** In the US, they are brought in with a "just-in-time attitude" and, in Japan, they tend to get work of a "seasonal" nature.

Q27.3 – C: Few men take on a share of household chores. The text says that "men...traditionally, are not sharing the burden of such responsibilities". Looking at the other options:

- **A: Age-related pay is common in companies.** The text says that the pay is seniority-related (i.e. linked to how many years you have worked in the company) rather than age-related. This message is reinforced by the rest of the paragraph, which discusses the issues faced by women who leave work and then come back.

- **B: Three-quarters of part-time workers are men.** The text mentions that a quarter of women work part-time. All we can conclude from that is that three-quarters of women don't work part-time. Without knowing the percentage of part-timers who are women we cannot conclude anything about the percentage of part-timers who are men.

- **D: Part-time workers rarely get paid for their overtime hours.** Nothing in the text suggests that.

Q27.4 – B: Few US part-timers are likely to buy a house. This is given in the text by "Why would anyone struggling with part-time work want to commit to buying a home? Long-term purchases are pushed off into the future." Looking at the other options:

- A: In the US, there are more part-timers than full-timers. All we know is that the number of part-timers is near record highs. There is no indication of how that relates to the number of full-timers.

- C: There are no accurate employment records in Japan. There is nothing in the text to suggest that.

- D: Most Japanese women whose children have left home tend to mostly work full-time. The text says that many women go part-time so that they can bring up their children. We cannot deduce from it that they go full-time again once the children have left, and in fact the text suggests that this is one of the difficulties that women encounter.

VR28 – Antibiotics

Q28.1 – C: Lack of research into new antibiotics. The text suggests that research is taking place and makes no link between a potential lack of research and overuse of antibiotics. The text is firmly placing the blame in three areas:

- A: Doctors giving in to patients' insistent requests. "Doctors are being reproached to be a 'soft touch' by…rapidly wilting under patient demand."

- B: Self-medication by patients. "Antibiotics are simply available over the counter without the need for a prescription or seeing any kind of health professional."

- D: Lack of patient understanding of the purpose of antibiotics. The text states that there is a good awareness of the dangers of overusing antibiotics; however, this does not mean that there is a universal understanding. The fact that people insist that the doctors should prescribe them even when antibiotics would be inappropriate means that some do not understand their purpose and effects (accounting for part of the 10 million inappropriate prescriptions).

Verbal Reasoning – Practice

Q28.2 – A: Patients with a cold may spend longer recovering from it. The text only mentions that antibiotics would not work on colds. It says nothing about worsening its effects. The other three options are, however, possible consequences of antibiotics overuse:

- **B: There is a constant need to develop new antibiotics.** The text explains that, as people become more resistant to antibiotics, those fail to work as effectively; a response from society has been to intensify research to find new classes of antibiotics.

- **C: Some patients may die.** This is stated at the end of the second paragraph.

- **D: It is possible for people who have never used antibiotics to treat an illness to become resistant to them.** The penultimate paragraph discusses the dangers of antibiotics entering the food chain and people consuming them unknowingly.

Q28.3 – B: Criminalising inappropriate prescriptions by doctors. The text tells us at the beginning of paragraph 3 that a prescription from a doctor is needed in order to obtain antibiotics in the UK. Therefore by criminalising inappropriate prescriptions, the practice would essentially stop. Looking at the other options:

- **A: Stepping up research efforts into new antibiotics.** This would resolve the issue of being able to continue to combat disease following the neutralisation of old antibiotics. It would not resolve the issue of overuse; if anything, it might actually encourage it because people would know that new types of antibiotics might be found and so they can overuse them without fear.

- **C: Making antibiotics available over the counter.** This would make antibiotics more freely available and would therefore encourage overuse.

- **D: Running an awareness campaign amongst the population.** This may have an effect though the text suggests that, despite a good awareness, the problem is still prominent. It certainly would not have as drastic an effect as criminalising inappropriate prescriptions.

Note that criminalising doctors may not necessarily be the most moral or socially appropriate/acceptable option. But we are not asked to exercise a moral judgement. We are only asked for the answer that would best resolve this particular problem amongst the options presented.

Q28.4 – D: Antibiotics do not kill viruses. The end of paragraph 2 is clear that antibiotics do not work on viral infections. Looking at the other options:

- **A: Antibiotics are addictive.** The text does refer to patients being criticised for an 'addiction' to the drugs but this refers to the fact that they just use antibiotics indiscriminately rather than their potential addictive qualities. Nothing in the text suggest that antibiotics are addictive in the way that nicotine might be.

- **B: Antibiotics can be deadly, even at normal dose.** Nothing in the text suggests that antibiotics themselves are deadly at all. The only link between mortality and antibiotics is through the decreasing effectiveness of antibiotics, which may result in untreated illness potentially leading to death.

- **C: Antibiotics should not be taken whilst driving.** There is no mention of the side effects of antibiotics at all in the text.

Q28.5 – C: Doctors need to be firmer with demanding patients. One cause of antibiotic overuse is the fact that doctors are a "soft touch" and "rapidly wilting under patient demand". Therefore, adopting a firmer stance would help resolve the problem. Looking at the other options:

- **A: If left untreated, colds simply resolve themselves.** The text mentions "viral infections (colds, sore throats) or conditions which would resolve themselves without any treatment". There is no suggestion that colds belong to the latter or that there is an overlap between the two.

- **B: A quarter of doctors wrongly prescribe antibiotics.** All we are told is that a quarter of antibiotics prescriptions (10 million out of 40 million) are deemed inappropriate. Nothing can be concluded about the number of doctors concerned.

- **D: Most doctors prescribe antibiotics inappropriately because they are unable to reach the correct diagnosis.** The text suggests that the reason is simply that they give in to patients' demands too easily rather than anything to do with their clinical diagnostic abilities.

Verbal Reasoning – Practice

Q28.6 – TRUE. We are told that antibiotics are given to patients when they will not in fact work (e.g. for viral conditions). The text attributes this to the fact that doctors are a "soft touch" and "rapidly wilting under patient demand", which indicates that they are prescribing them reluctantly and/or despite the fact they know they will not work.

VR29 – Eighty Hours

Q29.1 – D: Amnesty is granted to doctors who speak up. The text clearly states that "statutes do not provide whistle-blower protection to residents who report work hour violations". The penultimate paragraph leaves no doubt about the fact that some doctors work over the limit (Option A), that many doctors report a lower number of hours than they actually work (Option B) and that residents caught working over the limit risk losing their accreditation (Option C).

Q29.2 – C: A doctor cannot work more than 3 nights in any week. There can't be night shifts more than once in 3 nights, which, if stated alone, would indeed mean that doctors could not work more than 3 nights in any week (e.g. Monday, Thursday, Sunday); but since this is calculated as an average over 4 weeks it is possible for a doctor to work nights for a full week provided he/she makes up for it in subsequent weeks. This statement is therefore incorrect. Looking at the other options:

- **A: It is possible for a doctor to work over 80 hours in a week.** This is correct since the 80-hour weekly limit is averaged over 4 weeks.

- **B: Doctors can be on shift for up to 30 continuous hours.** This is correct since we know that the limit is 24 hours to which can be added an extra 6 hours for continuity of care and education. Total: 30 hours.

- **D: A doctor finishing work at 8pm must not start his next shift before 6am the next day.** This is correct since there must be a 10-hour rest period between shifts.

Q29.3 – B: Residents are not usually adhering to the regulations. The reason mortality figures have not dropped is that "actual duty hours (as opposed to reported duty hours) have not changed substantially". In other words, doctors are lying on their timesheets about the actual hours they work and work a lot more than they are declaring. Consequently, it looks on paper as if they are complying when in reality they are not. Looking at the other options:

- **A: Doctors did not work over 80 hours/week before anyway.** This implies that doctors were working within the new standards before they were implemented, which is not correct.

- **C: The mortality rate calculations are flawed.** Nothing in the text supports this.

- **D: The regulations are not mandatory.** The text states clearly that, although the limits are voluntary, they are mandated for accreditation. Therefore, they are pretty much mandatory for most doctors. If they were not mandatory in some way, doctors would not feel the need to lie about the hours they actually work. In a context where most doctors have accepted those limits, it is their non-compliance with those limits that is the cause of the issue. In other words, even if the limits were fully mandatory, doctors would still find ways to get around them.

Q29.4 – C: Long hours act as a deterrent to future medical school applicants. This can be concluded from the sentence "The phenomenon exists in order to create a higher entry barrier", which essentially means that the authorities are deliberately keeping the hours long to reduce the number of applicants to medicine. Looking at the other options:

- **A: Making fewer doctors work longer hours is more expensive than making more doctors work fewer hours.** The text states that making people work longer hours reduces costs. We can therefore infer that having more doctors working fewer hours would be more expensive, which directly contradicts Option A.

- **B: Non-trainees also have to adhere to the regulations.** This is unlikely to be true since we are told that the limits are voluntary except for accreditation [of residency programmes].

- **D: The regulations risk decreasing the standard of training.** Nothing in the text suggests that. In fact we are told that long hours affect learning, so the new regulations should lead to increased standards of learning.

Q29.5 – CAN'T TELL. The text only mentions a higher risk of cardiovascular disease in relation to night work, not necessarily long hours (e.g. if those hours are in daytime).

Verbal Reasoning – Practice

VR30 – Science Funding

Q30.1 – D: Government funding has not increased in line with charity funding. Paragraph 1 explains that, whilst charity funding has increased, government funding has been frozen, which means that it is no longer sufficient to cover the overheads. Looking at the other options:

- **A: Government funding has been withdrawn.** The text talks about a freeze and not a withdrawal.

- **B: There is a lack of medical researchers.** Nothing in the text suggests this is the case.

- **C: Charities struggle to raise funds from the general public.** Paragraph 5 talks about fundraising as a way of plugging the deficit. However, there is no indication that this is a struggle or that the lack of fundraising is causing universities to drop projects. In any case the question is asking for the main cause, which remains a relative drop in government funding.

Q30.2 – B: Charities are increasingly redirecting their funds abroad. The text states that some members of the AMRC have already been spending their research funds abroad but that the trend has not increased over the past five years. Looking at the other options:

- **A: Some research centres are finding other ways to make up the funding shortfall.** Paragraph 4 talks about fundraising.

- **C: Some research centres are running at a loss.** The end of the text says that "more medical science divisions have started to run a deficit".

- **D: The Wellcome Trust is refusing to increase funding to compensate for a relative drop in government funding.** The penultimate paragraph says that the Wellcome Trust "wouldn't fund the full economic costs of research in universities".

Q30.3 – B: Smaller charities often deal with different diseases than larger charities. This can be concluded from the second paragraph which explains that if universities only accept funding from large organisations then this will impact on the range of diseases being researched. If small charities dealt with similar diseases to large charities then there would be no impact on the range. From the text we can see that universities will tend to favour funding from large charities (which means that Option A is not correct). There is no indication that smaller charities send their funds abroad more than large charities (Option C): the text only refers to "some members of the association". There is nothing in the text that helps raise any conclusion with regard to fundraising abilities (Option D); the only reference to fundraising is in relation to universities and not charities.

Q30.4 – C: The funding gap issue is affecting mostly the smaller research centres. The text does not differentiate between small and large research centres. The only mention of size is in relation to the fact that grants from smaller charities are more likely to be rejected, but this does not relate to the size of the recipient of the grant. Looking at the other options:

- **A: Charities are threatening to redirect their funds abroad.** This is addressed in the last line of paragraph 3.

- **B: Universities will consider not taking charitable grants because they cannot afford to cover the related overheads.** This is the whole premise of the text.

- **D: Lack of funding may make research centres stagnate instead of developing.** This is addressed in the last paragraph.

VR31 – Children's Books

Q31.1 – C: Liz Pichon. In the first paragraph Liz Pichon's *Tom Gates* is listed as an example of a new type of book that replaces classics. And, in the same paragraph, the phrase "Only the prolific Roald Dahl remains sandwiched between the bookends..." indicates that Roald Dahl (Option A) is the only classics writer who is still being read. Jules Verne (Option B) and Charles Dickens (Option D) are described as writers of "challenging classics" in the last paragraph.

Q31.2 – C: The style of his books is similar to that of newer books. The last sentence of the second paragraph ("you only have to look at Dahl's work to see that there is nothing new here in taste or in style") indicates that his style is similar to that of newer books. In the first paragraph, we are told that Roald Dahl's books are the only ones which "remain sandwiched between the bookends", meaning that they are still being read (hence Option

Verbal Reasoning – Practice

A is incorrect). The sentence "And when it comes to the 19th century classics", straight after having discussed Roald Dahl's books, means that Dahl is not a 19th century author (Option B). Finally, *Treasure Island* (Option D) was written by Stevenson as indicated in paragraph 3.

Q31.3 – C: Parents prefer their children to read modern stories. The text mentions in the third paragraph that one of the reasons why children still read classics is because parents buy them on their behalf. There is no indication, however, that the success of modern books is due to parents preferring their children to read them (Option C). Paragraph 2 explains that the mix of cartoons and text is an important factor to make the text more approachable (Option A) and that, in modern books, adults tend to be non-existent, evil or weak in comparison to the young protagonists (Option D). The last sentence of the text complains that classics are not borrowed because they are often not made available in electronic format (Option B).

Q31.4 – C: Some classics are too hard for children to read in their original versions. The start of paragraph 4 explains that some of the more challenging classics need to be abridged and enriched with graphics, which we can deduce is to make them more approachable, i.e. they are too hard to read. Looking at the other options:

- **A: Children like them so much that publishers are reprinting them in their original format.** The classics are indeed being reprinted but the text is suggesting that a likely explanation is because parents are buying them on behalf of (i.e. forcing them on to) their children, not necessarily because their children love them.

- **B: Complex words and phrases put children off reading them, even in their abridged versions.** The text actually explains that some of the harder classics need to be abridged and illustrated but says nothing about children being put off reading classics by the complexity of the wording being a factor. The main argument earlier in the text is actually the lack of illustration rather than complexity of words.

- **D: They are mostly bought by libraries.** The only mention of libraries is in relation to unborrowed books, not in respect of volume of purchase.

Q31.5 – CAN'T TELL. All we are told is that they are classics of children's literature. There is no mention of any publication date.

VR32 – Dismaland

Q32.1 – B: The Banksy bemusement park reached full visitor capacity across the five-week run. We are told that there was room for 4,500 paying customers every day and that each day those at the back of the queue never made it to the front despite seamless organisation. That implies that the venue had reached its capacity. Looking at the other options:

- **A: More people visited the Hockney exhibition than the Banksy bemusement park across their respective runs.** We are told that the Hockney exhibition attracted 7,512 visitors a day (compared to 4,500 for Dismaland) but we are not told how many days it lasted; therefore we cannot conclude which exhibition welcomed the most visitors over the respective runs.

- **C: Beaches had to close to make space for queuing.** All we know is that queuing took place along the beaches. There is no mention of closures.

- **D: The queuing system for Dismaland was disorganised.** We are told it was seamless.

Q32.2 – C: Hotels in the area are not normally full in September. The third paragraph states that "the major benefit was that every B&B and hotel bed was full throughout September", which implies that they wouldn't be full, were it not for Dismaland.

- **A: The exhibition was reserved solely for locals.** The fact that people had to stay in hotels means that they were not locals.

- **B: Children were banned from visiting the exhibition.** The only reference to children is that Banksy billed the attraction "a family attraction unsuitable for children". This contradiction seems more of a joke than a statement of fact and, in any case, nothing in the text suggests children were banned.

- **D: The exhibition opened its doors early September.** The first sentence says that the attraction is closing its doors 'today' in an article dated 27 September. The fourth line says that it had a five-week run. This means that it opened its doors in August and not September.

Verbal Reasoning – Practice

Q32.3 – C: Banksy has a connection with Bristol. The text refers to the "elusive Bristolian". Looking at the other options:

- **A: Some tourists visited the attraction more than once.** All we know is that some have said they would return to the town.

- **B: Banksy was born in Weston-super-Mare.** All we know is that he has a personal connection with the town. That could mean a lot of different things.

- **D: McQueen was alive at the time of the exhibition of his work.** Nothing in the text suggests this was the case. All we know is that the exhibition was on Alexander McQueen.

Q32.4 – B: Banksy's art is often found outdoors. Nothing in the text suggests this is the case. Paragraph 4, however, explains that many artists felt empowered to make their own art more political (Option A), that Banksy's art is easily accessible (Option C) and that Banksy conveys a message (often political or social) through his art (Option D).

Q32.5 – B: The exhibition was a one-off. There is no hint in the text that anyone knows of any further plans to hold another exhibition, whether as part of a tour (Option A), in a larger venue (Option C) or in Bristol (Option D). The author states in the final paragraph that it is unlikely that other parks would open in other areas of the country because Weston-super-Mare had been chosen due to its connection with Banksy. But there is no hint anywhere of any further exhibition taking place, even in places connected with Banksy, in future.

VR33 – Indian Rugby

Q33.1 – C: There is at least one England v. Scotland match each year. The text refers to "Calcutta Cup, the annual game played between England and Scotland". There is nothing in the cup explaining whether the Calcutta Cup is part of the Six Nations Tournament (Option A) or is played in Kolkata (Option B). Equally, the decade 1870s refers to the year the Calcutta Cup started and not the year rugby was invented (Option D).

Q33.2 – C: Rugby is not popular because its tournaments lack a show business element. The text explains that rugby would be made more popular if there was more of it on television. Part of the issue is that not enough international rugby is being played on television, but the author also explains that other, more popular sports, have adopted a more television-friendly format, with more music and razzmatazz. Therefore we can conclude that the author would agree that having a more festive element would mean more television airtime for rugby. Accordingly this would attract more sponsors and make the sport more attractive.

We know that the Rugby World Cup is shown on Indian TV (therefore Option A is untrue). There is no suggestion that the Indian team is not participating in international tournaments (Option B) or that the sport is considered dangerous (Option D).

Q33.3 – D: Hockey is more popular than football. The list "football, hockey and badminton" at the start of paragraph 3 is given in decreasing order of popularity. Therefore hockey is less popular than football. Looking at the other options:

- **A: Rugby is seen as an old-fashioned and elitist sport.** The sport is described as "stuffy" and "carry[ing] an air of elitism".

- **B: Rugby is less popular than badminton.** In the text, it is suggested that rugby could learn from the experience of badminton and other sports in improving its image and popularity. The author is therefore likely to conclude that rugby is less popular than badminton.

- **C: Football is less popular than cricket.** The text states that "cricket remains the most popular sport in India".

Q33.4 – B: Increasing the appeal of rugby would attract more sponsors. The text explains that the lack of understanding of rugby is putting sponsors off. Therefore increasing its appeal would attract more sponsors. Looking at the other options:

- **A: Rugby needs to attract a different kind of sponsor.** The issue does not appear to be that rugby attracts the wrong sort of sponsors. It is struggling to attract sponsors at all.

- **C: Birla Tyres is currently the only sponsor of rugby in India.** Birla Tyres is only quoted as an example of a sponsor. There may well be others.

- **D: International cricketers want to play for India because they like the spectacle surrounding the game.** The text explains that the entertaining spectacle attracts international players by making it financially viable. In other words it is not the spectacle itself that matters, but the fact that it makes the sport more attractive to audiences and therefore generates revenue.

Q33.5 – B: They should broadcast more international rugby games. This is stated explicitly at the end of the second paragraph. There is no suggestion in the text that TV stations should recruit international players as commentators (Option A) or that they should find wealthier advertisers (Option D) since advertisers are not put off by the cost but by the value they would get in return. With regard to Option C, the Rugby World Cup is already being broadcast in India (last sentence of paragraph 3).

VR34 – Plastic Bags

Q34.1 – B: The policy is not the same in different parts of the UK. The text states at the beginning that "unlike schemes in other parts of the UK, paper bags are exempt from a charge". Looking at the other options:

- **A: Plastic bags do not actually harm wildlife.** The text explicitly states that plastic bags can harm seabirds and other animals.

- **C: Cotton bags take less time to degrade than plastic bags.** Nothing in the text helps conclude that this is true. Cotton bags are deemed to be better because they are "reusable" and so therefore less easily discarded, but that says nothing about their degradability.

- **D: Plastic bags degrade faster in landfill than on beaches.** Nothing in the text deals with this issue.

Q34.2 – D: This policy may increase the sale of bin liners. The text explains that plastic bags were not as bad as first thought since, for example, people reused them as bin liners. It therefore follows that if people no longer have access to free plastic bags then there will be fewer "free" bin liners and therefore they may need to purchase some. Looking at the other options:

- **A: The money raised by the government through the tax will be used to promote environmental schemes.** We are told that the money is not passed to the government but kept by the retailers.

- **B: 5p is not a high enough amount to make people switch away from plastic bags.** The text mostly debates whether there is a point in imposing the 5p tax but says nothing with regard to whether the 5p level is sufficient to achieve its aim.

- **C: Retailers will feel compelled to donate the money to charity.** Nothing in the text hints that this will happen.

Q34.3 – D: Online shopping is more environmentally friendly than physical shopping. The very end of the text states that "The 5p charge may also push people to shop online more as retailers will deliver to your door without using bags, whilst also reducing the number of car journeys made." Looking at the other options:

- **A: Reusable bags play an important role in reducing landfill waste.** The text gives evidence that in some cases people ended up discarding larger numbers of paper bags, or threw away more heavy-duty reusable plastic bags, thus increasing landfill waste.

- **B: Reusable bags are more environmentally friendly than standard plastic bags.** The text explains that cotton bags for example would need to be used a very large/unrealistic number of times to be better in terms of global warming, without even talking about the effect of washing them. The author believes that they are therefore less environmentally friendly than standard plastic bags.

- **C: Reusable plastic bags do not need to be washed.** The risk of harbouring bacteria means that they do.

Q34.4 – A: Cotton bags are a potential infection risk to shops. This is explained clearly in the second paragraph.

Nothing in the text suggests that reusable plastic bags are more hygienic than cotton bags (Option B) or that it is nearly impossible to clean cotton bags (Option C). With regard to placing goods directly in the car boot being a hygienic solution (Option D), this may circumvent the issue of infecting bags with bacteria. However, the text does explain that the boot is a breeding ground and therefore this would contaminate the food itself, thus making this approach unhygienic.

DECISION MAKING

TIPS & TECHNIQUES

+

206
PRACTICE QUESTIONS & ANSWERS

12 Decision Making
Format, Purpose & Key Techniques

FORMAT

The decision-making section of the UCAT consists of 29 questions associated with text, charts, tables, diagrams or graphs. The questions are varied in nature, and some of them may contain several stems. You are given 31 minutes to answer them all.

Most of these questions are essentially logical reasoning questions and will test your problem-solving abilities. Some of them are virtually indistinguishable from verbal reasoning or quantitative reasoning questions asked in other parts of the exam. Overall, you will see questions of the following types:

Type 1 – Logical puzzles (also referred to as Einstein questions). These questions tend to give you a list of facts from which you need to deduce information. The facts are often confusing and mixed up and require the drawing of a diagram or table to make sense of them, e.g. "George's house is red but is not next to Andrew's house. Laura's house is not blue and is on the left of Andrew's house, etc."

Type 2 – Syllogisms. These are questions of the type "Most mice are wrinkly, no wrinkly animal has black eyes, some black-eyed animals have short teeth. Can we conclude that wrinkly mice have short teeth?" These questions require a degree of mental gymnastics.

Type 3 – Data interpretation. These questions will present you with a graph or a table, from which you will need to deduce facts. They are fairly similar to the quantitative reasoning questions which contain graphs and tables, except that instead of calculating a number you may be asked to indicate whether a particular fact is true or not. So instead of asking "How many people watched the BBC on Saturday night?" questions will be of the type "More people watched the BBC on weekdays than they did on weekends. YES/NO".

Type 4 – Assumption recognition. These questions will ask you whether it would be a good idea to implement a particular solution to a given problem, e.g. "Should the government reintroduce wild wolves in forests in order to control the spread of rabbits?". You are then presented with two arguments, usually two in favour and two against, from which you must select the strongest. The topics discussed are usually contentious and will often be topics on which you have your own ideas (e.g. should schools lecture parents on how they raise their children, etc.). These questions are therefore a key test of whether you can look at issues objectively.

Type 5 – Diagrams. You are presented with a Venn or Euler diagram and asked to deduce information based on the shape of the diagram and the numbers it contains. In some cases, you are presented with wordy information and need to select which shape of diagram would best match the information given.

Type 6 – Probabilities. These are usually simple statistics problems but with a twist. And rather than just calculating an answer, you will need to select the option that best explains that answer.

PURPOSE

Throughout your career, you will need to interpret information and reach conclusions to formulate a management plan for your patients. Sometimes, you will need to do this at short notice and without all the information you need. Quick wit and strong analytical / deduction skills will therefore be crucial.

Introduced in 2017, the decision-making section is designed to test your ability to reason and deduce from information given to you.

KEY TECHNIQUES

The main problem with this section is that, unlike the others, each question may need to be approached differently depending on its type and on the information provided; as such we have made sure that we have provided full workings for each answer. However, there are still several things you can do to ensure that you can answer questions quickly and accurately.

You may not need to resolve the full problem to answer the question
Many questions involve several logical steps. At each step you can often discount one of the options. That also means that you don't need to get scared if a question contains a lot of data; you may not need all of it. Proceeding by elimination can save you a lot of time.

Practise your logical reasoning
"A" leads to "B" means that *"Not B" leads to "Not A"*. "All mice are white" means that if an animal is not white then it cannot be a mouse. It does NOT mean that all animals that are not mice are also not white. And it does not mean that all animals that are white are mice.

Some questions may use made-up words or ridiculous relationships just to make sure that you cannot guess the answer (e.g. you may be given relationships of the type "All pineapples are monkeys"). So it is crucial that you can manipulate those concepts well. This book contains a lot of practice on this type of question.

Also, watch out for words such as "several", "many", "not all". "Several mice are white" could mean that only some are white, but it may also be that they all are (because if all mice are white then it is also true that "some" mice are white). Do not make assumptions.

Revise your basic probabilities
The level you need to have is fairly basic; essentially you just need to be able to calculate the probability of taking something out of a bag.

Watch out for your bias in the assumption recognition questions
The assumption recognition questions are not difficult to answer once you understand what they are looking for. These questions deal with an ambiguous topic for which there may be several answers, depending on which side of the argument you sit.

So, for example, if the question were "Should we ban fox hunting in England and Wales?", everyone might have their own reasons to agree or disagree. However if you compare two arguments such as:

Argument A: "Yes, because it may be that the hunt traumatises the fox."
and
Argument B: "No, because even if it were banned, those who engage in it would probably ignore the ban."

Decision Making – Practice

you can see that Argument B is the weaker of the two because it does not really justify why a ban should not be implemented (it is a bit like saying there is no point having a law since many people will disobey it), but also it is entirely speculative. So whether you disagree or not with the actual point made, Argument A is put across more strongly and is more relevant than Argument B.

Similarly, if the point to discuss were "Should we reintroduce wild wolves in forests in order to control the rapidly growing rabbit population", you could be faced with various arguments:

Argument A: "Yes, because rabbits are causing damage to vital crops"
Argument B: "No, because wolves may also multiply out of control"
Argument C: "No, because wolves may not target rabbits specifically"
Argument D: "Yes, because it would save the wolves from becoming an endangered species".

You can see that:

- Argument A directly plays into the issue at heart. The rapidly growing rabbit population ravages important crops.
- Argument B is unlikely but, in any case, speculative. And even if that were true, it does not mean a solution to that problem cannot be found.
- Argument C is also speculative.
- Argument D is not really addressing the point.

So, Argument A would be the strongest here.

Draw tables and diagrams
Some problems can be solved simply in your head, but many will require you to draw something or create a grid/table to set out the information and see what you can conclude from it. Make full use of your whiteboard.

Don't be complacent in your logic
Some exercises will be worded in a way that is designed to confuse. For example: "100 people play tennis, badminton and football, with some playing more than one sport. 20 play badminton and football.". The fact that 20 play badminton and football does not mean that some of them do not play tennis.

Another example is: "At least 25% of men play tennis". That does not necessarily mean that more than 25% play tennis. It could be exactly 25%.

Practise, practise, practise
Once you start practising, you will soon realise that the decision-making questions are all variations on similar themes. You will start recognising patterns in the wording of the questions, and you will also soon see that the same traps are being laid for you question after question. Doing repetitive practice will therefore help greatly. But, before rushing into timed practice, work first at your own pace to ensure that you understand the logic underlying each question. Once you have understood the logic you can start worrying about timing.

IMPORTANT WORD ABOUT TIMING

There are two types of questions: multiple choice (i.e. you have to choose an answer amongst the four proposed options) and YES/NO. Most questions will have only one stem, but the YES/NO questions will include five stems.

The exam allows just over one minute per question. That is usually more than sufficient for the multiple-choice questions but is very tight for the YES/NO questions since you need to answer all five stems within that time frame.

We would therefore recommend that you target a response time of 55 seconds per multiple-choice question, and 100 seconds per question containing five YES/NO stems (there are usually four or five of these in each exam). This will give you 20 seconds for each YES/NO stem. In total this will add up to 24 questions x 55s + 5 questions x 100s = 30 minutes 20 seconds.

13 Decision Making Practice Questions

In this section you will find 206 practice questions (94 scenarios containing between 1 and 12 questions each).

The questions have been carefully chosen to represent the different numerical reasoning approaches and levels of difficulty that you may encounter in the live exam. We have deliberately provided more questions per scenario than you would have at the exam to enhance your learning experience. At the end of the section we have also set out detailed explanations on how the answers can be derived. Where relevant, we have provided several possible ways of getting to the answer.

Depending on your way of learning and working, you may decide to answer the questions in real time (in which case you would need to allocate an average of 55 seconds per multiple-choice question and 20 seconds per YES/NO question) or to approach the questions at your own pace in order to build your awareness of the difficulties that you may encounter. The answers to all questions can be found from page 461 onwards.

Once you have practised answering all 206 questions, you should be ready to confront the mock exam at the back of the book under exam conditions. You may want to wait until you have practised all sections in this book before going ahead with the mock exam.

1300 UCAT Practice Questions

DM 1 Practice — Professional Chefs

Not all chefs are professionally trained, but all chefs who are professionally trained have excellent knife skills. It is fair to say that some professionally-trained chefs don't know how to season their food properly.

Answer YES if the conclusion follows and NO if it does not.

Q1.1 Some of the chefs who know how to season their food properly also have excellent knife skills. | YES | NO |

Q1.2 Some of the chefs with good knife skills are professionally-trained chefs who know how to season their food properly. | YES | NO |

Q1.3 All chefs with good knife skills are professionally-trained chefs or know how to season their food properly, or both. | YES | NO |

Q1.4 Not all chefs with good knife skills know how to season their food properly. | YES | NO |

Q1.5 All chefs who know how to season their food properly and have excellent knife skills are professionally trained. | YES | NO |

DM 2 Practice — Vaccination

Q2 This year, 40% of the population received the flu vaccine. Despite this, 70% of the population caught the flu. Which of the following must be true?

A. At most 10% of those vaccinated caught the flu.
B. At least 25% of those vaccinated caught the flu.
C. At most 10% of the population was vaccinated and caught the flu.
D. At least half of those who were not vaccinated stayed healthy.

408

DM 3 Practice — Table Etiquette

A host has organised a dinner party. The table has been set by his children very haphazardly. Each guest should have been provided with a fork, a knife, a spoon and a napkin. Instead, the host finds that some guests are missing one or more of those items.

The diagram below shows the allocation of items amongst guests, with labels and numbers deliberately excluded. Note that if two areas are inside the same set of shapes then they are considered to be the same sector, even if they are disconnected on the diagram (e.g. a and b below).

Q3.1 If the only guests who were given both a knife and a spoon are those who possess all four items, which shapes have been used to represent the knife and the spoon (in any order)?

A. Arrow and Rectangle
B. Arrow and Triangle
C. Ellipse and Rectangle
D. Triangle and Rectangle

Q3.2 If the number of guests in each sector is equal to 1, how many items (cutlery and napkins) have been placed on the table in total by the children?

A. 13   B. 18   C. 22   D. 24

DM 4 Practice
Orchestra Politics

Q4 Tracy, Simon, Paul, William and Victoria are five musicians, who all play different instruments: violin, oboe, percussion, flute and clarinet.

Paul, Victoria, Simon and the flute player live in the same town. The clarinet player likes to have dinner with Paul, Simon and Tracy after concerts but cannot stand the presence of the oboe player.

Simon and Victoria are friends of the violinist, but William and the oboe player don't like each other.

Which of the following must be true?

A. William plays the flute
B. Simon plays percussion
C. Tracy plays the violin
D. Victoria plays the clarinet

DM 5 Practice
Gardeners' Question Time

Q5 A gardener installs eight boxes of flowers around a tree, in a square configuration (see diagram). In each box he places a different number of flowers. The number of flowers in a box ranges from 1 to 8, and no two boxes contain the same number of flowers. The box in the top-left corner contains one single flower. Each side of the square contains 14 flowers.

How many flowers are there in the box at the bottom right corner?

A. 2   **B.** 3   **C.** 4   **D.** 5

410

Decision Making – Practice

DM 6 Practice — Nuts and Seeds

All biscuit brands produced in a biscuit factory, with the exception of the biscuits sold under the brand NoNut, contain nuts. Several biscuit brands produced in the factory contain seeds.

Answer YES if the conclusion follows and NO if it does not.

Q6.1 Some biscuits contain both nuts and seeds. YES | NO

Q6.2 There are seeds in NoNut biscuits. YES | NO

Q6.3 If a biscuit is picked at random from the factory's stock and is found not to contain nuts, then it must be a NoNut biscuit. YES | NO

Q6.4 If two biscuits of two different brands are picked at random from the factory and both contain seeds, then one of them has to be a NoNut biscuit. YES | NO

Q6.5 If a biscuit does not contain nuts, then it must contain seeds. YES | NO

DM 7 Practice — Fitness Crowd

Q7 Jenny, Bob, Marc and Peter each practise a different activity from this list: swimming, judo, dance, and rugby.

- Jenny and Peter enjoy watching their friend practise judo.
- The rugby player and the dancer went to Peter's for dinner.
- Jenny and Marc don't live in the same town as the dancer.

Which one plays rugby?

A. Jenny
B. Bob
C. Marc
D. Peter

411

DM 8 Practice — Card Game

Q8 Allan, Bob, Charles, David, Elvis and Frank play cards in three teams of two people.
- Allan plays with Elvis or Frank.
- If Allan is with Frank, then David is with Elvis.
- If Bob is with Charles or David, then Allan is not with Elvis.
- If David is with Charles, then Bob is not with Frank.

Which of the following must be true?

- **A.** Allan plays with Elvis
- **B.** Bob plays with Frank
- **C.** David plays with Elvis
- **D.** David plays with Charles

DM 9 Practice — Rota Management

Q9 In a hospital, 30 doctors are discussing their plans for taking time off on key holidays: Christmas, Easter, and August bank holiday. They all wish to claim at least one of these.

6 doctors want to take Christmas off only
5 doctors want to take Easter off only
6 doctors want to take only Christmas and August bank holiday off
8 doctors want to take only Christmas and Easter off
1 doctor wants to take Easter and August bank holiday off

How many doctors want to take the August bank holiday off altogether?

A. 4   **B.** 7   **C.** 11   **D.** 15

Decision Making – Practice

DM 10 Practice — PE Practice

Q10 In a class of 34 students, 16 students reported playing basketball, 15 volleyball and 14 football. 7 play basketball and volleyball, 4 play volleyball and football, and 5 play football and basketball.

The person who gathered the statistics cannot remember if, when students said that they played two sports, it meant they played two sports only or whether the figures included those who played all three sports.

Which of the following diagrams represents the information given?

A

B

C

D

413

DM 11 Practice — Round table

Q11 Last night, Claire and her husband invited their neighbours (two male/female couples) for dinner around a round dinner table.
- David sat on the left of the woman who sat on the left of the man who sat on the left of Barbara.
- Paula sat on the left of the man who sat on the left of the woman who sat on the left of the man who sat on the left of the woman who sat on the left of Claire's husband.
- Ahmed sat on the left of the woman who sat on Robert's left.
- Claire did not sit next to her husband.

What is the name of Claire's husband?

    A. Ahmed
    B. David
    C. Robert
    D. Cannot be determined using the information provided

DM 12 Practice — Sweets

At school, Johnny has only two friends to whom he gives sweets. George gives sweets to Johnny, who reciprocates. All school children give sweets to Lydia.

Answer YES if the conclusion follows and NO if it does not.

Q12.1	If a child is given sweets by Johnny, then he/she must be either George or Lydia.	YES | NO
Q12.2	All children receive sweets from George.	YES | NO
Q12.3	If a child receives sweets from Adam, then that child must be Lydia.	YES | NO
Q12.4	Johnny reciprocates only with George.	YES | NO
Q12.5	Lydia gives sweets to all children.	YES | NO

DM 13 Practice — Adding Up

Q13 Consider the following equations:

$$\triangle + \triangle = \blacklozenge + \blacklozenge + \blacklozenge$$
$$\blacksquare = \bullet + \blacklozenge$$
$$\blacksquare + \bullet = \triangle$$

How many circles is one square equal to?

A. 2   B. 3   C. 4   D. 5

DM 14 Practice — Teachers

Q14 Mrs Amin, Mrs Begum, Mrs Cook and Mrs Debono teach at the same school the following subjects: maths, history and chemistry.

Each teacher teaches only two different subjects:

- Two teachers, Alisha and Mrs Debono, teach history.
- There are two teachers for chemistry and only one for maths.
- Three teachers teach English. Debbie is not one of them.
- Carole teaches chemistry.
- Mrs Amin does not share a subject with Betty or Mrs Cook.

What is Alisha's surname?

A. Amin   B. Begum   C. Cook   D. Debono

DM 15 Practice — Disorientation

Q15 From my house I can drive to four different supermarkets: A, B, C and D. Distances are as follows:

- Home to A: 3 miles
- Home to B: 5 miles
- Home to C: 6 miles
- Home to D: 8 miles.
- B to A: 2 miles
- B to C: 11 miles

Assuming that any road linking two points is straight, which of the following must be true?

A. A and D are five miles apart.
B. The road from Home to B passes in front of C.
C. The road from Home to B passes in front of A.
D. B could be as little as 2 miles away from D.

DM 16 Practice — Shop Samples

Q16 A local shop owner has decided to hand out free samples of its food to 500 people who live in the area. He offers each adult six food samples and each child four samples.

If only half of the adults and three quarters of the children accept the samples, how many samples will he have given in total?

A. Can't be calculated without being given either the number of adults or the number of children who entered the shop.
B. 1500
C. 2500
D. 3000

DM 17 Practice: Venn v. Euler Diagrams

Not many people know the difference between Venn and Euler diagrams.

A Venn diagram consists of several intersecting circles and must show all possible combinations; if an intersection contains no item then it is shown as shaded.

However, a Euler diagram will be drawn in such a way that only the intersections which are not empty are shown; this means that as the number of contours increase, Euler diagrams are typically less visually complex than the equivalent Venn diagram, particularly if the number of non-empty intersections is small.

Answer YES if the conclusion follows and NO if it does not.

Q17.1 A Euler diagram will contain fewer sectors than a Venn diagram representing the same problem. | YES | NO |

Q17.2 If a diagram contains a sector with an empty intersection, then it is a Venn diagram and not an Euler diagram. | YES | NO |

Q17.3 A Euler and a Venn diagram for the same problem can look the same. | YES | NO |

Q17.4 The greater the number of empty sections in a Venn diagram, the simpler the equivalent Euler diagram will look. | YES | NO |

Q17.5 If a Euler and a Venn diagram look the same, then it means that there are no empty intersections in the Venn diagram. | YES | NO |

DM 18 Practice — Charity

Q18 A charity representative asks people in the street if they have 5 minutes to spare to answer a few questions. When a passer-by agrees, she asks whether he/she would be willing to contribute £5 to the charity as a one-off cash payment. In the course of a week, the representative finds that 30% of those she talked to gave £5.

Can she conclude that 30% of the population is willing to give to charity?

A. Yes, because the number of people she will have talked to is a representative sample.
B. Yes, because that is the percentage of people she talked to who agreed to make a donation.
C. No, because only those with time to spare could stop to answer her questions.
D. No, because the amount that people were asked to donate was fixed by her.

DM 19 Practice — Unemployment

Q19 The unemployment rate is defined as the proportion of the labour force (i.e. those in work + those looking for work) that is unemployed. The employment rate is defined as the percentage of the working age population that is in work. The unemployment rate in the UK is 5%, whilst the employment rate is 75%.

What statement can be concluded from the above text?

A. 25% of the working age population is unemployed and not looking for work.
B. 95% of the working age population has a job.
C. Under 5% of the working age population is unemployed.
D. 25% of the working age population is looking for work.

DM 20 Practice — Mandatory Training

All NHS employees must attend a number of mandatory training sessions every calendar year. This includes training on Health and Safety, Fire Safety, Patient Moving and Handling, Infection Control, and Basic Life Support. All mandatory training sessions are independent from one another and last an hour. Staff must book their course places with the HR department. Though people may cancel attendance (e.g. if unwell), they must ensure that no more than 12 months have elapsed since they last attended the same course. No courses run on weekends, national holidays and bank holidays, e.g. New Year's Day, May Bank Holidays, etc.

Answer YES if the conclusion follows and NO if it does not.

Q20.1 Staff have five hours of mandatory training per year. | YES | NO |

Q20.2 Drug Administration is not mandatory training. | YES | NO |

Q20.3 People who have not cancelled attendance at a course are exempt from the 12-month rule. | YES | NO |

Q20.4 At least five days of the year will be affected by mandatory training requirements. | YES | NO |

Q20.5 An employee could attend the same course two days in a row in order to satisfy requirements. | YES | NO |

DM 21 Practice — Bus Ride

Q21 Angie, Ben, Carol, Dan and Elliott are the only five students at the bus station. They each independently and randomly choose one of four empty buses to board. What is the average number of students in the bus that Ben chooses to board?

   A. 1.25 as there are five students for four buses.
   B. 2 as the other four students will average 1 per bus, + 1 for Ben.
   C. 2 as the 5 students will split between an average of 2.5 buses.
   D. 2.6 as the other 4 will split between an average of 2.5 buses + 1 for Ben.

419

DM 22 Practice: Hair

Q22 The average number of hairs on a person's head is 100,000. Hair grows at a rate of about 6 inches per year and lasts about 6 years before falling out. Two friends have 222,222 strands of hair between them, with one having 20% more hair than the other.

Which of the following statements must be true?

- A. They both have a number of hairs that is above average.
- B. They both have a number of hairs that is below average.
- C. Only one has a number of hairs below average.
- D. More information is needed to determine whether their respective numbers of hairs is below or above average.

DM 23 Practice: Siblings

Q23 Boys Andrew, Elliott and Fred and girls Belinda, Carol and Davina are six siblings born in six successive years, albeit in a different order.

Andrew and Elliott were born four years apart
Fred is two years older than Andrew
The three girls were born in alphabetical order of their first name.

Which of the following cannot be concluded?

- A. The sex of a newborn was always the opposite of sex of the previous year's newborn.
- B. Andrew is younger than Carol.
- C. Belinda is younger than Elliott.
- D. Carol is younger than Elliott.

DM 24 Practice — Family Food

Q24 A mother and her two children enjoy various foods. Their likes are as follows:

Mother:	Child 1	Child 2
• Pizza	• Pizza	• Salad
• Salad	• Pasta	• Pizza
• Curry	• Burger	• Burger

The following diagram is a representation of the situation, with each dotted shape representing a member of the family.

Which of the shapes represent the burger?

A. The triangle or the arrow
B. The diamond or the circle
C. The square or the circle
D. The square or the diamond

DM 25 Practice — Loaded Dice

Q25 Dan has two dice, both with six faces. The first die is normal. The second die is loaded so that the number 3 appears twice as often as each other number but the other five outcomes are equally likely.

What is the probability that when Dan throws both dice together he obtains a double 3?

A. 1/18 – The chance of obtaining a double three with two normal dice is 1/6 x 1/6 = 1/36. But because one die has a double probability, the odds are 2/36 = 1/18.

B. 1/18 – The probability of landing a 3 with the loaded die is 2/6, which we must multiply by 1/6 for the normal die.

C. 1/21 – The loaded die has a probability of 2/7 of landing a 3, whilst the other die has a probability of 1/6.

D. 1/36 – The probability is not affected by the loaded die since we are looking at obtaining the same number on both dice.

DM 26 Practice — Free Museum Entry

Q26 Should entry to museums be made free to the public in order to increase the number of visitors? Select the strongest argument from the statements below.

A. YES. Most museums are funded by donors or other subsidies. Loss of entrance fee would not significantly affect their finances.
B. YES. It would make visits to museums affordable to those with little disposable income.
C. NO. Admission fees contribute to meeting museums' running costs.
D. NO. It will mostly lead to people who usually visit museums visiting more often.

DM 27 Practice — Pharmacy

A pharmaceutical company provides drugs in the following formats only:
- All liquid drugs are sold in bottles or vials.
- All non-liquid drugs come in packages weighing more than 250 g.
- All drugs sold in bottles come with a syringe doser.
- All drugs sold in packages or containers of more than 250 g come with a patient information leaflet setting out the side-effects.

Answer YES if the conclusion follows and NO if it does not.

Q27.1 A powdered drug must come with a leaflet. | YES | NO |

Q27.2 A drug coming with a syringe doser always comes in a bottle. | YES | NO |

Q27.3 If a drug comes with a leaflet then it must be non-liquid. | YES | NO |

Q27.4 A syrup in a 525 g bottle comes with a syringe doser and a patient information leaflet. | YES | NO |

Q27.5 If a drug comes in a 200 g package then it must be liquid. | YES | NO |

DM 28 Practice — Civic Education

Q28 Should the government introduce a compulsory civic awareness day in order to teach all 18-year-olds about politics, the workings of society and their civic responsibilities? Select the strongest argument from the statements below.

A. YES. Unless they have an interest in the topic, teenagers tend to enter adulthood without such knowledge.

B. YES. This would help increase turnout at elections.

C. NO. A one-day course would only address such issues superficially and its content would quickly be forgotten.

D. NO. It would make teenagers miss a day off school or work.

DM 29 Practice — Recall

A car manufacturer makes three models: Basic, Intermediate and Premium. It has made the decision to recall all its Basic and Premium models manufactured in September 2016. All Basic models have developed a fault, whereas only some of the Premium models have.

Answer YES if the conclusion follows and NO if it does not.

Q29.1   A car with no fault cannot have been manufactured in September.   YES | NO

Q29.2   A car with a fault must have been manufactured in September.   YES | NO

Q29.3   Intermediate cars made in August 2016 have no fault.   YES | NO

Q29.4   A car made in September, which has no fault, is a Premium model.   YES | NO

Q29.5   More Basic models will be recalled than Premium models.   YES | NO

DM 30 Practice — Greedy

Jane is taking 7 orange tarts, 6 apple tarts and 3 lemon tarts to Annie's house. On the way, Jane eats three of the tarts.

Answer YES if the conclusion follows and NO if it does not.

Q30.1   There is at least one lemon tart left for Annie.   YES | NO

Q30.2   Annie will have more apple tarts than lemon tarts.   YES | NO

Q30.3   Annie will have the same number of each tart.   YES | NO

Q30.4   Annie could be left with the same number of apple tarts as orange tarts.   YES | NO

Q30.5   Annie will have fewer lemon tarts than orange tarts.   YES | NO

DM 31 Practice
Multilinguals

The following diagram shows the number of students who speak a variety of languages. Each of the five shapes represents a different language: English, French, Italian, Japanese and Spanish. The lower a language appears in alphabetical order, the fewer people speak that language, i.e. English is the least spoken language, followed by French, etc. Spanish is the most spoken language.

Q31.1 How many students speak two languages only?

A. 37   B. 43   C. 46   D. 53

Q31.2 How many students speak four languages only?

A. 0   B. 18   C. 25   D. 43

Q31.3 Only one of the five languages is never spoken in isolation (i.e. it is spoken by people who also speak at least one other language). Which one?

A. French   B. Italian   C. Japanese   D. Spanish

DM 32 Practice — Mobile Phones

Q32 Should schools ban children from bringing their mobile phones to school in order to enhance concentration and learning? Select the strongest argument from the statements below.

A. YES. Some students use smart phones to access the internet during lessons.

B. YES. Students can use phones to cheat in exams.

C. NO. Students may feel safer if they have a phone on them after school is finished.

D. NO. Some schools have shown that, if used with a strict set of rules, mobile phones do not interfere with lessons.

DM 33 Practice — Which Language?

In my year at school, there are only 10 students who study Spanish. They are all in Class 8A1, which has 24 students in total. All students study one language and one only.

Answer YES if the conclusion follows and NO if it does not.

Q33.1 John is in my year. He studies Spanish and so he is in Class 8A1. | YES | NO |

Q33.2 Allison is in Class 8A1 so she is studying Spanish. | YES | NO |

Q33.3 Paul is in my year and studies French, so he cannot be in Class 8A1. | YES | NO |

Q33.4 Faheem must be in Class 8A1 because he studies Spanish. | YES | NO |

Q33.5 Fatima is in class 8A3 so she must study French. | YES | NO |

Decision Making – Practice

DM 34 Practice — Cosmopolitan Travellers

Q34 In a train travelling from London to Leeds, all travellers are either tourists, students or doctors. All travellers are also either German, Japanese or British.

Between London and Leeds, the train stops twice.

- At the first stop, only the tourists who are not British leave the train.

- At the second stop, only the Germans who are not students, the British doctors and the Japanese doctors leave the train.

Which of the following must be incorrect?

A. None of the doctors reach Leeds.
B. All students reach Leeds.
C. Out of all tourists, only the British ones reach Leeds.
D. Out of all Japanese travellers, only the tourists reach Leeds.

DM 35 Practice — Three Daughters

Q35 Ben, who has three daughters, is chatting with his neighbour Paul. Paul asks how old Ben's daughters are. Ben replies the following:

- The product of their ages is 36.
- The sum of their ages is equal to my house number.

Upon hearing this, Paul is still unable to determine the three daughters' ages. Which additional piece of information would help Paul conclusively determine the three daughter's ages?

A. Two of them are twins.
B. None of them are twins.
C. The eldest is blonde.
D. All daughters are below the age of 10.

DM 36 Practice — Clothes Shopping

Q36 Albert, Barbara, Cassandra and Denise went shopping. Each bought a different type of item: shirt, hat, trousers or shoes. The labels showed the following prices (in no particular order): £35, £45, £50 and £60.

- Barbara did not buy the shoes.
- Denise bought black trousers.
- Denise spent £10 more than Barbara.
- The blue shirt was bought by a woman for £45.

Which of the following must be correct?

A. The shoes cost £35.
B. Barbara bought the shirt.
C. Albert bought the hat.
D. Cassandra bought the shoes.

DM 37 Practice — Cat and Mouse Games

Q37 When it rains, the cat is either in the bedroom or in the cellar.

When the cat is in the bedroom, the mouse is hiding behind the fridge and the cheese is in the fridge.

When the cheese is on the table and the cat is in the cellar, the mouse is in the bedroom.

Right now, the cheese is on the table and it is raining. Which of the following statements must be true?

A. The cat and the mouse are in the bedroom.
B. The cat is in the bedroom and the mouse is behind the fridge.
C. The cat is in the cellar and the mouse is behind the fridge.
D. The cat is in the cellar and the mouse is in the bedroom.

Decision Making – Practice

DM 38 Practice	Blind Spot

Q38 In a dark room, three blue hats and two green hats sit on a table. Three people, the last of whom is blind, enter the room. Each of the three people takes a hat at random without being able to see what colour it is and places it on its own head. The two hats which have not been drawn are taken out of the room.

The light is switched on and each person is asked to say whether they can guess the colour of the hat they are wearing.

The first person says NO. The second one says NO. The blind man speaks last.

Which of the following must be true?

A. The probability that the blind man's hat is blue is 60%.
B. The blind man is wearing a blue hat.
C. The blind man is wearing a green hat.
D. The probability that the blind man's hat is green is 20%.

DM 39 Practice	Café Crème

Q39 One cup contains 150 ml of coffee and another cup 150 ml of milk. One spoonful of milk is taken from the milk cup. It is emptied into the coffee cup and the resulting liquid is thoroughly mixed. The same spoon is then used to take liquid from that cup. This is poured into the milk cup. Each cup now contains 150 ml of liquid.

Ignoring the volume of the spoon itself, which of the following must be true?

A. There is more coffee in the milk than milk in the coffee.
B. There is less coffee in the milk than milk in the coffee.
C. There is as much coffee in the milk as milk in the coffee.
D. Both cups have a capacity of more than 150 ml.

DM 40 Practice — Commuting

Q40 A study looks at the commuting distances of all working inhabitants of towns A and B. The pie charts below show the number of inhabitants in each town and how far they need to travel to get to work.

Town A
1600 people

Town B
2000 people

- 0-10 miles
- 10-20 miles
- 20-30 miles
- 30-40 miles

Town A: 40%, 15%, 20%, 25%
Town B: 50%, 10%, 20%, 20%

Based on the data provided, which of the following must be true?

A. More people in Town A than in Town B live less than 20 miles away from their workplace.

B. If the two towns were located 30 miles apart then some people would be counted in both pie charts.

C. Town B inhabitants who commute less than 30 miles commute on average 17 miles.

D. The average commuting distance for Town A inhabitants is equal to or greater than 19 miles.

430

DM 41 Practice: Football

Q41 Three medical school football teams played a mini-championship amongst one another. Each team played only once against each of the other teams.

The (incomplete) results table is as follows:

Team	No. of games played	No. of games won	No. of games lost	No. of games drawn	No. of goals scored by that team	No. of goals scored against that team
X	2		1		3	2
Y			1	1	0	
Z						1

Based on the data provided, which of the following must be false?

A. Team X only won once.
B. Team X beat Team Y with a score of 2 goals to 1.
C. Team X scored more goals than the other two teams.
D. The match between Team Y and Team Z ended in a draw.

DM 42 Practice: Pets for Children

Q42 Should children be encouraged to keep pets to gain a sense of responsibility and care towards others?

Select the strongest argument from the statements below.

A. YES. Scientific consensus is that owning a pet reduces stress.
B. YES. Pets require regular duties of care.
C. NO. Some children are allergic to pets.
D. NO. Many children are not disciplined enough to look after animals.

DM 43 Practice — Blue Eyes

Q43 In a group of X students, we note that they have three different eye colours: brown, green and blue; and two different hair colours: blonde and black.

- 20 students have blue eyes and blonde hair.
- 60 students have green eyes and black hair.
- 42 students have blonde hair.
- 50 students have brown eyes.
- 72 students have green eyes.

Based on the data provided, which of the following must be true?

A. (X − 120) students have blue eyes.
B. There are at least 152 students.
C. There are fewer students with black hair than with blonde hair.
D. The percentage of students with brown eyes and black hair is 40/X %.

DM 44 Practice — Ties

Q44 Three friends are discussing another friend's tie collection:

Ali: "Steve has at least 100 ties in his collection."
Julia: "No way! I am sure he has fewer than 100 ties."
Tony: "I am quite sure he owns at least one tie."

Assuming that only one of the three friends is correct, which option most accurately represents the number of ties that Steve owns?

A. 0
B. Between 0 and 50
C. Between 50 and 100
D. Between 1 and 100

DM 45 Practice — Glassware

Q45 A restaurant is planning to host a dinner for 100 people. They have been warned by the client that diners should be given a maximum of two glasses of wine each. This maximum applies to each diner and diners are not allowed to use the unused allowance of one of the other diners (i.e. if someone does not drink then no one can drink their glass instead as their third glass).

The client sent an email to the restaurant to say that X% of the diners will require only one glass of wine and that half of the remaining diners will require two glasses. Some will not require any since they won't be drinking.

Unfortunately, the client has forgotten to state what X is and he cannot be reached before the day of the dinner, when it will be too late to change anything. Only one type of wine is served throughout the evening and one bottle of wine can serve 6 glasses.

Based on the data provided, which of the following must be true?

A. The restaurant owner will need to buy 34 bottles in order to satisfy the client's demands.

B. When all guests have been served, one bottle will be left open. That bottle will be 1/3 full.

C. The number of glasses that will be served can be as low as 0 and as high as 200.

D. The probability that the restaurant owner will order the correct quantity of wine is below 1%.

DM 46 Practice — End of Year Bonus

A Human Resources director announced that "One condition for an employee to be eligible for a bonus is that the employee must have participated in the Orion project."

Answer YES if the conclusion follows and NO if it does not.

Q46.1 All those who receive a bonus will have participated in the Orion project. | YES | NO |

Q46.2 All those who participated in the Orion project will receive a bonus. | YES | NO |

Q46.3 Those who do not receive a bonus will not have participated in the Orion project. | YES | NO |

Q46.4 Those who did not participate in the Orion project will not receive a bonus. | YES | NO |

Q46.5 Some employees who participated in the Orion project may not receive a bonus. | YES | NO |

DM 47 Practice — Average Earnings

Q47 The average salary of a factory's 3000 employees is £2,000. The average salary of the men is £3,000 whereas for women it is £1,500. The 10% of women who are the least well paid have an average salary of £1,000. The highest paid male employee earns £10,000. Based on this data, which of the following must be true?

A. There are more male employees than female employees.
B. The highest paid employee is a man.
C. The 10% of women who are least well paid earn less than 4% of the total payroll.
D. The least well paid man earns less than the least well paid woman.

Decision Making – Practice

DM 48 Practice — Medical School Marathon

Vicky, Wolfgang and Yvonne are students at three medical schools: King's, Warwick and Birmingham. They are all participating in an inter-medical school marathon and finish in the first three places. They each travelled to the marathon using a different means of transport: car, bike and bus.

- Vicky, who did not travel by car, finished second.
- Yvonne studies at King's.
- The Warwick student went by bus and finished before the Birmingham student.
- The King's student finished the race well behind the others.

Answer YES if the conclusion follows and NO if it does not.

Q48.1 The Warwick student finished second.   YES | NO

Q48.2 Vicky studies in Birmingham.   YES | NO

Q48.3 Wolfgang used the bus.   YES | NO

Q48.4 The student who rides a bike won the race.   YES | NO

Q48.5 Yvonne finished third.   YES | NO

DM 49 Practice — Health Cards

Q49 Should everyone carry a card containing a chip with their health information to ensure accurate and up-to-date information is readily accessible at every healthcare encounter?

Select the strongest argument from the statements below.

A. YES. Not everyone remembers their medical history well.
B. YES. This could also be used as an ID card system
C. NO. This would be too costly to implement.
D. NO. If lost, the information could be read by others.

| DM 50 Practice | Three Presents |

Q50 Helen, Stephanie and Nishali have each received a present.

The present is either a pen, a watch or a bracelet. They were wrapped in paper that was either red, blue or green.

- Helen received the red-wrapped present.
- The watch was not in green paper and did not go to Helen.
- Nishali received the bracelet.

Which of the following statements must be true?

A. Helen did not receive the pen.
B. The watch was not in the blue paper.
C. Stephanie received the pen.
D. The blue present did not go to Nishali.

| DM 51 Practice | Syllogisms |

Q51 Which of the following syllogisms is incorrect?

A. No baker is tight-fisted. All the people living in this house are bakers. Therefore no one in this house is tight-fisted.

B. All peacocks are proud. All birds in this park are peacocks. Therefore all birds in this park are proud.

C. Caterpillars are not edible. Some worms are edible. Therefore some worms are not caterpillars.

D. All good speakers are talkative. Some clowns are good speakers. Therefore some clowns are not talkative.

Decision Making – Practice

DM 52 Practice — Brothers

Q52 Joseph, Arthur and Les are three brothers of different ages and heights.

- Out of the three brothers, Joseph is smaller than the oldest.
- Arthur, who is not the youngest, is not the smallest.
- Les is younger than the smallest of the three.

Which of the following statements must be true?

A. The youngest is also the tallest.
B. Les is smaller than Arthur.
C. The oldest is also the smallest.
D. Joseph is not the youngest.

DM 53 Practice — Toys

Q53 A survey carried out amongst 100 families about the toys they own from this list: car, bicycle and roller skates, shows the following results:

- 30 families have a car
- 90 families have a bicycle
- 50 families have roller skates
- 10 families have all three toys
- 50 families have a bicycle but no roller skates
- 15 families have only roller skates and a car.

Which of the following statements must be true?

A. 70 families have exactly two toys.
B. 5 families only have roller skates.
C. 15 families have only a car and a bicycle.
D. 5 families have only a car.

1300 UCAT Practice Questions

DM 54 Practice — Coloured Cubes

Q54 Two identical cubes have sides of different colours: red, green, blue, black, yellow, and white.

The first cube has three visible sides: yellow, blue and green.
The second cube has three visible sides: black, white, and blue.

Which colour is on the opposite side of the red side?

A. Green
B. Blue
C. Yellow
D. White

DM 55 Practice — Wooden Tables

In this country, we can proudly assert that:

- Strong tables are made of wood.
- All carpenters are bald.
- Only carpenters build strong tables.
- All bald people wear a hat.

Answer YES if the conclusion follows and NO if it does not.

Q55.1 People who wear a hat can build strong tables. YES | NO

Q55.2 All wooden tables are built by bald people. YES | NO

Q55.3 A carpenter who builds a strong table does not necessarily wear a hat. YES | NO

Q55.4 All people who wear hats are carpenters. YES | NO

Q55.5 A flimsy table can't have been built by a carpenter. YES | NO

DM 56 Practice — Lineage

Q56 In John's family, in each of the past five generations, there has been one offspring, who was male. John has a son, who is also an only child. John has just one grandchild, who is also a boy.

John looks at a family photo and says "The grandfather of this man's son is my grandfather's grandchild."

Who is the man in the picture?

A. John's grandfather
B. John's father
C. John
D. John's son

DM 57 Practice — Library

Consider the following statements:
- All books in English have a red cover.
- All books in a foreign language have more than 200 pages.
- All and only the books with illustrations have red covers.
- All and only the books with an index have more than 200 pages.

Answer YES if the conclusion follows and NO if it does not.

Q57.1 Foreign books can have a red cover. YES | NO

Q57.2 Some books with illustrations have an index. YES | NO

Q57.3 An 85-page book in English has an index. YES | NO

Q57.4 A 600-page book with a red cover has no index. YES | NO

Q57.5 All English books have illustrations. YES | NO

DM 58 Practice — Friday 13th

Q58 Every Friday 13th, Veronica announces what day of the week the last day of the month will be.

One month she made a mistake. Which of the following is the mistake that she made?

"Today, Friday 13th, I can guarantee that ...

- **A.** ... the last day of the month will be a Friday."
- **B.** ... the last day of the month will be a Saturday."
- **C.** ... the last day of the month will be a Sunday."
- **D.** ... the last day of the month will be a Monday."

DM 59 Practice — Labels

Q59 In the diagrams below, all shapes are labelled either A, B or C.

In this box, there are more Bs than As

In this box there are 2 As, 2 Bs and 2 Cs

- All shapes labelled A are round.
- All shapes labelled C contain a dot.

What label is associated to the black square with a dot?

- **A.** A
- **B.** B
- **C.** C
- **D.** It can be B or C

Decision Making – Practice

DM 60 Practice — Order

Q60 Consider the following pieces labelled A to F.

    A   B   C   D   E   F

You have been asked to lay the pieces out in a line in an order that satisfies the following requirements:

- No. 2 has at least one square
- No. 3 has at least one triangle
- No. 6 has one star
- No. 1 has two circles
- No. 4 has two black objects
- No. 5 has two white objects
- No. 3 has at least one black shape

What is Piece F's position?

A. 3
B. 4
C. 5
D. 6

DM 61 Practice — Tokens

Q61 Five tokens of different colours (blue, green, yellow, red and white) are aligned. The blue token is on the right of the yellow token. The blue token is on the left of the white token and on the right of the green token. There are two tokens between the white and the red.

Which of the following statements is true?

A. The yellow token is at one extremity.
B. The blue token is at one extremity.
C. The white token is not at an extremity.
D. The left-hand token is either yellow or green.

1300 UCAT Practice Questions

DM 62 Practice — Xanias and Zazas

All Xanias are Yogos. All Zazas are Yogos.

Answer YES if the conclusion follows and NO if it does not.

Q62.1   All Xanias are Zazas   YES | NO

Q62.2   All Zazas are Xanias   YES | NO

Q62.3   No Xania can be a Zaza   YES | NO

Q62.4   Some Zazas can be Xanias   YES | NO

Q62.5   All Yogos are Xanias   YES | NO

DM 63 Practice — Student Life

Q63   Consider the following diagram:

○ Total population

▢ Males

◖ Students

△ Enjoy sport

▷ Under age 25

What does the letter A represent?

A. Female non-students below age 25 who don't enjoy sport.
B. Male students over the age of 25 who don't enjoy sport.
C. Female students below age 25 who enjoy sport.
D. Female students over age 25 who enjoy sport.

442

DM 64 Practice — Food Allergies

Q64 A hundred people are all allergic to at least one of the following ingredients: garlic, tomatoes, pasta, cheese. Not all are allergic to the same combinations.

- Those allergic to tomatoes can eat garlic or cheese, but some of them cannot eat pasta.
- All those allergic to cheese are also allergic to garlic.
- Some people who are allergic to pasta are also allergic to cheese.

Which diagram best represents the information above?

A

B

C

D

DM 65 Practice — Student Athletes

60% of students play football.
50% of students play cricket.
30% of students play rugby.

Answer YES if the conclusion follows and NO if it does not.

Q65.1 At most 10% of students play football and cricket. | YES | NO |

Q65.2 At least 20% of students play neither cricket nor rugby. | YES | NO |

Q65.3 Some students play all three sports. | YES | NO |

Q65.4 At most 10% of students do not play football or rugby. | YES | NO |

Q65.5 At most 30% of students play all three sports. | YES | NO |

DM 66 Practice — Rectangular Table

Q66 Mary, Damian, Patrick, Louisa, Karl, and Rob are sitting around a rectangular table.

- Damian is sitting opposite Louisa.
- Karl is not sitting next to Damian.
- Patrick is sitting on Louisa's right.
- The two women are not sitting side by side.
- Mary is occupying Seat 1.

```
    (2)   (3)
(1)           (4)
    (6)   (5)
```

Which of the following statements must be true?

A. Damian is sitting in Seat 2 or Seat 6.
B. Karl is not sitting opposite Rob.
C. Karl sits in Seat 6.
D. Patrick is sitting next to Rob.

Decision Making – Practice

DM 67 Practice — False Positives

Q67 A laboratory can use Test A to determine whether a particular protein is contained in a blood sample. The probability that an individual's blood contains the protein in question is 0.1%. Test A has the following characteristics:

- If the protein is in the blood, Test A always detects it.
- When Test A gives a negative result, it is 100% accurate, i.e. it means the person does not have the protein in their blood.
- When 100 people with no protein in their blood were tested, for 5 of them the test showed a positive result.

The laboratory predicts that the probability that an individual who tests positive has the protein is very low (of the order of 2%). Which of the following applies?

A. No, it should be 95% since the test only gets it wrong in 5% of cases.
B. No, the probability should be far higher since the test has a low failure rate. But it is not 95%.
C. Yes, this is because the low prevalence of the protein presence makes the test very unreliable.
D. The lab cannot calculate a percentage using the data provided.

DM 68 Practice — Speed Humps

Q68 Should speed-reducing road humps be introduced in all town centres and residential areas?

A. YES. This would help raise awareness of the dangers of the road amongst drivers.
B. YES. People hit by vehicles at lower speeds sustain less serious injuries.
C. NO. More emphasis should be placed instead on educating pedestrians on the dangers of the road.
D. NO. Road humps could damage cars.

1300 UCAT Practice Questions

DM 69 Practice — Asthmatic Nurses

No nurse has asthma.
Many smokers become asthmatic.

Answer YES if the conclusion follows and NO if it does not.

Q69.1   No nurse is a smoker.   YES | NO

Q69.2   Some smokers are nurses.   YES | NO

Q69.3   No asthmatic is a nurse.   YES | NO

Q69.4   All smokers are asthmatic.   YES | NO

Q69.5   An asthmatic smoker cannot be a nurse.   YES | NO

DM 70 Practice — Who Lives Where?

Q70   Martin, George, Phil, and Steve each live in a different city: London, Pontefract, Manchester and Birmingham.

If Phil lives in London or Pontefract, then George lives in Manchester.
If Martin does not live in London, then Steve lives in Pontefract.
If Steve does not live in Birmingham, then Phil lives in Birmingham.
If George lives in Pontefract, then Phil lives in London.
If Martin does not live in Birmingham, then George does not live in Manchester.

Which of the following MUST be true?

A. Martin lives in Birmingham.
B. George does not live in Pontefract.
C. Phil lives in Pontefract.
D. George lives in Manchester.

DM 71 Practice — Coding

Q71 Consider the following numbers:

12478 – 34852 – 75261 – 57123 – 86514

Those same numbers are encoded such that each digit is replaced by another digit in a unique way. Here are the same numbers after they have been encoded, presented in a random order:

68479 – 86734 – 53642 – 92567 – 47285

Which number, when coded, would give 75324?

A. 28614
B. 28641
C. 79862
D. 86972

DM 72 Practice — Guilty Or Not Guilty

Q72 After a recent robbery, it has been established that one or more of four suspects are guilty.

- If Fred is guilty then they are all guilty.
- If Theo is guilty then he has two accomplices.
- If Eddie is innocent, then Theo isn't.
- If Victor is guilty then there are only two guilty suspects.

Which of the following must be true?

A. Eddie is guilty.
B. Eddie alone is guilty.
C. Victor is guilty.
D. Eddie or Victor is guilty but not both.

DM 73 Practice — Fertility Study

Q73 A study on fertility based on 1000 women shows the following:

- 20% of women have no child.
- 25% of women have one child.
- 25% of women have two children.
- 15% of women have three children.
- 10% of women have four children.
- 5% of women have more than four children.

Which of the following must be true?

A. 50% of women who have at least one child have at least three children.

B. These 1000 women collectively have over 1850 children.

C. The probability that one woman chosen at random has at least 3 children is greater than 35%.

D. 55% of children have at least one brother and one sister.

DM 74 Practice — Curious Food Lovers

Q74 All curious people are nice. No food lover is beyond reproach. Some food lovers are curious.

Which of the following statements contradicts the above statements?

A. Some food lovers are nice.
B. Some nice people are beyond reproach.
C. All nice people are beyond reproach.
D. Some curious people love food.

Decision Making – Practice

DM 75 Practice — Colourful Bouquet

Q75 A florist has 1000 flowers split between three varieties: roses, tulips and pansies. Those flowers can be of three different colours: red, white and yellow.

- Half of all flowers are pansies, of which 180 are white.
- There are as many red flowers as there are yellow flowers.
- One quarter of white flowers are roses.
- 30% of white flowers are tulips.
- 20% of roses are red, which represents 60 flowers.
- There are as many red tulips as there are yellow tulips.

Which of the following statements cannot be true?

A. There are 400 red flowers.
B. There are as many yellow pansies as there are white tulips.
C. There are 300 roses.
D. There are fewer yellow flowers than there are white flowers.

DM 76 Practice — Movie Munchies

Q76 Saria goes to the cinema with her younger brother and two older sisters Suneeta and Varunee (the eldest). One buys salty popcorn, one buys nachos, one buys candy floss, and one buys nothing.

- The eldest picks a savoury snack.
- Saria doesn't like nachos.
- The youngest girl has a savoury snack.
- One of the girls picks no snack.

Which one chooses the candy floss?

A. Saria
B. Suneeta
C. Varunee
D. Saria's brother

DM 77 Practice — Supporting Colours

Q77 Four friends, Sushama, Keith, Grace and Vijay, live in Binbury and each support a different football team, either: Newtown United, Weston City, Binbury City or Binbury United. United teams have a single-coloured scarf; other teams' scarves are multi-coloured.

- Keith supports a United team.
- Grace wears a multi-coloured scarf.
- Vijay and Sushama do not support a home team.

Which of the following MUST be true?

A. If Keith's team plays Grace's team both sides will have multi-coloured scarves.
B. If Keith's team plays Vijay's team both sides will have single-coloured scarves.
C. Keith does not support Newtown United.
D. Sushama supports Weston City.

DM 78 Practice — Youth Travel

Q78 Last summer, Ann, Ben, and Carole each visited a different country. Each tells the truth twice and lies once.

Ann: I visited England, Carole visited Italy, Ben visited Germany
Ben: I visited Germany, Carole visited Italy, Ann visited England
Carole: I visited England, Ann visited Austria, Ben visited Germany

Which country did Ann visit?

A. Austria
B. England
C. Germany
D. Italy

DM 79 Practice — Golf Club

The following information relates to guests invited to a reception:

- All guests wearing a black jacket are golf players.
- All guests with brown hair have a hearing aid.
- None of the dishonest people wear glasses.
- None of the guests who wear a black jacket have a beard.
- All guests with a bowler hat wear glasses.
- All golf players have blue eyes.
- All guests who wear white socks wear a bowler hat.
- Many of the dishonest guests have brown hair.

Answer YES if the conclusion follows and NO if it does not.

Q79.1 Those who wear white socks are dishonest. YES | NO

Q79.2 Guests who don't have blue eyes have no beard. YES | NO

Q79.3 Guests who wear a bowler hat are dishonest. YES | NO

Q79.4 All those who wear glasses are honest. YES | NO

Q79.5 Some people with brown hair do not wear glasses. YES | NO

Q79.6 No bearded guest wears a black jacket. YES | NO

Q79.7 Those who do not play golf do not have beards. YES | NO

Q79.8 All guests with a black jacket have blue eyes. YES | NO

Q79.9 Guests with no bowler hat don't wear white socks. YES | NO

Q79.10 Some people with glasses have brown hair. YES | NO

Q79.11 Guests with no hearing aid do not have brown hair. YES | NO

Q79.12 Many dishonest guests have a hearing aid. YES | NO

DM 80 Practice — Coded Language

Q80 In a certain code language:

- "Economics is not money" is written as "ka la ho ga"
- "Demand and supply economics" is written as "mo ta pa ka"
- "Money makes only part" is written as "zi la ne ki"
- "Demand makes supply economics" is written as "zi mo ka ta".

What is the code for "supply" in the given code language?

- A. Only "ta"
- B. Only "mo"
- C. Either "pa" or "mo"
- D. Either "ta" or "mo"

DM 81 Practice — Going South

Q81 Ashok started walking towards South.

After walking 50 metres he took a right turn and walked 30 metres.

He then took a right turn and walked 100 metres.

He again took a right turn and walked 30 metres and stopped.

How far and in which direction was he from the starting point?

- A. 50 metres North
- B. 50 metres South
- C. 150 metres North
- D. 180 metres East

DM 82 Practice — Going Round In Circles

Q82 A, B, C, D, E, F, G and H are sitting around a round table.
- F is third to the right of C and second to the left of H.
- H is sitting next to A.
- D is not an immediate neighbour of C or H.
- E is on the immediate right of A.
- A is second to the right of G.

Who sits between G and D?

A. B   **.** F   **C.** Both B and F   **D.** H

DM 83 Practice — Extra-Terrestrial Foliage

On the planet Oribot, to measure height, there are seven Farinks in a Jobobum. A tree is classified as being a plant life that grows to at least half a Jobobum high, otherwise it is classified as a flower. All plant life produces fruits known as Zechbodies, which are either red or blue. Kendu trees have either leaves or needles. All Guruk flowers have both leaves and suckers. Red Zechbodies never grow on trees where needles are present.

Answer YES if the conclusion follows and NO if it does not.

Q83.1 Kendu trees are more than 3 Farinks high. | YES | NO |

Q83.2 You will never see a red Kendu tree with needles. | YES | NO |

Q83.3 Any Kendu tree with leaves will have red fruit. | YES | NO |

Q83.4 Plants with suckers are under 0.5 Jobobum high. | YES | NO |

Q83.5 If you see a red Zechbody on a plant, then you can expect to find leaves or suckers on it too. | YES | NO |

DM 84 Practice — Foodie's Delight

Maria is arranging the programme for the final day of a community food festival. There are three back-to-back one-hour sessions from 9am and three back-to-back 45-minute sessions starting at 1:15pm. There are five types of sessions running at fixed durations: cake competition, wine tasting and three types of food demonstration: bread, fish, and vegetables.

There has to be at least 45 minutes between any food demonstration. The cake competition and the wine tasting run only once. The cake competition takes place in the afternoon. The fish demonstrator has to leave by 1:30pm. The bread demonstration takes only 45 minutes. The vegetable and fish demonstrations run for different lengths of time.

Answer YES if the conclusion follows and NO if it does not.

Q84.1 The wine tasting lasts a full hour. | YES | NO |

Q84.2 If Maria has the venue until 5pm she will have just one hour to clear up. | YES | NO |

Q84.3 The vegetable demo is definitely at 1:15pm. | YES | NO |

Q84.4 The fish demo is repeated. | YES | NO |

Q84.5 The cake competition and the bread demo run one after the other in any order. | YES | NO |

DM 85 Practice — Double Winners

Q85 Andrea, Ben and Charles play a game using only pound coins. The game involves several rounds. Each round is won by two people. The two winners double their pot of money at the expense of the loser. At the end of the 5th round, Andrea has £4, Ben £18 and Charles £5. How much did Charles start the whole game with?

A. £1   B. £2   C. £9   D. £18

DM 86 Practice — Alarm Clocks

Q86 John's alarm clock is neither next to Anna's nor next to Lydia's. John's and Brendan's alarm clocks show that it is not yet 2:45. Animesh's alarm clock is on the immediate left of Lydia's. What time does Lydia's alarm clock show?

A. 02:32   B. 03:00   C. 02:48   D. 02:55   E: 02:40

DM 87 Practice — Births, Marriages and Deaths

Q87 If John died before Paul's birth and Michael got married after Paul's birth, which of the following must be true?

A. Michael got married when Paul was alive.
B. Michael got married after Paul's death.
C. Michael got married before Paul's death.
D. None of the above.

DM 88 Practice — Light Weights

Q88 If A is lighter than B and C, and if D is heavier than B, which of the following must be true?

A. D is lighter than A.
B. D is heavier than C.
C. D could be lighter than C.
D. None of the above.

DM 89 Practice — Relationships

Consider the following relationships:
- A + B means that A is the father of B
- A x B means that A is the sister of B
- A $ B means that A is the wife of B
- A % B means that A is the mother of B
- A / B means that A is the son of B

For the purpose of this exercise, assume that:
- The parents of the same child(ren) are married.
- Siblings have the same parents.
- There are no same sex relationships.

Q89.1 Which of the following implies that A is C's mother-in-law?

A. A % B x C   B. A % B / C   . B / A / C   D. A % B x D $ C

Q89.2 What is C's relationship to A if the following is true: A + B x C x D.

A. Father   B. Son   C. Daughter   D. Daughter-in-law

Q89.3 Which expression can be deduced from A / B $ C?

A. A + C   B. C % B   C. C + A   D. C / B x A

Q89.4 What should come in the place of the question mark to establish that J is the brother of T in this expression? J / P % H ? T

A. x   B. /   C. $ D. either + or %

Q89.5 Which of the following statements is true if I + T % J x L / K is true?

A. L is the daughter of T
B. K is the son-in-law of I
C. I is the grand-mother of L
D. T is the father of J
E. J is the brother of L

DM 90 Practice
Cuppa Anyone?

Liang owns a shop. Her product catalogue lists over 100 options for tea that customers can buy. Her teas come from at least six different countries.

- Teas can be either "single origin" which means that they originate from the same estate, or "blends", which means that leaves from different estates have been mixed.
- The tea subtypes she sells are: black, green and oolong.
- No blend can contain more than one subtype.
- The tea produced in Kenya is always black.
- All green teas are single origin.
- Most of her Taiwanese teas are oolongs.
- The majority of her teas are from China.
- Her most expensive teas are oolongs.
- All her Japanese tea is green.
- She has more teas from India than Taiwan.
- Both blends and single origin teas can be scented with perfumes.

Answer YES if the conclusion follows and NO if it does not.

Q90.1	Most teas from China are blends.	YES | NO
Q90.2	Most tea from Taiwan is expensive.	YES | NO
Q90.3	Most expensive teas contain a green/oolong blend.	YES | NO
Q90.4	Chinese teas are cheaper than Taiwanese.	YES | NO
Q90.5	A blend may contain teas from several countries.	YES | NO
Q90.6	Kenyan teas can be scented.	YES | NO
Q90.7	Liang has more non-black tea than black tea.	YES | NO
Q90.8	Liang has some Japanese and Kenyan blends.	YES | NO
Q90.9	Some of her teas do not come from Taiwan, Japan, China, India or Kenya.	YES | NO
Q90.10	Taiwanese tea production is expensive.	YES | NO

DM 91 Practice — Garden Gnomes

Q91 One hundred garden gnomes have various features (boots, glasses, hat and beard), though not all of them the same.

- All those with boots wear glasses.
- Those with a beard do not wear boots or a hat.

Which of the following diagrams is a possible representation of the group of gnomes?

A

B

C

D

DM 92 Practice — House Features

Q92 The following diagram shows the features that can be found in 100 houses located in the same neighbourhood. All houses have at least one of the features.

Red bricks   Chimney   Front garden

(Venn diagram with values: 10, 5, 7, 9, 8, 9, A, B, 12, 15, 5)

Driveway

Which of the following statements is true?

A. There are more houses with a chimney than with a driveway.
B. There are 20 houses with a driveway, a chimney but no front garden.
C. There are 40 houses with exactly one feature.
D. The number of houses with all four features cannot be determined.

DM 93 Practice — Guidebooks

Q93 Out of 50 people, 30 have never travelled abroad. However, 35 possess a guidebook for Greece and 20 possess a guidebook for Spain. Which of the following statements must be true?

A. At least 15 people do not have any guidebook.
B. All those who travelled abroad have at least one guidebook.
C. At least 5 people who travelled abroad possess both guidebooks.
D. At least a quarter of those who travelled abroad have one or more guidebooks.

DM 94 Practice — Big Spender

A group of shoppers are being interviewed about their shopping habits during the previous week.

The following information has been gathered:

- On average people shopped twice during the week.
- The average number of high street shopping trips made by a shopper is three, the maximum being five.
- A number of people shopped online, though no one shopped exclusively online.

Answer YES if the conclusion follows and NO if it does not.

Q94.1 Some people who have visited a high street shop have also shopped online. | YES | NO |

Q94.2 Those who have shopped only once during the week did their shopping in a high street shop. | YES | NO |

Q94.3 All those interviewed went shopping at least once. | YES | NO |

Q94.4 The number of people who shopped once is equal to the number of people who shopped five times. | YES | NO |

Q94.5 All those who shopped twice did some of their shopping online. | YES | NO |

Q94.6 No one shopped more than five times. | YES | NO |

Q94.7 No one who shopped in a high street shop did any online shopping. | YES | NO |

Q94.8 Most people visited a high street shop three times. | YES | NO |

14 Decision Making Answers to Practice Questions

DM 1 – Professional Chefs

Q1.1 – YES. We know that all professionally trained chefs have excellent knife skills. We also know that some of the professionally trained chefs don't know how to season their food properly, from which we can infer that some DO know how to season their food properly. Therefore, there are chefs who can both season their food properly and have excellent knife skills. Note that, though we cannot demonstrate that this is true for non-professionally trained chefs, we do not actually need to demonstrate it since the question does not ask to differentiate between professionally or non-professionally trained chefs.

Q1.2 – YES. The reasoning as for Q1.1 above helps us also conclude that some of the chefs with good knife skills are professionally trained chefs who know how to season their food properly.

Q1.3 – NO. We know that, among those who have good knife skills, there will be professionally trained chefs. So, those will satisfy the statement. However, we know nothing about the non-professionally trained chefs who have good knife skills because the text simply does not deal with them at all. As such we are not able to conclude whether all the non-professionally trained chefs with good knife skills know how to season their food properly and so the statement cannot be concluded using the information present in the text alone.

Q1.4 – YES. The text is quite clear that all professionally trained chefs have good knife skills but that not all of them know how to season their food properly. As such it is clear that not all chefs with good knife skills know how to season their food properly.

Q1.5 – NO. The fact that all professionally trained chefs have good knife skills does not mean that there can't be non-professionally trained chefs with good knife skills as well. Similarly, it is possible that some non-professionally trained chefs know how to season their food properly. As such there may be non-professionally trained chefs who have excellent knife skills and know how to season their food properly.

DM 2 – Vaccination

Q2 – B: At least 25% of those vaccinated caught the flu
This type of question is often best solved by using simple graphs:

Graph 1: Vaccination graph

40% vaccinated	60% non-vaccinated

Graph 2: Flu infection graph

70% caught flu	30% had no flu

Graph 3: Same as Graph 2 but inverted

30% had no flu	70% caught flu

Then by juxtaposing graphs in accordance with each option, you can determine whether each statement is correct or not.

From Graphs 1 and 3, we can see that those who caught the flu have to represent at least 40% – 30% = 10% of the population. This is equivalent to 10/40 = 25% of the vaccinated population.

Looking at the other options:

A: At most 10% of those vaccinated caught the flu.
You can see from Graphs 1 and 2 that it is possible that all 40% vaccinated caught the flu. Therefore, it cannot be deduced that most 10% of those vaccinated caught the flu since it could be as high as 100%.

C: At most 10% of the population was vaccinated and caught the flu.
We know from the reasoning used for A above that this could be as high as 100%. What is true, however, is that AT LEAST 10% of the population was vaccinated and caught the flu.

D: At least half of those who were not vaccinated stayed healthy.
Graphs 1 and 3 show that it is possible that all non-vaccinated people caught the flu. What is true, however, (based on Graphs 1 and 2) is that AT MOST half of those who were not vaccinated stayed healthy.

Decision Making – Practice

DM 3 – Table Etiquette

Q3.1 – B: Arrow and Triangle
If the only guests who have both a knife and a spoon are those who have four items, it means that when the two corresponding shapes overlap, no other shapes interfere and this overlap is made up of one sector only. So, for example, if we take option A: Arrow and Rectangle, we can see that the overlapping area consists of three sections. Similarly, with option D: Triangle and Rectangle, there are also three sections.

The only pair of shapes which has an overlap made up of one section only is the Arrow and the Triangle.

Q3.2 – D: 24
If the number of people in each sector is 1, then we simply need to add up the number of overlaps per sector. There are four sectors with just one item, i.e. where the guest will have received just one item. There are five sectors with two items (note that on either side of the arrow there are two areas where the ellipse overlaps the rectangle only, which should just count as one because they represent the same thing), two sectors with three items and one sector with four items.

4 x 1 + 5 x 2 + 2 x 3 + 1 x 4 = 4 + 10 + 6 + 4 = 24.

DM 4 – Orchestra Politics

Q4 – B: Simon plays percussion
Since Simon and Victoria are the most mentioned individuals, it seems sensible to focus on those two. From the text we can deduce that:

1 – Simon does not play the flute, the clarinet or the violin since he socialises with those who play these three instruments.

2 – Simon does not play the oboe since the clarinet player likes to have dinner with Simon but cannot stand the presence of the oboe player.

Therefore Simon plays percussion.

Note: using similar logic we can also conclude that Victoria plays the oboe, but that only serves to dismiss option D.

DM 5 – Gardeners' Question Time

Q5 – C: 4

We are starting from this position:

1		
	■	

We know that each side adds up to 14, therefore we are missing 13 from both the top row and the left-hand column. The only way we can make 13 from the remaining numbers, 2 to 8, is as follows: 8 + 5, or 6 + 7. Therefore one combination can go at the top and the other one on the left. Since the grid is symmetrical, it does not matter which goes where.

If we apply 8 + 5 to the left column there are two possibilities: the bottom left square is an 8 or a 5. If the bottom left square is a 5, then we get:

1	6/7	6/7
8	■	c
5	a	b

Since the bottom row must add up to 14, then squares a and b must add up to 14 – 5 = 9. But the only digits we can use are 2, 3 and 4, this is not possible to achieve. Therefore the bottom left digit must be an 8.

Similarly the top right digit can be a 6 or a 7. If it is a 6, then b + c has to be equal to 14 – 6 = 8, which cannot be achieved with just the digits 2, 3 and 4. Hence the top right digit is a 7.

We now have:

1	6	7
5	■	c
8	a	b

b + c must equal 7, which can only be done with 3 + 4, and a + b must equal 6, which can only be done with 2 + 4.

Therefore b = 4.

Decision Making – Practice

DM 6 – Nuts and Seeds

Q6.1 – YES
Only the brand NoNut contains no nuts. Therefore, the only way that there could be no brand of biscuits that contains both nuts and seeds would be if NoNut were the only brand that contains seeds. However, we are told that several biscuit brands contain seeds; hence it can be deduced that some biscuits contain both nuts and seeds.

Q6.2 – NO
All we know is that all biscuits except NoNut contain nuts and that some brands contain seeds. Nothing helps us conclude that NoNut actually contains seeds.

Q6.3 – YES
We are told that NoNut is the only brand not to contain nuts. So any biscuit with no nuts has to be a NoNut biscuit.

Q6.4 – NO
The text does not preclude more than one brand of nutty biscuits from containing seeds. As such, as long as there are more than two brands, there is no obligation for one of the biscuits to be a NoNut.

Q6.5 – NO
Nothing points to the fact that NoNut biscuits contain seeds.

DM 7 – Fitness Crowd

Q7 – A: Jenny
With this type of exercise, the easiest starting point is often the item which is most often mentioned – in this case: Peter or Jenny.

We know that Peter does not practise judo, rugby or dance. So he must be the swimmer.

Jenny is not a dancer and does not practise judo. Since Peter is the swimmer, then Jenny must be the rugby player.

DM 8 – Card Game

Q8 – C: David plays with Elvis
Allan is the most mentioned person so it makes sense to start with him. We know that Allan plays with Elvis or Frank. Looking at both possibilities:

- If Allan plays with Frank, then we know that David plays with Elvis and therefore that the other two, Bob and Charles, play together. We are told that if Bob is with Charles then Allan is not with Elvis, which is consistent with our original assumption which was that Allan was with Frank anyway.

- If Allan plays with Elvis, then it means that Bob must be playing either with Charles, or David, or Frank. We know that if Bob is with Charles or David then Allan is not with Elvis, which contradicts our original assumption. Therefore Bob has to be with Frank and it then follows that David is with Charles. However we are told that if David is with Charles then Bob is not with Frank, which also contradicts our earlier finding. Therefore, since no combination of players works, it cannot be possible for Allan to be with Elvis.

Therefore the only viable option is the first one, i.e. Allan + Frank, David + Elvis and Bob + Charles. Hence only option C can be true.

DM 9 – Rota Management

Q9 – C: 11
The easiest approach is to draw a Venn diagram. The data enables us to produce the following:

In the diagram A and B are two unknowns. However, we know that:
A + B + 5 + 8 + 1 + 6 + 6 = 30, i.e. A + B = 30 − 26 = 4

Therefore the number of doctors who want to take the August bank holiday off altogether is A + B + 1 + 6 = 4 + 7 = 11

DM 10 − PE Practice

Q10 − Diagram B
Only diagrams B and D contain a total number of students equal to 34. Diagram A has 32, and Diagram C has 23.

Counting the number of students within each individual circle and therefore each sport, Diagram B has: 16, 15 and 14 students respectively, whereas Diagram D has 13, 12 and 11. Therefore only Diagram B matches the requirements.

DM 11 − Round Table

Q11 − C: Robert
From the second statement, we can deduce the following placement:

Woman	Man	Woman	Man	Woman	Man
Paula					Claire's Husband

We know that Claire is a woman and that she is not sitting next to her husband, therefore we can place her in position 3, which means that the woman sitting next to her husband has to be Barbara. So we obtain:

Woman	Man	Woman	Man	Woman	Man
Paula		Claire		Barbara	Claire's Husband

From the first statement we can then deduce that David is sitting between Paula and Clare.

Woman	Man	Woman	Man	Woman	Man
Paula	David	Claire		Barbara	Claire's Husband

The third statement says that Ahmed is sitting two places to the left of Robert and so we can conclude that Claire's husband is Robert.

DM 12 – Sweets

Q12.1 – YES. We know that Johnny gives sweets to only two children. We know that all children give sweets to Lydia therefore one of the two has to be Lydia, and we also know that Johnny and George swap sweets. Therefore Johnny shares sweets only with Lydia and George.

Q12.2 – NO. All we can deduce from the text is that George gives sweets to Johnny and to Lydia but we cannot conclude anything definite about whether he gives to all children. The question is not whether this could be true (and it could!), but whether it follows from the text (which it does not!).

Q12.3 – NO. We know that Lydia will be receiving sweets from Adam since she receives sweets from all children. However the question implies that she is the only one who would be receiving sweets from Adam, which cannot be concluded from the text.

Q12.4 – NO. The only other child (other than George) whom Johnny gives sweets to is Lydia. We can't tell from the text whether she also gives sweets to Johnny and so we cannot conclude whether George is the only child that Johnny reciprocates with.

Q12.5 – NO. All we know is that Lydia receives sweets from all children. There is no indication she reciprocates.

DM 13 – Adding Up

Q13 – D: 5
If we call T = Triangle; C = Circle; D = Diamond; S = Square, we can write the three equations as:

(1) 2T = 3D   (2) S = C + D   (3) S + C = T

Substituting T from (3) into (1) we get: 2(S + C) = 3D

Equation (2) states that S = C + D, and therefore D = S – C. Since we are looking to express S as a function of C, we can substitute D from (2) into the new equation as follows:

2(S + C) = 3(S – C) i.e. 2S + 2C = 3S – 3C i.e. 2C + 3C = 3S – 2S
i.e. 5C = S. Hence the number of circles is 5, i.e. option D.

Decision Making – Practice

DM 14 – Teachers

Q14 – C: Cook
Since Debbie does not teach English, we can deduce that Alisha, Betty and Carole all teach English.

We also know that Mrs Amin does not share a subject with Betty or Mrs Cook. Therefore, since Debbie is the only one who does not teach English, her surname must be Amin.

Alisha and Mrs Debono teach history, and we know they also teach English. Therefore, there are only two topics left for Debbie Amin to teach: maths and chemistry.

Because Carole also teaches chemistry, she cannot be called Debono (who teaches history and English) or Cook (who does not share a topic with Mrs Amin). Therefore Carole's surname is Begum.

Betty and Mrs Cook are different people; Alisha and Mrs Debono are also different people; so the others are called Alisha Cook and Betty Debono.

DM 15 – Disorientation

Q15 – C: The road from Home to B passes in front of A
The distance between Home and A is 3 miles and between Home and B is 5 miles. The distance between A and B is two miles, which is the difference between the two distances. Hence Home, A and B are all aligned in that order. Looking at the other options:

Option A: A and D are five miles apart. That would be true if Home, A and D were on the same line in that order, but this is not necessarily the case.

Option B: The road from Home to B passes in front of C. The distance from B to C is equal to the sum of the individual distances between Home and B / C. Therefore B and C are actually on totally opposite sides of Home.

Option D: B could be as little as 2 miles away from D. If B is 5 miles from home and D is 8 miles from home, then the distance from B to D is between $8 - 5 = 3$ miles and $8 + 5 = 13$ miles.

DM 16 – Shop Samples

Q16 – B: 1500
If half the adults accept the samples then on average an adult will take: 0.5 x 6 = 3 samples. If three quarters of children accept the samples, then on average a child will take: 0.75 x 4 = 3 samples. Therefore we know that the total number of samples given will be 3 x 500 = 1500 regardless of the number of adults and children.

DM 17 – Venn v. Euler Diagrams

Q17.1 – NO. An Euler diagram will only contain fewer sectors than a Venn diagram if some intersections in the Venn diagram are empty. They will both contain the same number of sectors if there are no empty sectors in the Venn diagram.

Q17.2 – YES. Only Venn diagrams can show empty sectors.

Q17.3 – YES. That is the case if the Venn diagram has no empty sectors.

Q17.4 – YES. This is actually explained in the last part of the text. A Venn diagram will be clogged up by empty sectors, whereas the Euler diagram can ignore them altogether.

Q17.5 – YES. If there were empty intersections, the Euler diagram would have fewer sections.

DM 18 – Charity

Q18 – C: No, because only those with time to spare could stop to answer her questions.
There are several problems which invalidate her conclusion. The first is that she is extrapolating to the population from a small sample in a particular street of a particular town. As such her sample is unlikely to be representative and so option A is incorrect, and, by extrapolation, option B is also incorrect. The second is that her sample consists exclusively of people who decide whether or not they have time to discuss charity donations and as such those who answer are self-selecting. With regard to option D, is it possible that the amount of £5 she imposes may put some people off. It is equally possible that some people simply don't have the cash on them. And

Decision Making – Practice

in any case, there may be people who are perfectly willing to give to charity but just not to her on that day. Since her conclusion does not mention the amount of £5, option D is not strong enough an option to consider.

DM 19 – Unemployment

Q19 – C: Under 5% of the working age population is unemployed.
The easiest way to handle this question is to write formulae with the different relevant portions of the population. There are:

- A = People who are in employment
- B = People who are unemployed and are looking for work
- C = People who are unemployed and are not looking for work

```
          A                    B    C
```
The sum A + B + C is equal to the working age population.

From the text we know that:

- Employment rate = A/(A + B + C) = 75%
- Unemployment rate = B/(A + B) = 5%

In other words, the unemployment rate ignores the population which is unemployed but not looking for work.

Option C is stating that B/(A+B+C) is under 5%. We know that B/(A+B)= 5%. We also know that C is not equal to zero, otherwise the employment and unemployment rate would add up to 1. Therefore B/(A+B+C) must be below 5%. Hence option C is the correct answer.

With regard to the other options:

- Option A and option D are incorrect because the 25% of the working age population which is unemployed will contain people who are looking for work and people who are not.

- Option B is incorrect because the 95% figure would be a proportion of those who are in employment or looking for work, and not the total working age population.

DM 20 – Mandatory Training

Q20.1 – NO. The five courses listed are examples of courses that need to be attended. There may be more.

Q20.2 – NO. Same reason as 20.1. The fact that a course is not listed in the text does not mean it is not mandatory.

Q20.3 – NO. The text in fact implies that the 12-month rule applies to everyone. It merely mentions that although there is a possibility to cancel, the rule still needs to be respected.

Q20.4 – NO. That would only be true if all courses take place on different days. The text does not suggest this is the case.

Q20.5 – NO. That would be true if courses could run on 1 January (since the calendar year is the period of reference). But we are told they can't.

DM 21 – Bus Ride

Q21 – B: 2 as the other four students will average 1 per bus, + 1 for Ben.
Ignoring Ben to start with, the other four students will board the four buses randomly and independently, therefore there will be an average of one student per bus.

Once Ben boards a bus, this will add 1 to the average for that particular bus.

DM 22 – Hair

Q22 – A: They both have a number of hairs that is above average.
If we call X the number of hairs of the friend with the fewest hairs, then the other friend will have 1.2X hairs.

So X + 1.2X = 222,222. Hence X = 222,222/(1+1.2)= 101,010.

Hence they both have an above-average number of hairs.

Decision Making – Practice

DM 23 – Siblings

Q23 – C: Belinda is younger than Elliott
We know that Andrew and Elliott were born four years apart so there will be three other siblings between them. Since we do not know which one is the younger of the two, there are four possible options:

Scenario	Older	2	3	4	5	Younger
1	Elliott	?	?	?	Andrew	?
2	?	Elliott	?	?	?	Andrew
3	Andrew	?	?	?	Elliott	?
4	?	Andrew	?	?	?	Elliott

However we know that Fred is two years older than Andrew, therefore scenarios 3 and 4 can be excluded. Since we are told that the girls were born in alphabetical order, there are therefore only two possibilities:

Scenario	Older	2	3	4	5	Younger
1	Elliott	Belinda	Fred	Carol	Andrew	Davina
2	Belinda	Elliott	Carol	Fred	Davina	Andrew

Therefore the only statement which cannot be concluded is that Belinda is younger than Elliott.

DM 24 – Family Food

Q24 – D: The square or the diamond
There are several ways in which you can find the answer. Some involve actually working out which shape corresponds to whom, which can take up valuable time. The quickest way to get to the answer is as follows:

Pizza is liked by three people, salad and burger are each liked by two people, and curry and pasta are each liked by one person. Therefore the circle represents pizza (as it overlaps three dotted shapes), the square and the diamond represent salad and burger (as each overlaps two dotted shapes) and the triangle and the arrow represent curry and pasta (as each overlaps one dotted shape).

So the burger must be the square or the diamond.

DM 25 – Loaded Dice

Q25 – C: 1/21 – The loaded die has a probability of 2/7 of landing a 3, whilst the other die has a probability of 1/6.
The calculation is done as normal by multiplying the probabilities for each die, but the loaded die has twice as much chance of landing a 3 than any other number, therefore number 3 has 2 in 7 chances of coming up whereas all other numbers only have 1 in 7 chances. (The total probability needs to add up to 1). 2/7 x 1/6 = 2/42 = 1/21.

DM 26 – Free Museum Entry

Q26 – B: YES. It would make visits to museums affordable to those with little disposable income.
This directly addresses the mechanism by which the number of people would increase.

Looking at the other options:

A: YES. Most museums are funded by donors or other subsidies. Loss of entrance fee would not significantly affect their finances. This addresses the affordability of the scheme and not the mechanism by which the number of visitors would increase.

C: NO. Admission fees contribute to meeting museums' running costs. Though this statement is probably correct, it is not to say that museums depend on those admission fees nor that they could not find alternative sources of income to make up the difference.

D: NO. It will mostly lead to people who usually visit museums to visit more often. That is entirely speculative. And even though it may indeed be the case that some people will just visit museums more often, it does not mean that new visitors won't be attracted by free entry.

DM 27 – Pharmacy

Q27.1 – YES. A powdered drug is a non-liquid and therefore will be sold in a package weighing over 250 g. So it will automatically include a leaflet.

Q27.2 – NO. We know that all drugs sold in bottles come with a syringe doser but the converse is not necessarily true.

Q27.3 – NO. We know that all non-liquid drugs weigh over 250 g and therefore come with a leaflet. But the converse is not necessarily true. For example, the drug in question could be a liquid drug in a 300 g container.

Q27.4 – YES. All bottles come with a syringe doser and since it is over 250 g it will also come with a leaflet.

Q27.5 – YES. Non-liquid drugs come in packages over 250 g therefore a package weighing under 200 g must be liquid.

DM 28 – Civic Education

Q28 – A: YES. Unless they have an interest in the topic, teenagers tend to enter adulthood without such knowledge.
There is little scope for teenagers to come across information on civic duties. This statement is generalised but the use of the word "tend" makes it realistic. Also, the statement gives a valid and direct reason to justify organising a one-day course. Looking at the other options:

B: YES. This would help increase turnout at elections.
Nowhere does it state that the aim is to increase turnout at elections. So though this may be part of the agenda, the statement is only asking whether organising such a course would help increase awareness. As such this statement is too specific to be the best answer.

C: NO. A one-day course would only address such issues superficially and its content would quickly be forgotten.
This is entirely speculative. And even if that were correct, one could argue that some knowledge/awareness is better than none.

D: NO. It would make teenagers miss a day off school or work.
That may be true for some teenagers but not all (e.g. this could be arranged at times which are suitable for each individual such as weekends or days off). But, in any case, the statement is irrelevant for our purpose here. The question is whether organising a civic awareness day would be of use to enhance civic awareness, and not whether it may be difficult to implement; there will be ways to get round the logistical issues, which will form an entirely different debate.

DM 29 – Recall

Q29.1 – NO. We know that only some Premium models have a fault, meaning some don't. As such, it cannot be concluded that a car with no fault can't have been manufactured in September.

Q29.2 – NO. We know nothing about cars manufactured in other months. As such it is possible that some cars manufactured outside of September may have faults.

Q29.3 – NO. The text says nothing about Intermediate cars, other than that they exist.

Q29.4 – NO. Since we know nothing about Intermediate cars, it is possible that some of them may have no fault.

Q29.5 – NO. All we know is that the proportion of Premium models with a fault is lower than the proportion of Basic models with a fault (which is 100%). But we know nothing about absolute numbers.

DM 30 – Greedy

Q30.1 – NO. Jane could actually eat all three lemon tarts.

Q30.2 – NO. There are 6 apple tarts and 3 lemon tarts. In the worst-case scenario, Jane will eat 3 apple tarts and Annie will get an equal number of both. Therefore, though in most scenarios it can be concluded that Annie will have more apple tarts than lemon tarts, there is one scenario where the number will be equal. As such the statement does not always hold true.

Q30.3 – NO. If Jane eats 3 orange tarts, there will be 4 left. This compares to 3 lemon tarts.

Q30.4 – YES. If Jane ate 2 orange tarts and 1 apple tart, Annie would be left with 5 of each. One example is enough to prove the point.

Q30.5 – YES. At worst, Jane will eat 3 orange tarts, leaving 4 orange tarts and 3 lemon tarts.

Decision Making – Practice

DM 31 – Multilinguals

Q31.1 – D: 53

The areas where two shapes only overlap are highlighted above.
2 + 5 + 13 + 16 + 10 + 7 = 53

Q31.2 – A: 0
There is no area where four shapes overlap.

Q31.3 – B: Italian
The number of people who speak each language is as follows:
- Diamond: 2 + 5 + 9 + 13 + 18 = 47
- Triangle: 5 + 18 + 13 + 8 + 16 + 10 + 25 + 5 = 100
- Ellipse: 2 + 18 + 16 + 25 = 61
- Square: 10 + 25 + 5 + 7 + 15 = 62
- Pentagon: 12 + 5 + 7 = 24

Therefore the languages are as follows:
- English: Pentagon (24, the lowest number)
- French: Diamond (47, the second lowest number)
- Italian: Ellipse (61)
- Japanese: Square (62)
- Spanish: Triangle (100, the highest number)

The ellipse (i.e. Italian) is the only shape overlapped entirely by other shapes.

DM 32 – Mobile Phones

Q32 – D: NO. Some schools have shown that, if used with a strict set of rules, mobile phones do not interfere with lessons.
This argument explains directly how it is possible to allow mobile phones and maintain concentration and learning. As such, it sets out why a ban would not necessarily be required. Looking at the other options:

A: YES. Some students use smart phones to access the internet during lessons. This option does not make a link between using the internet and losing concentration or diminishing learning. It may be that students are looking up relevant facts on the internet, or only use it briefly. This argument is a bit vague. It would be a good option if there was not a better alternative.

B: YES. Students can use phones to cheat in exams. The question deals with concentration and learning, not exams.

C: NO. Students may feel safer if they have a phone on them after school is finished. The question we are trying to answer is whether banning mobile phones would be effective at enhancing learning, not whether, considering all sides, on balance, we would recommend a ban or not. This argument makes total sense but does not deal with the enhanced learning part of the question.

Here are examples of answers that would have been correct if they had been part of the list:

- **YES. The instantaneous nature of social media means that children find it hard to leave their phone alone for more than a few minutes.** This directly addresses the issue of concentration. The mention of social media also clearly makes it a distraction.

- **YES. Message notification, even through a 'vibrate' option, can be distracting to the user and others.** This directly addresses the link between use of phones and distraction.

DM 33 – Which Language?

Q33.1: YES. All those studying Spanish are in Class 8A1.

Q33.2: NO. There are 14 students in Class 8A1 who don't study Spanish.

Decision Making – Practice

Q33.3: NO. He could be one of the 14 students who don't study Spanish.

Q33.4: NO. He might be in a different year group.

Q33.5: NO. We don't know if French is the only alternative to Spanish.

DM 34 – Cosmopolitan Travellers

Q34 – D: Out of all Japanese travellers, only the tourists reach Leeds.
The easiest way to solve the problem is to draw a small table and write the data provided in the text:

	British	German	Japanese
Students			
Tourists		1	1
Doctors	2	2	2

In this table, 1 and 2 denote at which stop those people left the train.

From the table we can see that A, B and C are correct and that D is incorrect. Indeed, out of all the Japanese travellers, only the students (and not the tourists) reach Leeds.

DM 35 – Three Daughters

Q35 – C: The eldest is blonde.
If the product of the three ages is 36 then there are 8 possible ways in which that can happen. The table below shows the possible options and also the sum of all three ages:

36x1x1	18x2x1	12x3x1	9x4x1	9x2x2	6x6x1	6x3x2	4x3x3
38	21	16	14	13	13	11	10

If after taking account of both the product and the sum, Paul is still unable to work out the ages, then it means that there are several possible answers. That would happen when both sums are 13.

Therefore the ages are either 9, 2 and 2; or 6, 6 and 1.

In both cases there is a set of twins, therefore option A would not help. Option B would make the problem unsolvable. And since, in both cases, all daughters are below age 10, option D would be pointless. Hence only option C would help. Indeed, if we know there is an eldest then the ages must be 9, 2 and 2.

DM 36 – Clothes Shopping

Q36 – A: The shoes cost £35.
Among the four people involved, there are three women and one man. Since Denise bought black trousers then it means that the blue shirt, which was bought by a woman, was bought either by Barbara or Cassandra.

We know that Denise spent £10 more than Barbara therefore, looking at the prices given, Barbara spent either £35 or £50. Since the blue shirt was bought for £45 then it means that the blue shirt was not purchased by Barbara and must therefore have been purchased by Cassandra.

We now know that Barbara did not buy the shirt or the trousers. Since we are told she did not buy the shoes then it means that she bought the hat.

Denise paid £10 more than Barbara and so must have spent either £45 or £60. Since £45 was the price paid for the shirt by Cassandra, we can deduce that Denise spent £60. In turn it means that Barbara spent £50.

Therefore Albert spent £35.

We can therefore deduce the following table:

Albert	Barbara	Cassandra	Denise
Shoes	Hat	Shirt	Trousers
£35	£50	£45	£60

DM 37 – Cat and Mouse Games

Q37 – D: The cat is in the cellar and the mouse is in the bedroom
We know that it is raining and so the cat is either in the bedroom or in the cellar (Statement 1)

If we assume that the cat is in the bedroom, then the mouse is hiding behind the fridge and the cheese is in the fridge (Statement 2). However, we are told that the cheese is on the table, therefore this is contradictory and the cat must be in the cellar instead.

If the cat is in the cellar, and the cheese is on the table (which we are told), then we know from Statement 3 that the mouse is in the bedroom.

DM 38 – Blind Spot

Q38 – B: The blind man is wearing a blue hat.
There are only seven possible combinations of hats using two green (G) and three blue (B) hats, as follows:

Scenario 1: BGG. That is not possible. Indeed, since there are only two green hats, the first person would have seen the other two wear a green hat and would have known straight away he was wearing a blue one.

Scenario 2: GBG. Similar to Scenario 1, the second person would have known he was wearing a blue hat. Therefore this scenario is not possible.

Scenario 3: BBG. The second person knows that if he and the blind man had both been wearing green then the first one would have known he was wearing a blue hat and would therefore have answered YES. Since the first person answered NO and the blind man is wearing a green hat, then the second person would have known he was himself wearing a blue hat. Therefore this scenario is also not possible.

The remaining four scenarios are BGB, GGB, GBB and BBB, all of which have the blind man wearing a blue hat.

DM 39 – Café Crème

Q39 – C: There is as much coffee in the milk than milk in the coffee.
Let's assume that after the double manoeuvre, the proportion of coffee and milk in what used to be the coffee cup is 80% coffee and 20% milk (for the sake of argument, it will work with any value). Since the quantity of liquids on both sides are the same (150 ml) then it means that in the other cup must be the missing 20% of coffee and 80% of milk. Therefore the proportions are perfectly reversed from one side to the other (option C).

Note that option D is incorrect since, after the first spoon is emptied, the milk cup will never need to contain more than 150 ml (liquid is taken out of it and then put back in). The coffee cup however will need to contain more than 150 ml (liquid is first added to it then taken away). Therefore it is not necessary that both cups have a capacity of more than 150 ml.

DM 40 – Commuting

Q40 – D: The average commuting distance for Town A inhabitants is equal to or greater than 19 miles.
The minimum possible commuting distance for Town A inhabitants is calculated as: 15% x 0 + 20% x 10 + 25% x 20 + 40% x 30 (i.e. you need to assume everyone lives at the lower end of their band) = 2 + 5 + 12 = 19.

Looking at the other options:

A: More people in Town A than in Town B live less than 20 miles away from their workplace. Town A: (15% + 20%) x 1600 = 560. This compares to Town B: (10% + 20%) x 2000 = 600.

B: If the two towns were located 30 miles apart then some people would be counted in both pie charts. In reality this would make no difference because the pie charts record people according to where they live. So someone living in Town A and working in Town B would be recorded only in the Town A chart.

C: Town B inhabitants who commute less than 30 miles commute on average 17 miles. Without knowing individual commuting distances for all inhabitants, or at least an average for each band, we are unable to calculate any average at all.

DM 41 – Football

Q41 – B: Team X beat Team Y with a score of 2 goals to 1
We know that Y lost one game and drew another one. Since each team can play only two games, it means that Y never won a game.

We know that X lost one game. Since Y never won a game, then X must have lost against Z.

X had 2 goals scored against it. Those goals cannot have been scored by Y (since Y never scored) therefore they were scored by Z during the X–Z match. Similarly, Z had 1 goal scored against it. That goal cannot have been scored by Y therefore it was scored by X in the X–Z match. Hence the X–Z match ended in a 2–1 win for Z.

We know that X scored 1 goal against Z, out of a total of 3 goals that it scored. Therefore X must have scored 2 goals against Y. Hence the match X–Y ended in a 2–0 victory for X.

We know that Y drew in one of its matches. Since it lost to X, then it has to have drawn against Z. And since it scored no goal then the score was 0–0.

The final scores were therefore:

- X(1), Z(2)
- X(2), Y(0)
- Y(0), Z(0)

Hence:
- Team X only won once, against Team Y (option A)
- Team X scored more goals than the other two teams, since it scored three goals, Team Y scored none and Team Z scored two (option C)
- The match between Team Y and Team Z ended in a draw (option D)

DM 42 – Pets for Children

Q42 – B: YES. Pets require regular duties of care
The argument is that by encouraging children to look after pets, they will gain a sense of responsibility. The fact that pets require regular duties of care means that children would indeed be exposed to the type of activities that would help achieve the stated goal.

Looking at the other options:

A: YES. Scientific consensus is that owning a pet reduces stress. The question has nothing to do with stress relief. Though this may be a welcome by-product, this is not relevant here.

C: NO. Some children are allergic to pets. The question does not talk about forcing children regardless of health issues. The fact some children are allergic to pets does not mean that those who are not allergic may not find the experience worthwhile.

D: NO. Many children are not disciplined enough to look after animals. The whole point is to teach them a sense of responsibility, so if anything this should be an argument in favour.

DM 43 – Blue Eyes

Q43 – D: The percentage of students with brown eyes and black hair is 40/X %.
The easiest way to resolve this question is to build a table. From the information provided we can write the following (numbers in bold are those given in the text):

	Green eyes	**Blue eyes**	**Brown eyes**	**Total**
Black hair	**60**	(X – 122) – 20 = X – 142	50 – 10 = **40**	X – 42
Blonde hair	72 – 60 = 12	**20**	42 – 20 – 12 = 10	**42**
Total	**72**	X – 50 – 72 = X – 122	**50**	**X**

The number of students with brown eyes and black hair is therefore 40, hence their proportion is 40/X %. Looking at the other options:

A: (X – 120) students have blue eyes. The number of students with blue eyes is X – 122 and not X – 120.

B: There are at least 152 students. Since all fields need to be positive, we can only conclude that X must be greater than 142 and not 152.

C: There are fewer students with black hair than with blonde hair. There are 42 students with blonde hair. As for black hair, we know that there are at least 142 – 42 = 100 (see answer above). Therefore this is incorrect. In any case, we can see that there are 60 students with black hair and green eyes and these alone are outnumbering the blonde-haired students.

DM 44 – Ties

Q44 – A: 0
Ali and Julia have complementary and mutually exclusive statements (one argues Steve has at least 100 ties and the other one that he has fewer than 100 ties). Therefore one of them has to be right.

If Ali is right in saying that Steve has at least 100 ties, then Tony (who states that Steve has at least one tie) is also correct. This contradicts the fact that only one of the friends is correct.

Therefore Julia must be telling the truth. And in turn it means that Ali and Tony are both incorrect.

Therefore we can conclude that:
- Steve has fewer than 100 ties (Julia and reverse of Ali).
- Steve has fewer than 1 tie (reverse of Tony).

Hence he MUST have no tie at all.

DM 45 – Glassware

Q45 – B: When all guests have been served, one bottle will be left open. That bottle will be 1/3 full.
From the text we can see that diners will be served 0, 1 or 2 glasses.

We know that X% of diners will be served just 1 glass. Half of the others will be served 2 glasses, meaning that the other half will therefore be served nothing. As such, the average number of glasses served to the rest of the diners will be 1 per person (50% with 2 glasses, and 50% with no glass). Hence over the entire population of diners, the average number of glasses served per person will be 1. This represents 100 glasses in total and will require 100/6 = 16.666 bottles. Hence one bottle will remain 1/3 full once everyone has been served.

Looking at the other options;

A: The restaurant owner will need to buy 34 bottles in order to satisfy the client's demands. He will actually only require 17.

C: The number of glasses that will be served can be as low as 0 and as high as 200. The number is constant at 100 as calculated above.

D: The probability that the restaurant owner will order the correct quantity of wine is below 1%. That probability is 100% if he knows how to calculate it. Otherwise it is just guess work.

DM 46 – End of Year Bonus

Q46.1 - YES. Participation in the Orion project is a condition of eligibility therefore all those who have received a bonus will have met that condition.

Q46.2 – NO. Though it is essential they have participated in the Orion project, we are not told whether other conditions may apply too.

Q46.3 – NO. It is possible that some people who have participated in the Orion project may not have received a bonus (e.g. if other conditions apply).

Q46.4 – YES. Participation is an essential requirement.

Q46.5 – YES. Same argument as Q46.2 and Q46.3.

DM 47 – Average Earnings

Q47 – C: The 10% of women who are least well paid earn less than 4% of the total payroll.
The total payroll is 3000 x 2000 = £6,000,000. If we call X the percentage of men then we can write the equation for the payroll as:

6,000,000 = 3000 x (3000X + 1500(1 – X)) i.e. 2000 = 3000X + 1500(1 – X) i.e. 2000 = 1500X + 1500 i.e. X = 2000/1500 – 1 = 0.3333 i.e. 1/3.

So there are 1/3 men and 2/3 women, i.e. 1000 men and 2000 women. Hence option A is incorrect.

The 10% least paid women would therefore represent 200 people. With an average salary of £1,000 their payroll would be £200,000.

200,000/6,000,000 = 0.0333 i.e. 3.33% i.e. less than 4%.

Options B and D are incorrect as this cannot be determined based purely on averages involving so many people.

Decision Making – Practice

DM 48 – Medical School Marathon

Q48.1 – NO. The Warwick student finished in front of the Birmingham student and the King's student was well behind the others, so the arrival order was Warwick (1st), Birmingham (2nd), King's (3rd).

Q48.2 – YES. Vicky finished second so she must be from Birmingham.

Q48.3 – YES. Since Vicky is from Birmingham and Yvonne is from King's then Wolfgang is from Warwick. Therefore he used the bus.

Q48.4 – NO. We know that the Warwick student won the race. We also know from 48.3 that Wolfgang is from Warwick and used the bus. Therefore the student who rides the bike cannot have won the race.

Q48.5 – YES. We know that Yvonne studied at King's and that the King's student finished third.

DM 49 – Health Cards

Q49 – A: YES. Not everyone remembers their medical history well. We are asked to determine whether carrying a health card would achieve the aim of accurate information being provided.

The most compelling argument to back up this claim is that some people can't keep track of their own medical history.

Looking at the other options:

B: YES. This could also be used as an ID card system. This may present another benefit but is not relevant to determine whether or not having the health card would ensure the goal of presenting more accurate information.

C: NO. This would be too costly to implement. This may be a valid argument, but it is not helping with the point we are trying to prove or disprove, which is whether having the card would ensure more accurate information being presented.

D: NO. If lost, the information could be read by others. Again, this may be a real problem, but it does not address the point of accuracy of information.

Here are a few possible arguments which could have been good answers if they had been part of the list:

- **YES. Medical information is far more detailed and complex than it used to be.** This would validate the need for an electronic support as few people would be able to remember specifics (e.g. test results, etc.).

- **NO. Hospitals use different IT systems which store the information in different ways. No single chip could be used universally.** This would essentially make the health cards pointless since the information would end up being incomplete or could not be read by all hospitals.

- **NO. IT failure or data corruption are still frequent occurrences.** This would essentially mean that the data cannot be read or may actually not be accurate.

DM 50 – Three Presents

Q50 – D: The blue present did not go to Nishali.
Helen did not get the watch; she did not get the bracelet either since it was given to Nishali. Therefore Helen received the pen. So we now know that Helen received the pen, Nishali received the bracelet and Stephanie received the watch.

The watch is not in a green paper, and we also know that, since it wasn't given to Helen, it wasn't in red paper. Therefore the watch was in the blue paper.

Hence the answer is:

Name	Helen	Stephanie	Nishali
Present	Pen	Watch	Bracelet
Colour	Red	Blue	Green

DM 51 – Syllogisms

Q51 – D: All good speakers are talkative. Some clowns are good speakers. Therefore some clowns are not talkative.
We are told that all good speakers are talkative; therefore we can conclude that the clowns who are good speakers will be talkative. However we know

Decision Making – Practice

nothing about people who are not good speakers; therefore we cannot conclude whether the clowns who are not good speakers are talkative or not. Looking at the other options:

A: No baker is tight-fisted. All the people living in this house are bakers. Therefore no one in this house is tight-fisted. If everyone is a baker and no baker is tight-fisted then we can safely deduce that no one is tight-fisted.

B: All peacocks are proud. All birds in this park are peacocks. Therefore all birds in this park are proud. If all birds are peacocks and all peacocks are proud then it follows that all birds are proud.

C: Caterpillars are not edible. Some worms are edible. Therefore some worms are not caterpillars. All we can really conclude from the first two points is that the worms that are edible can't be caterpillars. Nothing can be concluded about the worms that are not edible. The fact that two objects possess the same characteristics does not mean they are linked.

DM 52 – Brothers

Q52 – D: Joseph is not the youngest.
The first sentence (Joseph is smaller than the oldest) enables us to conclude that Joseph is neither the tallest nor the oldest. The second sentence states that Arthur is not the youngest nor the smallest. The third sentence (Les is younger than the smallest of the three) enables us to conclude that Les is not the oldest nor the smallest. Therefore we can conclude that the smallest brother is Joseph and that the oldest brother is Arthur.

Since Les is younger than the smallest (who is Joseph), and Arthur is the oldest brother, we can conclude that Les is the youngest, followed by Joseph, followed by Arthur. There isn't enough information to conclude who of Les and Arthur is the tallest.

The information can be summarised as:

Name	Les	Joseph	Arthur
Place	Youngest	Middle	Oldest
Height	?	Smallest	?

DM 53 – Toys

Q53 – B: 5 families only have roller skates
The information can be drawn as follows:

```
        CAR (30)              BICYCLE (90)
                    ┌──┐
                    │50│
                    └──┘
                    10
            5
         (15–10)
                       30
                    (90–10–50)
                    5
                (50–30–10–5)

            ROLLER SKATES (50)
```

The 50 families owning a bicycle and no roller skates cannot be apportioned between the two sections, so options A, C, and D cannot be definitely validated.

DM 54 – Coloured Cubes

Q54 – B: Blue
The colour blue appears in the description of both cubes. On the first, it is adjacent to yellow and green, and on the second it is adjacent to black and white.

Since the cubes are identical, we can conclude that the blue side is surrounded by yellow, green, white and black and therefore its opposite side must be red (the only colour left). Hence, the opposite side to red must be blue.

DM 55 – Wooden Tables

Q55.1 – NO. People who wear a hat don't have to be carpenters. If they are not carpenters, then they can't build strong tables.

Q55.2 – NO. That would be true of all strong tables (which are all made of wood) but a flimsy wooden table could be built by anyone.

Q55.3 – NO. All carpenters are bald and all bald people wear a hat. Therefore all carpenters wear a hat.

Q55.4 – NO. All carpenters wear a hat but not all hat-wearers are carpenters. In fact people who wear a hat don't even need to be bald.

Q55.5 – NO. "Only carpenters build strong tables" does not mean "Carpenters build only strong tables". It is possible for a carpenter to build a flimsy table.

DM 56 – Lineage

Q56 – D: John's son
"My grandfather's grandchild" is John himself. Therefore the sentence can be rephrased as "I am the grandfather of this man's son.". Therefore "This man's son" must be his grandson. Hence this man is his son.

DM 57 – Library

Q57.1 – NO. For a foreign book to have a red cover, it would need to have illustrations. We cannot determine that from the text.

Q57.2 – NO. We would need to show that books with illustrations have over 200 pages. All we know is that they have red covers.

Q57.3 – NO. All books with an index have over 200 pages.

Q57.4 – NO. Only the books with an index have over 200 pages. Therefore a 600-page book will have an index, regardless of its colour.

Q57.5 – YES. All English books have a red cover and only the books with illustrations have a red cover. Therefore all English books have illustrations.

DM 58 – Friday 13th

Q58 – A: The last day of the month will be a Friday
If the 13th is a Friday then so is the 27th of the month. Months have 28, 29, 30 or 31 days. Therefore months containing a Friday 13th will end either on a Saturday, a Sunday, a Monday or a Tuesday. But never on a Friday.

DM 59 – Labels

Q59 – D: It can be B or C
In the second box, the two plain hexagons are not round (and therefore cannot be A) and do not have dots (and therefore cannot be C); hence they are B. The second box contains two As. We know that As should be round. Therefore only the two circles (the plain black one and the white one with a dot) fit the criteria. From that box we can therefore conclude the following:

In the first box we know that the white circle with a black dot and the black circle are both labelled A (using the above information). If another one of the shapes were to be A, then there would be three As and it would not be possible to have more Bs than As. Therefore these are the only As in the box. Hence the other four shapes are either B or C; but since we know there must be more Bs than As then at least three of them are B. This leaves the door open for the fourth one to be either B or C.

DM 60 – Order

Q60 – C: 5
Piece 3 has at least one triangle and at least one black shape. So C = 3.
Other than C, A is the only piece that contains a star, so A = 6.
Other than A, E is the only piece that contains a square, so E = 2.
Other than E, D is the only piece that contains two black shapes, so D = 4.
Other than D, B is the only piece that contains two circles, so B = 1
Hence F = 5.

Decision Making – Practice

DM 61 – Tokens

Q61 – D: The left-hand token is either yellow or green.
Note that the fact that one token is on the right or the left of another token does not necessarily mean they are next to each other.

If the blue token is on the right of the yellow token, we start with the configuration: YELLOW – BLUE. The blue token is on the left of the white token; hence we get: YELLOW – BLUE – WHITE.

The blue token is on the right of the green token. This leads to two possibilities:

- GREEN – YELLOW – BLUE – WHITE
- YELLOW – GREEN – BLUE – WHITE

There are two tokens between the white token and the red token. Hence the red token cannot be on the right-hand side otherwise it would be next to the white token. Hence we are left with the two options:

- GREEN – RED – YELLOW – BLUE – WHITE
- YELLOW – RED – GREEN – BLUE – WHITE

DM 62 – Xanias and Zazas

Q62.1 – NO. The fact that two entities share the same characteristic does not mean that they are the same.

Q62.2 – NO. Same reasoning as Q62.1.

Q62.3 – NO. Two entities which share the same characteristic could be the same, though they don't have to be. So we cannot conclude either way.

Q62.4 – YES. See reasoning for 62.3. The use of the word 'can' is the key here.

Q62.5 – NO. The fact all Xanias are Yogos does not mean all Yogos are Xanias. Using an analogy: all cats are mammals but not all mammals are cats.

DM 63 – Student Life

Q63 – C: Female students below age 25 who enjoy sport.
A is outside of the square (hence not male) but is inside all the other shapes (hence students under age 25 who enjoy sport).

DM 64 – Food Allergies

Q64 – A
All those allergic to cheese are also allergic to garlic. The cheese circle must therefore be entirely included within the garlic circle. This excludes Diagram B.

Those allergic to tomatoes can eat garlic or cheese. So it means that the tomato circle is totally separated from the garlic circle (which contains the cheese circle). This excludes Diagram D.

So far we have the following:

We know that some people allergic to tomatoes cannot eat pasta so the pasta circle must cross the tomato circle, but the pasta circle cannot entirely contain the tomato circle otherwise it would mean that all those allergic to tomatoes are also allergic to pasta. Also we know that all those allergic to pasta are also allergic to cheese. So we get:

i.e. Diagram A.

Decision Making – Practice

DM 65 – Student Athletes

Q65.1 – NO. It is possible that all those who play cricket also play football. Hence the figure is 50%, not 10%.

Q65.2 – YES. The minimum percentage of students who play neither cricket nor rugby is 100 – 50 – 30 = 20%.

Q65.3 – NO. We have seen from Q65.2 that at least 20% of students do not play cricket or rugby. So it is possible that no one plays all three sports.

Q65.4 – NO. If all those who play rugby also play football, then 30% of students play both, 30% play football and not rugby, and 40% of students play neither. It is true however that AT LEAST (not at most) 10% of students do not play football or rugby.

Q65.5 – YES. If all those who played rugby also played cricket and football, then 30% of students would be playing all three sports. There can't be more, but there could be fewer (as few as zero, as we have seen from Q65.3).

DM 66 – Rectangular Table

Q66 – C: Karl sits in Seat 6.
Since Mary occupies Seat 1, and the two women are not sitting side by side, Louisa cannot be sitting in Seats 2 or 6. Also, since Damian is sitting opposite Louisa, Louisa cannot be sitting in Seat 4 either (since Seat 1 is occupied by Mary). Hence Louisa is sitting in Seats 3 or 5, as is Damian. With Patrick sitting on Louisa's right, we therefore have two possibilities:

```
          Patrick  Louisa                      Damian
            ②       ③                    ②       ③
   Mary  ①              ④            ①              ④  k
            ⑥       ⑤                    ⑥       ⑤
                 Damian                          Louisa
```

Karl is not sitting next to Damian; therefore this eliminates the first option since the only two seats left are next to Damian.

The layout is as follows:

```
              Rob   Damian
            ┌──────────────┐
            │  ②     ③    │
    Mary    │①            ④│  Patrick
            │  ⑥     ⑤    │
            └──────────────┘
              Karl  Louisa
```

DM 67 – False Positives

Q67 – C: Yes, this is because the low prevalence of the protein presence makes the test very unreliable.
We know that 0.1% of individuals will have the protein in question in their blood. So, if we take 1000 people, 1 person will have it and 999 will not.

Since the test accurately predicts the presence of the protein when it is there, we know that the 1 person who has it will have tested positive.

Out of the remaining 999 people, we know that 5% will wrongly be testing positive. So out of 1000 people, 1 + 0.05 x 999 = 51 people will have a positive test. But only one of them will actually have the protein. i.e. 1/51 i.e. about 2%.

We can see that the problem is that the low prevalence means that the numerator is only 1. Had the protein been more prevalent, the rate would be higher. For example, if the protein was present in 70% of people, then the calculation would be 700 / (700 + 0.05 x 300) = 700/715 = 98%.

DM 68 – Speed Humps

Q68 – B: YES. People hit by vehicles at lower speeds sustain less serious injuries.
This answer provides a practical consequence of implementing the speed humps. Looking at the other options:

A: YES. This would help raise awareness of the dangers of the road amongst drivers. This is a sensible answer, but it merely deals with awareness and not necessarily a change in behaviour (which, after all, would be the point of lowering the speed limit). As such we can only speculate that this argument would lead to a practical effect.

C: NO. More emphasis should be placed instead on educating pedestrians on the dangers of the road. That may well be the case, but the two are not mutually exclusive. In addition, educating pedestrians would help make them more careful but it would not reduce the severity of the accidents if any occurred. Option B would serve both purposes.

D: NO. Road humps could damage cars. This is a side issue and is in many ways speculative. The main problem is speed reduction, and one could argue that, if the humps are driven over at low speed, there should be no damage.

DM 69 – Asthmatic Nurses

Q69.1 – NO. Any smoker who hasn't got asthma could potentially be a nurse.

Q69.2 – NO. It is possible that some smokers could be nurses (if they don't have asthma) but nothing helps us conclude definitely that this is the case. If the question said: "Some smokers may be nurses" instead of the more definite "Some smokers are nurses", the answer would be YES.

Q69.3 – YES. We know that no nurse has asthma. So, if anyone has asthma, they cannot be a nurse.

Q69.4 – NO. We simply know that <u>many</u> smokers are asthmatic.

Q69.5 – YES. Like Q69.3 but with the added restriction of smoker, which makes no difference in this case since asthma is the determining factor.

DM 70 – Who Lives Where?

Q70 – B: George does not live in Pontefract.
From the third statement, we can see that Birmingham can only be home to either Steve or Phil. Hence option A is incorrect. Since Martin does not live in Birmingham, then it follows that George does not live in Manchester. Hence option D is incorrect. From the first statement we can conclude that, since George does not live in Manchester then Phil lives neither in Pontefract nor in London. Hence option C is incorrect. From the fourth statement we can conclude that since Phil does not live in London then George cannot live in Pontefract. Hence option B is correct.

DM 71 – Coding

Q71 – B: 28641

The key here is to try to identify patterns. An obvious starting point would be to look at whether two numbers have the same digit in the same position (e.g. two of them start with a '1' etc.) but that is not the case. Here we could start, for example, by noticing that 12478 starts with 12 and 1 and 2 are also the last and middle digit of 75261. So if we could find two numbers which satisfy this relationship and are unique in doing so then we can start the deducing.

Here we can see that 47285 starts with 47 and that 86734 has 4 and 7 in last and middle position. They are the only pair to satisfy that relationship. Hence 12478 is encoded as 47285; and 75261 is encoded as 86734.

Therefore:

1 becomes 4	6 becomes 3
2 becomes 7	7 becomes 8
4 becomes 2	8 becomes 5
5 becomes 6	

In turn it means that 34852 must be encoded as ?2567. The only number which matches this is 92567 and so 3 is encoded as 9.

Hence 75324 is the code for 28641. Make sure you use the code in reverse otherwise you will get the answer 86972. The number 75324 is the number once it has been coded, not before.

DM 72 – Guilty Or Not Guilty

Q72 – A: Eddie is guilty

If Fred is guilty then they are all guilty, therefore Victor is guilty. However, we know if Victor is guilty then there are only two guilty suspects. This is contradictory. Hence Fred must be innocent.

We are told that if Theo is guilty then he has two accomplices, which means that three people would be guilty. We know that Fred is innocent, so that would mean that Victor would be guilty. But we are told that if Victor is guilty then there are only two suspects. Hence this is contradictory and so Theo is not guilty.

Therefore, there are only two possible suspects left: Eddie and Victor. We know that if Eddie is innocent then Theo is not innocent (i.e. he is guilty). But we know that Theo is innocent, therefore Eddie cannot be innocent. Hence Eddie is guilty.

However, we are unable to determine whether Victor is also guilty or not. Indeed, if he were guilty then both he and Eddie would be guilty and that would be compatible with the fourth statement. No statement helps decide either way, hence options B, C and D cannot be concluded to be definitely true.

DM 73 – Fertility Study

Q73 – B: These 1000 women collectively have over 1850 children.
The minimum number of children will be calculated as:

1000 x (0 x 20% + 1 x 25% + 2 x 25% + 3 x 15% + 4 x 10% + 5 x 5%)
= 1000 x (0 + 25% + 50% + 45% + 40% + 25%)
= 1000 x 185% = 1850 children.

Note that the minimum is calculated by assuming that those who have more than four children have only five.

Looking at the other options:

A: 50% of women who have at least one child have at least three children. The percentage of women with at least one child is 80%. The percentage of women with at least three children is 15 + 10 + 5 = 30%. The ratio is 30/80 = 37.5%, well below 50%.

C: The probability that one woman chosen at random has at least 3 children is greater than 35%. The probability is 15 + 10 + 5 = 30% and so is lower than 35%.

D: 55% of children have at least one brother and one sister. No information is given about the gender of the children.

DM 74 – Curious Food Lovers

C: All nice people are beyond reproach.
Here we are looking for a statement that contradicts the facts given. So, the logic must lead you to conclude that the statement made is false and not simply that it cannot be proven. We know that some food lovers are curious and that all curious people are nice. So, we can conclude that some food lovers are nice. We also know that no food lover is beyond reproach. So, we can conclude that some food lovers are nice but not beyond reproach. Therefore, it is not true that all nice people are beyond reproach.

Looking at the other options:

A: Some food lovers are nice. We have demonstrated that above.

B: Some nice people are beyond reproach. All we know is that someone who is beyond reproach cannot be a food lover. Anyone who is nice could potentially be beyond reproach as long as they are not a food lover. There is not enough information to conclude that this goes against the information provided.

D: Some curious people love food. We have already established that some food lovers are curious. Therefore, there are some curious people who love food.

DM 75 – Colourful Bouquet

A: There are 400 red flowers.
We can summarise the information given in a table as follows:

	Roses	Tulips	Pansies	TOTAL
White	100 (a)	120 (a)	**180**	400 (a)
Red	**60**	40 (b)	200 =300-60-40	300 (c)
Yellow	140 =300-60-100	40 (b)	120 =500-180-200	300 (c)
TOTAL	300 (=60/0.2)	200 (1000-300-500)	500 (0.5 x 1000)	**1000**

Decision Making – Practice

(a) We are told that there are 180 white pansies, that one quarter of white flowers are roses and that 30% of white flowers are tulips. Therefore, the white pansies represent 1 – 25% – 30% = 45% of white flowers. Hence the number of white flowers is 180/0.45 = 400. This in turn means there are 100 white roses and therefore 120 white tulips

(b) There are 200 tulips in total including 120 white ones. We are told the red and yellow tulips are in a 50:50 ratio. So there are 40 of each type.

(c) There are 1000 flowers in total, 400 of which are white. Since there are as many red flowers as yellow flowers then there are 300 of each.

Important note: make sure that you check the options and eliminate them as you go along. You do not actually need to complete the whole table to get to the point where you can figure out that option A is incorrect. In a question like this, as soon as you find that one answer satisfies the criteria, you do not need to demonstrate that the others do not.

DM 76 – Movie Munchies

Q76 – D: Saria's brother
If there are three sisters and Saria has two older sisters, then she is the youngest girl. Therefore, she has bought a savoury snack. Since we are told she does not like nachos then she must have bought the salty popcorn. In turn, this means that the eldest (Varunee), who has bought a savoury snack, has bought the nachos. Since one of the girls picked no snack, it means that the candy floss was bought by the brother.

DM 77 – Supporting Colours

Q77 – C: Keith does not support Newton United.
The information can be summarised in a grid as follows:

	Binbury C	Binbury U	Weston C	Newtown U
Sushama	X	X		
Keith	X	YES	X	NO
Grace	YES	X	NO	X
Vijay	X	X		

X = information provided, YES and NO are deduced from that information.

Note that you can't resolve the whole grid and that is why answers B and D are incorrect. We cannot say for certain that they MUST be true.

DM 78 – Youth Travel

Q78 – A: Austria.
Ann and Ben are essentially saying the same thing, so they will be telling the same lies and truths and we can just ignore one of them.

If Ann is telling the truth when she says that she visited England, then it means that Carole is lying when she says that she (herself) visited England. And since one person can only tell one lie then it means that Carole must be correct when she is saying that Ann visited Austria. This contradicts our assumption that Ann visited England. Therefore, Ann has not visited England.

If Carole is telling the truth when she says she visited England, then it means that Ann is lying when she says she visited England. That would then mean that the other two statements made by Ann are correct, in particular that Carole visited Italy. This contradicts our assumption that Carole visited England. Hence neither Ann nor Carole visited England and they both lied in that regard.

Therefore their other statements are all correct and: Carole visited Italy, Ben visited Germany, and Ann visited Austria.

DM 79 – Golf Club

Q79.1 – NO. We know that those who wear white socks wear a bowler hat. We also know that all those with a bowler hat wear glasses. Therefore we can conclude that those who wear white socks all wear glasses. But we are told that none of the dishonest people wear glasses. Therefore someone with white socks cannot be dishonest.

Q79.2 – NO. We know that all golf players have blue eyes. Therefore we can deduce that those who do not have blue eyes are not golf players.

We know that all those who wear a black jacket are golf players. Therefore since those who do not have blue eyes are not golf players then we can conclude that they don't wear a black jacket.

We are told that those who wear a black jacket don't have a beard, but we know nothing about those who do not wear a black jacket. Therefore we cannot conclude either way.

Decision Making – Practice

Q79.3 – NO. Similar argument to Q79.1.

Q79.4 – YES. We know that none of the dishonest people wear glasses. Therefore, if someone wears glasses then it means they are honest.

Q79.5 – YES. We know that many of the dishonest guests have brown hair. We also know that none of the dishonest people wear glasses. Therefore, the dishonest guests with brown hair do not wear glasses.

Q79.6 – YES. We are told that none of those who wear a black jacket has a beard. Therefore, if someone has a beard, then they can't be wearing a black jacket.

Q79.7 – NO. We know that if someone does not play golf, it means that they cannot have a black jacket. We know that those who have a black jacket don't have a beard, but we don't know if that is the case for those who don't have a black jacket.

Q79.8 – YES. All guests with a black jacket are golf players. And all golf players have blue eyes.

Q79.9 – YES. If those who wear white sock wear a bowler hat, then someone who is not wearing a bowler hat can't have white socks.

Q79.10 – NO. Those with glasses will be honest (since dishonest guests do not wear glasses). We know nothing about the relationship between honest guests and brown hair.

Q79.11 – YES. All guests with brown hair have a hearing aid. That means that if someone has no hearing aid then they cannot have brown hair.

Q79.12 – YES. Many of the dishonest guests have brown hair. Since all guests with brown hair have a hearing aid, we can conclude that many of the dishonest guests have a hearing aid.

DM 80 – Coded Language

Q80 – D: Either "ta" or "mo"
"Economics" appears in sentences 1, 2 and 4, for which the only word in common is "ka". Hence "economics" = "ka". "Supply" appears in sentences

2 and 4, which have the words "mo", "ta" and "ka" in common. Since "ka" means "Economics" then "supply" is coded by "mo" or "ta". Because the word "demand" also appears in the same sentences as "supply" without appearing anywhere else, we are unable to determine which specific word corresponds to "supply".

DM 81 – Going South

Q81 – A: 50 metres North
See diagram below

```
          30 →
        ↑
  100   │
        │   │
        │   │ 50
        └───↓
          30
```

DM 82 – Going Round In Circles

Q82 – B: F
If E is on the immediate right of A and A is second to the right of G then we obtain the following:

If F is third to the right of C and second to the left of H then it means that C and H are five places apart with F in between, two places away from H. Since H is sitting next to A, then C is next to E and F is next to G.

Since D is not an immediate neighbour of C, D must be next to F. Hence F is sitting between D and G.

Decision Making – Practice

DM 83 – Extra-Terrestrial Foliage

Q83.1 – YES. Kendu are trees and we know that trees must be greater than half a Jobobum. A Jobobum is 7 Farinks so half a Jobobum is 3.5 Farinks.

Q83.2 – NO. Kendu trees can have needles. The limitation with the colour red is to do with the fruit, not the tree itself.

Q83.3 – NO. If a Kendu tree has leaves then it has no needles. We know that red Zechbodies (i.e. the fruit) does not grow on trees when there are needles, but it does not automatically follow that they grow systematically on trees with leaves. It is possible that the Kendu tree has blue fruits.

Q83.4 – NO. The text mentions that Guruk flowers have suckers but nothing precludes the existence of trees with suckers. Those would be over half a Jobobum high.

Q83.5 – NO. Similar to the previous question, we do not know what other plant life may exist on this planet and the text specifies 'Red Zechbodies never grow on trees where needles are present'. That doesn't mean you can't find <u>flowers</u> with needles and red Zechbodies.

DM 84 – Foodie's Delight

It helps if you sketch out the six time slots: three in the morning and three in afternoon (see diagram below). There are 5 types of sessions running so we know that one has to run twice. Since the cake competition and the wine tasting run just once we can say that the extra session has to be a food demonstration. Due to the cleaning time constraints, we can start to fill the grid:

9-10am	10-11am	11-12pm	1.15-2pm	2-2.45pm	2.45-3.30pm
Demo	Wine/cake	Demo	Demo	Wine/cake	Demo

We know that the cake competition is in the afternoon, so the wine tasting is in the morning and lasts one hour.

The fish demonstrator must leave by 1:30pm and so the fish demonstration can only take place in the morning. Since the vegetables demonstration and the fish demonstration run for different times, it means the vegetables demonstration is in the afternoon.

The bread demonstration takes 45 minutes and must therefore be in the afternoon. This now means that both the vegetable and the bread demonstrations have to be in the afternoon; and since there are only two demonstrations in the afternoon, they are both run only once. This means the fish demonstration has to run twice in the morning. So we now have:

9-10am	10-11am	11-12pm	1.15-2pm	2-2.45pm	2.45-3.30pm
Fish	Wine	Fish	Bread or Veg	Cake	Bread or Veg

Hence the answers are:

Q84.1 – YES
Q84.2 – NO. She has 1.5 hours from 3:30pm to 5pm, not just one hour.
Q84.3 – NO. It could also be at 2:45pm
Q84.4 – YES
Q84.5 – YES

DM 85 – Double Winners

Q85 – A: £1
At the end of the 5th round we have: Andrea = £4, Ben = £18 and Charles = £5. Since the two winners have just doubled their pot, it means that the winners are the two who have an even number of pounds, i.e. Andrew and Ben.

So at the end of round 4, they had: Andrew: 4/2 = £2 and Ben: 18/2 = £9. The £11 they collectively won in round 5 were therefore taken from Charles. So Charles had 5 + 11 = £16. We can then apply the same principle to all the other rounds, halving the pots of those with an even amount and adding the amount into the loser's pot. We get:

End of round	Andrea	Ben	Charles
5	4	18	5
4	4/2 = 2	18/2 = 9	5 + 9 + 2 = 16
3	2/2 = 1	9 + 1 + 8 = 18	16/2 = 8
2	1 + 9 + 4 = 14	18/2 = 9	8/2 = 4
1	14/2 = 7	9 + 7 + 2 = 18	4/2 = 2
Start of game	7 + 9 + 1 = 17	18/2 = 9	2/2 = 1

Hence Charles started the game with just £1.

Decision Making – Practice

DM 86 – Alarm Clocks

Q86 – C: 02:48

| A | B | C | D | E |

Since John's and Brendan's alarm clocks are not yet past 2:45 we know that they are A and E (though we don't know in what order). Animesh's alarm clock is on the immediate left of Lydia's, so it means that Animesh's clock is either B or C.

If Animesh is in C then Lydia is in D and Anna is in B. But that would mean that wherever John is (A or E) he would be either next to Anna or next to Lydia. This contradicts the information given.

If Animesh is in B then Lydia is in C and Anna is in D. Since John cannot be next to Lydia or Anna, it means John is in A. So we get:

A	B	C	D	E
John	Animesh	Lydia	Anna	Brendan

DM 87 – Births, Marriages and Deaths

Q87 – D: None of the above.
All questions relate to Michael and Paul and so the statement about John is irrelevant. All we know is that Michael got married after Paul's birth, but we don't know if Paul was still alive at that time. So, we cannot conclude that A, B or C are correct.

DM 88 – Light Weights

Q88 – C: D could be lighter than C.
We know that A is lighter than B, which itself is lighter than D. As for C, we simply know that it is heavier than A but we don't know where it fits in relation to B and D. It is possible that C is the heaviest of all.

DM 89 – Relationships

Q89.1 – D: A % B x D $ C
A is the mother of B who is the sister of D, who is the wife of C. Hence A is C's mother-in-law. Looking at the other options:
- **A:** A is the mother of B, who is the sister of C. So A is the mother of C
- **B:** A is the mother of B, who is the son of C. So A and C are mother and father, assuming they are different individuals.
- **C:** B is the son of A who is the son of C. So A is the son of C

Q89.2 – C: Daughter
C is a woman since she is the sister of D. She is also the sister of B, and A is the father of B. Hence C is A's daughter.

Q89.3 – C: C + A
A / B $ C means that A is the son of B, who is the wife of C. Hence C is A's father. Therefore the expression C + A is true.

Looking at the other options:
- **A:** A + C means that A is C's father, which is not true.
- **B:** C % B means that C is the mother of B. They are in fact married.
- **D:** C / B x A means that C is B's son, when in fact they are married.

Q89.4 – A: x
J / P means that J is the son of P.
P % H means that P is the mother of H.
So we can deduce that J and H are either the same person or siblings.
So for J to be the brother of T, we would need H and T to be siblings too. The only possibility is "x", i.e. H is the sister of T.

Q89.5 – B: K is the son-in-law of I
I + T means that I is the father of T and is a man. So option C is false.
T % J means that T is the mother of J. So that excludes option D.
J x L means that J is the sister of L. So that excludes option E.
L / K means that L is the son of K and so is male. That excludes option A.

This leaves option B. If you wanted to work it out by deduction rather than by elimination, here is the process: we know from above that T is the mother of J, who is the sister of L. Hence T is the mother of L. We know that L is the child of T and also of K. Since T is female, then K is male and T is married to K. I is the father of T, hence K is the son-in-law of I.

Decision Making – Practice

DM 90 – Cuppa Anyone?

Q90.1 – NO. There is nothing in the text that supports this.

Q90.2 – NO. Although her most expensive teas are oolongs that doesn't mean that most or all oolongs are expensive. So, even though most Taiwanese are oolongs it can't follow for sure that most Taiwanese teas are expensive.

Q90.3 – NO. You cannot make a blend with more than one subtype.

Q90.4 – NO. There is nothing in the text that supports this.

Q90.5 – YES. The operative word is 'may'. The only restriction is that a blend cannot contain more than one subtype. Since you can get some subtypes in more than one country (we know there are at least six countries and only three different subtypes), it is possible to build a blend from more than one country. Had the word 'may' been omitted, the answer would have been 'no'.

Q90.6 – YES. Both blends and single origin teas can be scented, which means in effect that all teas can be scented, including Kenyan tea.

Q90.7 – NO. Nothing in the text suggests it is the case. All we know is that the majority of her teas are from China but we don't know what subtype they are.

Q90.8 – NO. All Kenyan tea is black and all Japanese tea is green. Different subtypes cannot be blended, so a Japanese/Kenyan blend is not possible.

Q90.9 – YES. We know that her teas come from six different countries. So one of those countries is unnamed in the text.

Q90.10 – NO. The word 'expensive' used in the information provided does not necessarily translate into expensive production costs. It could simply be expensive because it is rare. Also, as in Q90.2, we can't conclude that Taiwanese tea is expensive in any case.

DM 91 – Garden Gnomes

Q91 – C
All those with boots wear glasses, so we expect one shape (for the boots) to be totally included within another (for the glasses). That is the case for A and C.

Each shape represents a feature. If those with a beard do not wear boots or a hat, then we expect one of the shapes to be detached from two others. This excludes A.

Therefore the answer is C.

DM 92 – House Features

Q92 – B: There are 20 houses with a driveway, a chimney but no front garden.
Houses with a driveway, a chimney but no front garden are represented by the two sections labelled A and B. Their number is therefore A + B.

We cannot estimate A and B individually, but since we know that there are 100 houses in total, then A + B will be the difference between 100 and the sum of the numbers shown on the diagram.

The sum of those numbers is: 10 + 5 + 7 + 9 + 8 + 9 + 12 + 15 + 5 = 80.

Hence there are 100 – 80 = 20 such houses.

Looking at the other options:

A: There are more houses with a chimney than with a driveway.
The numbers are 33 + A + B and 41 + A + B respectively so it is not true.

C: There are 40 houses with exactly one feature.
There are in fact 10 + 7 + 8 + 5 = 30.

D: The number of houses with all four features cannot be determined.
The four areas do not all intersect at the same time. Hence there is no house with all four features.

Decision Making – Practice

DM 93 – Guidebooks

Q93 – D: At least a quarter of those who travelled abroad have one or more guidebooks.
30 people never travelled abroad, yet 35 people have a guidebook for Greece. It means that at least 5 people who travelled abroad have a guidebook for Greece. Since there are 20 people who travelled abroad, that represents one quarter.

Looking at the other options:

A: At least 15 people do not have any guidebook.
It is possible that all of them have a guidebook since there are 55 guidebooks for 50 people. So this is incorrect.

B: All those who travelled abroad have at least one guidebook.
It is possible that 30 of the 35 Greek guidebooks belong to non-travellers and that all 20 Spanish guidebooks also belong to non-travellers. In this case, 15 of the travellers would have no guidebook at all.

C: At least five people who travelled abroad possess both guidebooks. Since the 20 Spanish guidebooks could belong to non-travellers, this is not correct.

DM 94 – Big Spender

Q94.1 – NO. All we know is that those who have shopped online must have also visited a high street shop. It is possible to have visited a high street shop and not have done any online shopping.

Q94.2 – YES. If they had done any online shopping, they would also have visited a high street shop since no one shopped exclusively online.

Q94.3 – NO. None of the information provided points to the fact that everyone went shopping.

Q94.4 – NO. Nothing in the text implies it.

Q94.5 – NO. This group could include people who did two trips to the high street.

Q94.6 – NO. The maximum of five is for high street shops. But if we add online shopping, this could go well above five times.

Q94.7 – NO. Those who did online shopping (and we know there are some) will also have gone to the high street. Therefore some high street shoppers have done online shopping.

Q94.8 – NO. An average of three could be achieved with no one visiting a high street shop three times.

SITUATIONAL JUDGEMENT

TIPS & TECHNIQUES

+

247
PRACTICE QUESTIONS & ANSWERS

15 Situational Judgement Format, Purpose & Key Techniques

PURPOSE AND FORMAT

The Situational Judgement section of the UCAT is designed to assess that you possess a range of skills expected of doctors, particularly integrity and an ability to show perspective in decision making, as well as an ability to work with people. It is designed to test whether you are guided by the right principles. For the purpose of the UCAT, you will be asked to answer a total of 69 questions, which relate to 22 different scenarios. One scenario will lead to between two and five questions. The time allocated is 26 minutes + 1 minute to read the instructions.

Given that it will take you about 30 seconds to read and understand each of the scenarios (thereby taking up 11 minutes of valuable time since there are 22 scenarios in total), you will be left with just about 15 minutes to understand and answer the 69 questions, i.e. about 22 seconds per question. You therefore need think fast because you won't have much time to debate which option to choose. In turn that means you need to acquire the ability to spot straight away what is being tested through each question and therefore how to best answer it.

One big issue with Situational Judgement tests is that the answers are not as clear cut as they might be for quantitative or verbal reasoning (where there is a definite correct answer). Indeed, Situational Judgement tests are often called SUBJECTIVE judgement tests because different people may allocate different levels of appropriateness to different courses of action. In practice, the questions are validated by asking 100 people to try them out. If more than, say, 90% of the people involved answer the same thing, then the question makes its way into the exam and their answer is taken as the correct answer. If a lower percentage of people answer the same thing, then the question is dismissed from the exam. So that means that you are being judged against what most people would answer. For that reason, the marking scheme recognises a degree of tolerance in favour of candidates who are not too far off the "correct" answer by allocating partial marks. So, for example, if you said that a course of action was "appropriate" but the answer was that it should be "very appropriate" then you would still score

Situational Judgement – Practice

some marks. However, if you said that it was inappropriate then you would score nothing.

In the UCAT, there are three types of question, both based on a central scenario.

TYPE 1 QUESTIONS
You are given a scenario and several courses of action. You are asked to ascertain the appropriateness or the importance of each:

Appropriateness options

A – A very appropriate thing to do. Usually that would be the case if a particular action helps resolve part or all of the problem in question in a suitable way (and most of the issues you will encounter will revolve around determining whether that way is actually suitable).

B – Appropriate, but not ideal. This is something that can be done but is not necessarily the most appropriate response.

C – Inappropriate but not awful. It shouldn't really be done but it would not be a terrible thing to do, for example, because the consequences are minor. An example of that would be asking a colleague to do one of your jobs for you because you are struggling to get everything done, in a context where you are not dealing with an emergency.

D – A very inappropriate thing to do. It should not be done and would make things worse. This applies to unethical behaviour or actions that place patients or other people at risk.

Importance options

A – Very important, i.e. it simply cannot be dismissed.

B – Important, i.e. it is not vital, but it may make a difference.

C – Of minor importance, i.e. it has some importance, but it won't hurt if you forget to take it into account. Essentially it is mildly relevant to the decision-making process.

D – Not important at all, i.e. it is either irrelevant or makes you think "Who cares?"

TYPE 2 QUESTIONS
You are given a scenario and a possible course of action. You simply need to decide if the given course of action is appropriate or not. Type 2 questions are essentially a cut-down version of Type 1 questions on appropriateness. The scenarios are usually easy to get right if you have some basic common sense.

TYPE 3 QUESTIONS
You are given a scenario and three possible actions. You need to decide which of the three actions is the most appropriate and which is the least appropriate.

KEY TECHNIQUES

Familiarise yourself with the issues that you are being tested on

The Situational Judgement section of the UCAT is designed to test that you have a good understanding of your responsibilities as a medical student and a future doctor. Those responsibilities are set out in a document called "Good Medical Practice" issued by the General Medical Council (GMC), which you can find here:

www.gmc-uk.org/guidance/good_medical_practice.asp

For dental applicants, the duties are very similar and are set out in a document called "Standards and guidance", which you can find here:

https://www.gdc-uk.org/information-standards-guidance/standards-and-guidance

These documents deal with a wide range of issues, and you should take some time to read them. However, it is true to say that most of the questions asked in the UCAT tend to relate to the following points:

Integrity
Anything that highlights a lack of integrity will essentially not be forgiven. It means that such behaviours will always be ranked as very inappropriate and nothing a person can do or say will ever make such behaviour acceptable. As such, in Type 2 questions, such excuses will always be considered as not important at all.

Situational Judgement – Practice

Examples of lack of integrity include:
- Lying to anyone if the intention is to mislead. So, for example, if you made a mistake, saying that someone made it and not you would be misleading. Similarly, telling a patient that their tests were ordered on time when in fact they were not would be misleading. However, some (rare) "white lies" may rank as "Appropriate, but not ideal" if the consequences of telling the truth would be more harmful to a patient. So, for example, imagine blood results had come back showing that a patient had a serious illness but you, as a medical student, would not be in a position to explain those results to a patient; if the patient asked you what the test results showed, you might say "I am not sure if they have come back yet", thinking that telling the patient they had come back without being able to answer their questions would actually make the patient become anxious.
- Cheating of any kind.
- Covering mistakes or problems up, even if it is by fear. That also means that you should feel confident in challenging another colleague if their behaviour is inappropriate.
- Stealing and, generally, doing anything criminal.
- Not recognising your limitations and, in particular, pretending that you know something that you don't know or "having a go" at something when you have no real expertise. Typically, this would involve scenarios where a patient is asking you to explain something you are unsure about, or where a colleague is asking you to do a procedure that you are not allowed or qualified to undertake. This applies whether you are under pressure or not. There is simply no excuse.
- Breaching confidentiality. This includes looking up patient records when they are none of your concern, as well as sharing information about patients with others, even if such sharing is accidental (e.g. you left some notes in a public place) and even if the patient is not identifiable.
- Discussing internal issues in a public forum (e.g. complaining about working conditions at the hospital on a bus, or on social media – this could undermine public confidence in the care provided there).
- Having relationships with patients.

Teamwork
Teamwork will involve making sure that you support your colleagues appropriately, that you do not impose burdens on them, that you involve them appropriately in relevant matters or discussions and that you respect them.

Examples of bad teamwork would include:
- Undermining a colleague in front of a patient (very inappropriate).
- Reporting colleagues to their supervisors without addressing the issue with the colleague first for simple issues with benign consequences (inappropriate but not awful). It is however appropriate to seek advice from someone you trust before discussing the matter directly with the colleague in question.
- Ignoring complaints from colleagues about your behaviour (usually very inappropriate – you may not change your behaviour after reflection, but you would at least need to acknowledge the issue and look into it).
- Pulling out of prearranged meetings without appropriate communication (inappropriate but not awful, unless the prearranged meeting was about patient care or with mandatory attendance, in which case it would be very inappropriate).
- Dumping your problems on to other people, such as asking another colleague to take on a more menial or boring task just because you have more interesting things to do (appropriate but not awful). Generally, you must demonstrate you can take responsibility for your own problems.
- Rudeness, even if provoked (inappropriate but not awful).

Bits and pieces
Here are a number of important points to remember:
- Listening to or reassuring a patient should always be ranked as "very appropriate" or "very important".
- You should prioritise clinical emergencies over anything else. A patient who is not an emergency (e.g. a sprained ankle) might be able to wait if something more pressing needs doing (e.g. dealing with a lost child). It's not ideal but it's appropriate.
- You should ensure timely communication with everyone.
- You should generally not do anything that may harm the patient (and this includes harm such as making them lose confidence in the health service or their doctor).

Answer according to what you SHOULD do, not what you WOULD do
When we are confronted with a problem, often the situation leads us to react in a way that may not be entirely by the book. However, the purpose of the Situational Judgement test is not to test what you would actually do, but whether you are aware of the "correct" way, i.e. what you SHOULD do.

Situational Judgement – Practice

For example, one scenario given on the official website talks about an A&E doctor who is dealing with a patient with a sprained ankle, when he/she notices a child who seems to have become separated from his mother. The question then asks whether it is appropriate for the doctor to ask the receptionist to take charge of the child whilst he/she deals with the patient with the sprained ankle.

Many people would think this would be a reasonable thing to do because the receptionist is not seeing patients and may have time to find the mother of the child; as such some may rate it as "A: Very appropriate". However, the official answer is that it is "Inappropriate but not awful" on the basis that the patient is not an emergency and it would not be right to make the receptionist deal with the child since she probably has other things to do. The premise is that both the doctor and the receptionist are equal members of the team and therefore there is no reason why one should dump his/her problems on to the other one. However, if the patient had been an emergency, then this would have been a "very appropriate" thing to do since the emergency patient would take precedence over the lost child and only the doctor could deal with that patient.

Judge each possible answer independently
For each scenario, you will be given a range of possible responses. You look at the question given to you without worrying about the others. It is perfectly possible that several courses of action may be very appropriate.

The option given should not be judged as if it is the only thing you do
In some situations, there may be several actions that need taking. For example, let's assume that a doctor has made a mistake and the wrong drug was given to a patient. The following will need to be done:

Step 1 – CLINICAL SOLUTION
Make sure the patient is fine by reversing the effects of the medication or just keeping an eye on them.

Step 2 – PATIENT COMMUNICATION
Be honest with the patient about the mistake, apologise and explain what happened.

Step 3 – COLLEAGUE COMMUNICATION
Make sure a senior doctor is alerted.

Step 4 – DOCUMENTATION
Document the mistake in the notes.

Step 5 – LEARN FROM THE MISTAKE
Raise it at a team meeting. If the same mistake keeps happening, then it may be worth doing an audit to see how frequent it is and change the way things are done within the department.

Each of those steps deals with different sides of the scenario. So:

- If you were given the action "Alert a senior colleague", this would be "Very Appropriate".

- If you were given "Apologise to the patient, explain what happened and reassure everything is now in hand ", this would be "Very Appropriate".

- If you were given "Discuss the mistake at a team meeting and organise an audit", that would also be "Very Appropriate".

However, be very careful:

If a statement relates to one category, then it will only be deemed "Very Appropriate" if it deals with the full picture for that category. So, for example, if the statement related to the communication with the patient, you should assume that whatever is in that statement is the entirety of the action taken for that step.

For example, in the case of the medication mistake described above, if the statement said: "Explain what happened to the patient" then this would only be ranked as "Appropriate, but not ideal" and not "Very Appropriate" because it would be missing the apology. The fact that the apology does not feature in the statement essentially means it is not given.

Practise and make sure you understand the logic
To be successful at Situational Judgement questions, it is vital that you practise on a lot of questions. Only then will you start to understand the patterns and apply them to various scenarios.

16 Situational Judgement Practice Questions

This section contains 54 scenarios, and a total of 247 practice questions. These questions are designed to help you develop an awareness of the different techniques and tips mentioned in the previous section and, as such, we have therefore generally included more questions per text than you would anticipate being asked to answer in the exam.

The answers to all questions, together with explanations, can be found from page 576 onwards.

Once you have practised answering all 247 questions, you should be ready to confront the mock exam, which features at the back of this book and replicates the actual exam's format.

You may want to wait until you have practised all the sections in this book before going ahead with the mock exam.

SJ 1 Practice — Scenario 1 – Aesthetics

Joshua is a medical student on a dermatology attachment. He is currently sitting in with a senior doctor and a nurse during a special rash clinic. Mr Andrews, a 75-year-old patient, presents with a nasty rash, complaining of severe itching; he mentions that he has previously been prescribed various ointments which all seemed to leave scars once the rash had disappeared.

Once the patient has left, whilst Joshua is still in the room, the senior doctor tells the nurse: "Honestly, at his age, aesthetics should be the least of Mr Andrews' worries." The nurse looks at Joshua and says: "Ignore him; he's always joking like that."

How appropriate are each of the following responses by **Joshua** in this situation?

1.1 Ask the senior doctor to apologise to the patient.

A – A very appropriate thing to do
B – Appropriate, but not ideal
C – Inappropriate but not awful
D – A very inappropriate thing to do

1.2 Politely ask the nurse to leave the room so that he can raise his concerns with the senior doctor before the next patient comes in.

A – A very appropriate thing to do
B – Appropriate, but not ideal
C – Inappropriate but not awful
D – A very inappropriate thing to do

1.3 Politely explain to the nurse and the senior doctor that he is not feeling well and withdraw from the clinic for the rest of the day.

A – A very appropriate thing to do
B – Appropriate, but not ideal
C – Inappropriate but not awful
D – A very inappropriate thing to do

1.4 Speak to the nurse privately after the clinic, making it clear that, joking or not, the comment was inappropriate, and ask her to speak to the senior doctor's supervisor about the incident.

A – A very appropriate thing to do
B – Appropriate, but not ideal
C – Inappropriate but not awful
D – A very inappropriate thing to do

SJ 2 Practice — Scenario 2 – Personal Statement

Two medical students in their first year, David and Sapna, are discussing the hard work they invested to gain entry into medical school. David mentions that he was fortunate that his uncle was a consultant in cardiology in a reputable hospital who also sat on interview panels; indeed, though David had not actually done any work experience, his uncle dictated to him a paragraph on work experience which would "push all the right buttons for the admission tutors". David is currently ranked in the top ten students of his class and is considered to be a very bright student who is always very honest.

How important to take into account are the following considerations for **Sapna** when deciding whether she should report the matter to a supervisor?

2.1 That David is now a top-ranking student.

A – Very important
B – Important
C – Of minor importance
D – Not important at all

2.2 That David's uncle's career may suffer if she discloses this information to anyone.

A – Very important
B – Important
C – Of minor importance
D – Not important at all

2.3 That this seems to be an isolated incident as David is now considered to be very honest.

A – Very important
B – Important
C – Of minor importance
D – Not important at all

2.4 That many other students in the school probably obtained some kind of help with their personal statement and may have lied or exaggerated a few things on it.

A – Very important
B – Important
C – Of minor importance
D – Not important at all

SJ 3 Practice — Scenario 3 – Staying Late

A junior doctor, Maryam, is working a shift which is meant to finish at 5:30 pm. At 5 pm, Maryam decides to use her last 30 minutes to check some blood test results on the computer. Unfortunately, she is unable to do so as the computer system is undergoing maintenance and will be unavailable for one to two hours.

Maryam then decides to contact another junior doctor (Rob) who is on call and will be looking after her patients from 5.30 onwards, to ask him to check the blood results when the system goes back online. Rob refuses point blank, telling Maryam that he would expect her to stick around for two hours to check the blood results herself. Maryam is working on a shift which starts at 7am early the next morning. She lives locally.

How appropriate are each of the following responses by **Maryam** in this situation?

3.1 Leave at 5:30 pm as planned and check the blood results in the morning if Rob has not done it before.

A – A very appropriate thing to do
B – Appropriate, but not ideal
C – Inappropriate but not awful
D – A very inappropriate thing to do

3.2 Contact Rob's supervisor before she leaves to make sure that Rob checks the results.

A – A very appropriate thing to do
B – Appropriate, but not ideal
C – Inappropriate but not awful
D – A very inappropriate thing to do

3.3 Acknowledge Rob's concerns, explaining that the situation is exceptional, and ask him to reconsider his position.

A – A very appropriate thing to do
B – Appropriate, but not ideal
C – Inappropriate but not awful
D – A very inappropriate thing to do

3.4 Stay until the computer system comes back online.

A – A very appropriate thing to do
B – Appropriate, but not ideal
C – Inappropriate but not awful
D – A very inappropriate thing to do

SJ 4 Practice — Scenario 4 – Needlestick Injury

Sartaj, a junior doctor on a ward, has been asked by a senior doctor to take blood from a patient, Mr Mushtaq, for an urgent test.

Sartaj is getting stressed. A few years ago, whilst at medical school, Sartaj accidentally pricked his finger with a needle when taking blood from a patient, and for a while lived in fear that he may have contracted a disease as a result. He developed a fear of needles and now panics at the thought of taking blood from patients. The senior doctor is aware of Sartaj's incident at medical school and that Sartaj has been accepted for a training post in a specialty where he will not be using needles again. That post will start next month.

How appropriate are each of the following responses by **Sartaj** in this situation?

4.1 Apologise to the senior doctor and explain that, given the fear of needles he has developed since medical school, the senior doctor may prefer to ask someone else.

A – A very appropriate thing to do
B – Appropriate, but not ideal
C – Inappropriate but not awful
D – A very inappropriate thing to do

4.2 Tell the senior doctor that he will try his best and, once he has left, ask around to see if anyone can do it instead.

A – A very appropriate thing to do
B – Appropriate, but not ideal
C – Inappropriate but not awful
D – A very inappropriate thing to do

4.3 Tell the senior doctor that he would be willing to take the blood but only if someone stayed with him to assist in case he panics.

A – A very appropriate thing to do
B – Appropriate, but not ideal
C – Inappropriate but not awful
D – A very inappropriate thing to do

4.4 Tell the senior doctor that it was unreasonable to ask him given what he knows of his past traumatic incident.

A – A very appropriate thing to do
B – Appropriate, but not ideal
C – Inappropriate but not awful
D – A very inappropriate thing to do

SJ 5 Practice — Scenario 5 – Chance Encounter

Dr Jones is a junior doctor who enjoys partying. One night, he goes to a bar with several of his friends, some of whom are doctors working in the same hospital, whilst the others are non-medics. That night, he spots a patient he has seen several times in clinic. The patient comes over to him and his group of friends and engages in basic pleasantries.

How appropriate are each of the following responses by **Dr Jones** in this situation?

5.1 Introduce the man to his friends as one of his patients and stick to basic conversation unrelated to the man's medical issues.

A – A very appropriate thing to do
B – Appropriate, but not ideal
C – Inappropriate but not awful
D – A very inappropriate thing to do

5.2 Take the patient aside. Tell him that his own career is at risk if they are seen socialising together and that he looks forward to seeing them soon in clinic for their next check-up.

A – A very appropriate thing to do
B – Appropriate, but not ideal
C – Inappropriate but not awful
D – A very inappropriate thing to do

5.3 Pretend he does not know the patient and ignore him.

A – A very appropriate thing to do
B – Appropriate, but not ideal
C – Inappropriate but not awful
D – A very inappropriate thing to do

5.4 Respond with basic pleasantries and take the patient aside to continue with a brief conversation.

A – A very appropriate thing to do
B – Appropriate, but not ideal
C – Inappropriate but not awful
D – A very inappropriate thing to do

5.5 Mention the incident to his senior manager and record it in the patient's notes.

A – A very appropriate thing to do
B – Appropriate, but not ideal
C – Inappropriate but not awful
D – A very inappropriate thing to do

SJ 6 Practice — Scenario 6 – Career Development

Dan and Thomas are two junior doctors working on a psychiatric ward. Dan enjoys the work, but Thomas finds the attachment disappointing. Thomas keeps disappearing when there are jobs to do which are seen as boring and Dan has just found out that Thomas attends theatre sessions instead of helping him. Though patient safety is not being affected by his disappearances, this is placing extra pressure on Dan, who is feeling increasingly frustrated. Dan confronts Thomas, who tells him that he wants to become a surgeon and that, although it will be over a year before he can apply for a surgical rotation, he takes every opportunity to attend surgical sessions in theatre whenever the surgeon can make space for a medical student.

How important to take into account are the following considerations for **Dan** when deciding how to respond to the situation?

6.1 That only a small part of the work they are doing in psychiatry is likely to be useful to Thomas in his future career as a surgeon.

A – Very important
B – Important
C – Of minor importance
D – Not important at all

6.2 That Thomas has not cleared his absences with a senior doctor.

A – Very important
B – Important
C – Of minor importance
D – Not important at all

6.3 That Thomas may fail his psychiatry attachment if his absences are reported by someone else.

A – Very important
B – Important
C – Of minor importance
D – Not important at all

6.4 That Thomas may be able to compensate for his absences by taking on more work at a later stage.

A – Very important
B – Important
C – Of minor importance
D – Not important at all

SJ 7 Practice — Scenario 7 – Venting Off

Rob is a well-established nurse within the elderly care department and has a reputation for frankness and a no-nonsense approach which many of his patients tend to like. Sandra is a medical student who just started her attachment in the elderly care department a couple of days ago. As she walks past a bed where a patient, Mrs Peacock, lies, Sandra overhears Mrs Peacock tell Rob with a frustrated voice that she has asked to see a doctor instead of a nurse many times and that none of them ever seem to come and see her. Rob replies that he has asked Dr Jones, a junior doctor in the unit, to speak to her many times, but that Dr Jones has a reputation for being a bit lazy, and he will see what he can do.

How important to take into account are the following considerations for **Sandra** when deciding how to respond to the situation?

7.1 That the patient may lose trust in Dr Jones as a result of Rob's allegations.

A – Very important
B – Important

C – Of minor importance
D – Not important at all

7.2 That Dr Jones's attachment will finish in two days' time, after which he will be working in a different hospital.

A – Very important
B – Important

C – Of minor importance
D – Not important at all

7.3 That Sandra may be regarded as a difficult colleague if she reports the conversation to her supervisor.

A – Very important
B – Important

C – Of minor importance
D – Not important at all

7.4 That Mrs Peacock seems to know Rob well and might lie to defend him if asked to confirm the details of the conversation.

A – Very important
B – Important

C – Of minor importance
D – Not important at all

Situational Judgement – Practice

SJ 8 Practice — Scenario 8 – Gift from Patient

Jonas is a junior doctor training to become a GP. He is currently doing an 18-month attachment in a GP practice, during which he sees many patients without supervision. One of his patients, Mr Skinner, is particularly grateful to Jonas about the support he gave him during a difficult period in his life and offers Jonas a small box of supermarket chocolates. Jonas is in two minds as to whether he should accept the box.

How important to take into account are the following considerations for **Jonas** when deciding how to respond to the situation?

8.1 That the gift is of small value.

A – Very important
B – Important
C – Of minor importance
D – Not important at all

8.2 That the patient is a regular in the practice and the gift is linked to a particular situation.

A – Very important
B – Important
C – Of minor importance
D – Not important at all

8.3 That refusing to accept the gift may upset the patient.

A – Very important
B – Important
C – Of minor importance
D – Not important at all

8.4 That other doctors seem to accept gifts from patients all the time.

A – Very important
B – Important
C – Of minor importance
D – Not important at all

8.5 That Jonas does not actually like chocolate.

A – Very important
B – Important
C – Of minor importance
D – Not important at all

SJ 9 Practice — Scenario 9 – Preoperative Questions

Sian is a medical student reaching the end of the shift at 6 pm. She is checking up on a patient, Mr Debono, who is meant to undergo a procedure at 8 am the next morning. The consultant and other doctors involved in the procedure have already seen the patient to explain the procedure in detail, to answer his questions and to seek his consent for the procedure. Mr Debono tells Sian that he is still anxious about some aspects of the procedure and would like to talk to one of the doctors again. Sian has tried to contact them on the phone several times, but none are available.

How appropriate are each of the following responses by **Sian** in this situation?

9.1 Explain to the patient that she has tried to reach the doctors on the phone, apologise for the inconvenience and let the patient know that there will be opportunities for him to ask questions when the doctors arrive at 7 am the next morning.

A – A very appropriate thing to do
B – Appropriate, but not ideal
C – Inappropriate but not awful
D – A very inappropriate thing to do

9.2 Inform the patient that the doctors he saw earlier are unavailable but that she will get another equally qualified doctor to answer his questions shortly.

A – A very appropriate thing to do
B – Appropriate, but not ideal
C – Inappropriate but not awful
D – A very inappropriate thing to do

9.3 Tell the patient that the team he has seen is not available but that she should be able to answer his questions.

A – A very appropriate thing to do
B – Appropriate, but not ideal
C – Inappropriate but not awful
D – A very inappropriate thing to do

9.4 Tell the patient that the team he saw is unavailable, but she may be able to address some of his concerns, and she will be able to get a doctor if some questions require more detailed input.

A – A very appropriate thing to do
B – Appropriate, but not ideal
C – Inappropriate but not awful
D – A very inappropriate thing to do

SJ 10 Practice — Scenario 10 – Busy Social Life

Robert and Campbell are two junior doctors working on a busy ward under the supervision of the same consultant. Just after arriving at work one Friday morning, Robert gets a call from Campbell, informing him that he is feeling rough and that he would rather not come to work that day. A week later, Robert sees on social media that Campbell has posted pictures of himself having a good time partying in Prague. The commentary clearly shows that the group flew out on the Friday morning when Campbell was meant to be off sick.

How appropriate are each of the following responses by **Robert** in this situation?

10.1 Monitor Campbell's social media prospectively. Decide to raise the issue with a senior colleague if it happens again.

A – A very appropriate thing to do
B – Appropriate, but not ideal
C – Inappropriate but not awful
D – A very inappropriate thing to do

10.2 Say and do nothing.

A – A very appropriate thing to do
B – Appropriate, but not ideal
C – Inappropriate but not awful
D – A very inappropriate thing to do

10.3 Approach Campbell in a non-confrontational manner, make it clear you are aware of the facts and let him know that you will have no choice but to raise the matter with a senior colleague if it happens again.

A – A very appropriate thing to do
B – Appropriate, but not ideal
C – Inappropriate but not awful
D – A very inappropriate thing to do

10.4 Discuss the matter privately with the supervising consultant.

A – A very appropriate thing to do
B – Appropriate, but not ideal
C – Inappropriate but not awful
D – A very inappropriate thing to do

10.5 Ask a secretary to raise the matter with one of the consultants.

A – A very appropriate thing to do
B – Appropriate, but not ideal
C – Inappropriate but not awful
D – A very inappropriate thing to do

SJ 11 Practice — Scenario 11 – No More Leaflets

Josie is a dental student currently on an attachment in a busy high street practice. As she walks into the waiting room to call the next patient, one of the other patients complains to her that the last time he attended the clinic he read an interesting leaflet about smoking cessation, but he has since lost it and would like another one. Unfortunately, the box normally containing the leaflets is completely empty. The patient says that the receptionist told him bluntly that the practice was out of leaflets and that he could pick one up next time he comes in, provided there are some in stock.

How appropriate are each of the following responses by **Josie** in this situation?

11.1 Apologise for the lack of leaflets and the fact the receptionist wasn't able to help. Advise the patient that she will see if she can download the leaflet from the NHS website and print one out for him. He can then pick up an original leaflet when he next comes back to the practice.

| A – A very appropriate thing to do | C – Inappropriate but not awful |
| B – Appropriate, but not ideal | D – A very inappropriate thing to do |

11.2 Send an email to the receptionist to inform her of the complaint, copying the practice manager in on it.

| A – A very appropriate thing to do | C – Inappropriate but not awful |
| B – Appropriate, but not ideal | D – A very inappropriate thing to do |

11.3 Ask the receptionist to come to a private room straight away for a quick chat and raise the comments made by the patient about her bluntness.

| A – A very appropriate thing to do | C – Inappropriate but not awful |
| B – Appropriate, but not ideal | D – A very inappropriate thing to do |

11.4 Have a quiet word with the practice manager about the patient's comment regarding the receptionist's bluntness.

| A – A very appropriate thing to do | C – Inappropriate but not awful |
| B – Appropriate, but not ideal | D – A very inappropriate thing to do |

SJ 12 Practice — Scenario 12 – Poor Presentation

A specialist doctor, Ahmed, has come across an interesting clinical case on his ward and would like to present it at a forthcoming conference. The patient was cared for mainly by two junior doctors, Barbara, and Sandra, under Ahmed's supervision, and he has asked them to prepare the presentation. At the initial briefing meeting, it was agreed that Barbara and Sandra would work on two separate halves of the presentation. Ahmed made it clear to Barbara and Sandra that time was of the essence and that, being very busy, he would have very few opportunities to review the final presentation before the conference. As work progresses, Barbara is confident that her part is very well polished, but she notices that Sandra's work is poor, that she is using misleading data and that she is misinterpreting facts.

How appropriate are each of the following responses by **Barbara** in this situation?

12.1 Do her own part of the presentation as well as possible and let Sandra get on with her own half of the work without interfering.

A – A very appropriate thing to do
B – Appropriate, but not ideal
C – Inappropriate but not awful
D – A very inappropriate thing to do

12.2 Arrange a progress meeting so that Ahmed can see for himself that Sandra's work is not up to the required standard.

A – A very appropriate thing to do
B – Appropriate, but not ideal
C – Inappropriate but not awful
D – A very inappropriate thing to do

12.3 Praise Sandra for the good work she has done up to now and ask her if she would welcome any input on her work so far.

A – A very appropriate thing to do
B – Appropriate, but not ideal
C – Inappropriate but not awful
D – A very inappropriate thing to do

12.4 Contact Ahmed to raise her concerns.

A – A very appropriate thing to do
B – Appropriate, but not ideal
C – Inappropriate but not awful
D – A very inappropriate thing to do

1300 UCAT Practice Questions

SJ 13 Practice — Scenario 13 – Heavy Burden

Jo is a medical student who shares her time between lectures and patient-related activities on various wards. She has been experiencing a whole range of personal issues which have been playing on her mind. In addition, the ward doctors are always finding interesting patients for her to examine, or interesting new tasks for her, well beyond normal expectations; this means that she has not been able to find the time she needs to study.

During one of her regular sessions with her academic supervisor, the supervisor points out that her academic results have gradually worsened to the point where they are starting to become a real worry.

How appropriate are each of the following responses by **Jo** in this situation?

13.1 Ask the supervisor to contact the ward consultant to see if he can alleviate her workload.

A – A very appropriate thing to do
B – Appropriate, but not ideal
C – Inappropriate but not awful
D – A very inappropriate thing to do

13.2 Tell her supervisor that unfortunately she feels compelled to prioritise patient-related work over her academic work and that she will need to take the consequences.

A – A very appropriate thing to do
B – Appropriate, but not ideal
C – Inappropriate but not awful
D – A very inappropriate thing to do

13.3 Ask her supervisor if she could take a few days off to sort out all her personal issues once and for all and then start afresh.

A – A very appropriate thing to do
B – Appropriate, but not ideal
C – Inappropriate but not awful
D – A very inappropriate thing to do

13.4 Tell the ward consultant that she will need to pull out of a number of projects and cases because she is overburdened.

A – A very appropriate thing to do
B – Appropriate, but not ideal
C – Inappropriate but not awful
D – A very inappropriate thing to do

Situational Judgement – Practice

SJ 14 Practice — Scenario 14 – Late Handover

Ron is a junior doctor on a busy Medical Assessment Unit. It is 5 pm and he is due to finish his shift at 5:30 pm. Ron needs to leave on time because he has a social engagement with his partner.

The colleague who is supposed to replace him, Saud, is supposed to start his shift at 5 pm, which allows for a 30-minute overlap for a verbal handover. (A handover is a meeting where the outgoing doctor explains to the incoming doctor what issues are still outstanding so that care continues to be provided to patients safely.)

Saud has just called to say that he will be 20 to 30 minutes late as he was delayed by traffic, but the road has now cleared. How appropriate are each of the following responses by **Ron** in this situation?

14.1 Call his partner to explain that he will be late.

A – A very appropriate thing to do
B – Appropriate, but not ideal
C – Inappropriate but not awful
D – A very inappropriate thing to do

14.2 Make a list of all outstanding test results and investigations to hand to Saud when he arrives.

A – A very appropriate thing to do
B – Appropriate, but not ideal
C – Inappropriate but not awful
D – A very inappropriate thing to do

14.3 Go round all the patients with outstanding issues, write detailed notes about those outstanding issues in the patient notes and leave at 5:30 pm.

A – A very appropriate thing to do
B – Appropriate, but not ideal
C – Inappropriate but not awful
D – A very inappropriate thing to do

14.4 Hand over all the relevant information to a more senior doctor, asking them to relay the information to Saud when he arrives.

A – A very appropriate thing to do
B – Appropriate, but not ideal
C – Inappropriate but not awful
D – A very inappropriate thing to do

SJ 15 Practice — Scenario 15 – Staying Late

Amy is a junior doctor currently working on a busy elderly care ward. Her shifts are normally meant to finish at 6 pm but every few days she has no choice but to finish at 8 pm just to complete a wide range of routine tasks. This has been going on for a couple of months and Amy is now finding it hard to get up in the morning and she starts the day being tired. She also has no social life to speak of. Her elderly care attachment is due to last another four months.

How important to take into account are the following considerations for **Amy** when deciding how to respond to the situation?

15.1 That her consultant might give her a bad reference if she does not complete all her tasks.

A – Very important
B – Important
C – Of minor importance
D – Not important at all

15.2 That her contract states that her shift finishes at 6 pm.

A – Very important
B – Important
C – Of minor importance
D – Not important at all

15.3 That she may make a mistake if she is constantly tired.

A – Very important
B – Important
C – Of minor importance
D – Not important at all

15.4 That not resting appropriately may impact on her wellbeing.

A – Very important
B – Important
C – Of minor importance
D – Not important at all

15.5 That her friends will get annoyed with her if she doesn't see them regularly.

A – Very important
B – Important
C – Of minor importance
D – Not important at all

SJ 16 Practice — Scenario 16 – Infection Control

John is working as a junior doctor on a ward. A few years ago, the hospital introduced an infection control policy stating that all members of staff with direct patient contact should wear only short-sleeved shirts or should roll their long sleeves up above the elbow. All staff starting a new post within the Trust are informed of that policy by the Infection Control Team as part of their mandatory induction process. John is on a 9 am to 5 pm shift with Lauren. At 10 am, John notices that Lauren, a fellow junior doctor, has her long sleeves down. This is the second time John has witnessed it in a week and, having raised the matter directly with Lauren the first time, John is now pondering whether he should raise the matter with the consultant.

How important to take into account are the following considerations for **John** when deciding how to respond to the situation?

16.1 That patients don't seem to mind.

A – Very important
B – Important
C – Of minor importance
D – Not important at all

16.2 That Lauren was unwell on that particular induction day and never received that information.

A – Very important
B – Important
C – Of minor importance
D – Not important at all

16.3 That Lauren may pass on an infection from one patient to another.

A – Very important
B – Important
C – Of minor importance
D – Not important at all

16.4 That Lauren has a scar on her forearm which she wants to hide.

A – Very important
B – Important
C – Of minor importance
D – Not important at all

16.5 That some senior colleagues often forget to roll up their sleeves.

A – Very important
B – Important
C – Of minor importance
D – Not important at all

SJ 17 Practice — Scenario 17 – Letter Mix-Up

Alfred is working as a junior doctor on a ward. He has recently discharged two patients who had the same procedure: Andrew Jones and Matt Jones. A day after the patients were sent home, Alfred realises that he has sent the wrong letter to each of the patients. The letter containing the name, address and clinical information for Matt Jones was sent to Andrew Jones, and vice versa.

How appropriate are each of the following responses by **Alfred** in this situation?

17.1 Call each patient and explain there has been an error and that a revised letter will be sent.

A – A very appropriate thing to do
B – Appropriate, but not ideal
C – Inappropriate but not awful
D – A very inappropriate thing to do

17.2 Ask each patient to come back to the hospital as soon as possible for a follow-up appointment. In the appointment, apologise, provide a revised letter, and ask them if they have any questions.

A – A very appropriate thing to do
B – Appropriate, but not ideal
C – Inappropriate but not awful
D – A very inappropriate thing to do

17.3 Alter the letters in each of the patients' records.

A – A very appropriate thing to do
B – Appropriate, but not ideal
C – Inappropriate but not awful
D – A very inappropriate thing to do

17.4 Do not contact the patients since they had similar procedures and therefore the letters will provide roughly similar information. But record the error in the respective patient notes.

A – A very appropriate thing to do
B – Appropriate, but not ideal
C – Inappropriate but not awful
D – A very inappropriate thing to do

17.5 Inform the consultant of the error.

A – A very appropriate thing to do
B – Appropriate, but not ideal
C – Inappropriate but not awful
D – A very inappropriate thing to do

SJ 18 Practice — Scenario 18 – Bad Atmosphere

Liz is a medical student and is currently working with a team of two senior doctors (Daniel and Raquel) and a junior doctor (Carlos).

When Raquel (one of the senior doctors) is around, everything works perfectly well. However, whenever Raquel is away, even for short periods of time, Daniel and Carlos adopt a sexist behaviour towards Liz, often criticising her openly in front of patients and leaving her out of important meetings.

How appropriate are each of the following responses by **Liz** in this situation?

18.1 Ask to be moved to a different ward.

A – A very appropriate thing to do
B – Appropriate, but not ideal
C – Inappropriate but not awful
D – A very inappropriate thing to do

18.2 Discuss her concerns with both Carlos and Daniel.

A – A very appropriate thing to do
B – Appropriate, but not ideal
C – Inappropriate but not awful
D – A very inappropriate thing to do

18.3 Wait a few weeks to see if their behaviour improves.

A – A very appropriate thing to do
B – Appropriate, but not ideal
C – Inappropriate but not awful
D – A very inappropriate thing to do

18.4 Seek advice from Raquel on how to improve team relations.

A – A very appropriate thing to do
B – Appropriate, but not ideal
C – Inappropriate but not awful
D – A very inappropriate thing to do

18.5 Document Daniel and Carlos's behaviour over a few weeks and give a copy of her log to the consultant so he can advise what to do.

A – A very appropriate thing to do
B – Appropriate, but not ideal
C – Inappropriate but not awful
D – A very inappropriate thing to do

SJ 19 Practice — Scenario 19 – Audit Data

As part of his educational programme at dental school, Joshua is required to carry out an audit. This exercise consists mainly of entering data collected from patient notes into a spreadsheet and then summarising and analysing the data to identify features which could be useful to improve the care given to patients. For this audit, he is using his own laptop.

It is Friday lunchtime and Joshua still needs to enter data from 25 patients into the spreadsheet. In view of his workload, he will not be able to collate all the remaining data by the end of the day. He is unable to stay late and the clinic where he works will be closed at the weekend; hence the patient notes that he needs will be inaccessible.

The results of the audit need to be presented to his supervisor on Monday morning. How appropriate are each of the following responses by **Joshua** in this situation?

19.1 Take the relevant patient notes home with him and continue the data input at the weekend.

A – A very appropriate thing to do
B – Appropriate, but not ideal
C – Inappropriate but not awful
D – A very inappropriate thing to do

19.2 Ask the supervisor to postpone the meeting until Tuesday.

A – A very appropriate thing to do
B – Appropriate, but not ideal
C – Inappropriate but not awful
D – A very inappropriate thing to do

19.3 Photocopy the relevant pages from the patients' notes, removing any patient-identifiable data and take the photocopies home.

A – A very appropriate thing to do
B – Appropriate, but not ideal
C – Inappropriate but not awful
D – A very inappropriate thing to do

19.4 Look at the average profile of the patients already entered into the database and create 25 new patient data matching the average profile.

A – A very appropriate thing to do
B – Appropriate, but not ideal
C – Inappropriate but not awful
D – A very inappropriate thing to do

SJ 20 Practice — Scenario 20 – Exam Cheat

Sarah has been asked to provide a series of lectures to final year dental students. One of the students, Ellen, whom she knows well, has somehow managed to get hold of a photocopy of a forthcoming exam paper and asks Sarah to make sure she addresses all the relevant issues in her teaching sessions. When probed, Ellen explains that the paper came from a previous final year dental student, who said that the exam was always the same and this sheet of paper has been handed down for at least the past 5 years.

How appropriate are each of the following responses by **Sarah** in this situation?

20.1 Confiscate the paper and report the matter to the deanery, keeping Ellen's name confidential.

A – A very appropriate thing to do
B – Appropriate, but not ideal
C – Inappropriate but not awful
D – A very inappropriate thing to do

20.2 Advise Ellen to throw away the paper without looking at it.

A – A very appropriate thing to do
B – Appropriate, but not ideal
C – Inappropriate but not awful
D – A very inappropriate thing to do

20.3 Inform Ellen that, in order to make sure the process is fair, she should ensure that all the other students are also given a copy.

A – A very appropriate thing to do
B – Appropriate, but not ideal
C – Inappropriate but not awful
D – A very inappropriate thing to do

20.4 Tailor the teaching material to the questions set in the paper.

A – A very appropriate thing to do
B – Appropriate, but not ideal
C – Inappropriate but not awful
D – A very inappropriate thing to do

20.5 Ask the deanery for the contact details of all students who have taken the exam in the past five years so that she can inform them that the matter is being looked into.

A – A very appropriate thing to do
B – Appropriate, but not ideal
C – Inappropriate but not awful
D – A very inappropriate thing to do

SJ 21 Practice — Scenario 21 – Quiet Attachment

Ishtiaq is a junior doctor on a surgical training rotation. He does not find the work very challenging. He also finds that he can complete all the work required of him (and sometimes more) well within the hours he is contracted to work. He has a lot of spare time.

How appropriate are each of the following responses by **Ishtiaq** in this situation?

21.1 Ask a senior doctor if he (Ishtiaq) can offer to help other junior doctors who work on busier wards during his spare time.

A – A very appropriate thing to do
B – Appropriate, but not ideal
C – Inappropriate but not awful
D – A very inappropriate thing to do

21.2 Ask the Programme Director to move him to a busier team with more training opportunities.

A – A very appropriate thing to do
B – Appropriate, but not ideal
C – Inappropriate but not awful
D – A very inappropriate thing to do

21.3 Ask a senior doctor to involve him more in some of the team's non-clinical activities such as audit and teaching.

A – A very appropriate thing to do
B – Appropriate, but not ideal
C – Inappropriate but not awful
D – A very inappropriate thing to do

21.4 Use his spare time to set up a revision course for medical students who want to prepare more intensely for their medical finals.

A – A very appropriate thing to do
B – Appropriate, but not ideal
C – Inappropriate but not awful
D – A very inappropriate thing to do

21.5 Tell the Programme Director that the post in which he works should be reassessed for training as it is too quiet and future students would not benefit from it.

A – A very appropriate thing to do
B – Appropriate, but not ideal
C – Inappropriate but not awful
D – A very inappropriate thing to do

SJ 22 Practice — Scenario 22 – Conflict of Opinion

Rosie is a junior doctor on a medical rotation. One of the patients on her ward is being reviewed by the consultant. The consultant sets out a management plan which involves Rosie and other junior doctors carrying out a number of investigations and performing a number of tasks. Once the consultant has left, one of the senior trainees tells Rosie that he thinks the consultant got it wrong and that she and the others should implement a different management plan. There is no urgency in implementing either plan.

How important to take into account are the following considerations for **Rosie** when deciding which plan to implement?

22.1 That the consultant has been a consultant for over 20 years.

A – Very important
B – Important
C – Of minor importance
D – Not important at all

22.2 That, should there be a problem, she can claim she was simply following orders because she is a very junior doctor.

A – Very important
B – Important
C – Of minor importance
D – Not important at all

22.3 That the other junior doctors agree with the senior trainee's plan.

A – Very important
B – Important
C – Of minor importance
D – Not important at all

22.4 That the senior trainee is the one signing off some of her procedures and assessments for her training portfolio.

A – Very important
B – Important
C – Of minor importance
D – Not important at all

22.5 That both proposed management plans will not cause any harm or inconvenience to the patient if they are not fruitful.

A – Very important
B – Important
C – Of minor importance
D – Not important at all

| SJ 23 Practice | Scenario 23 – Struggling Colleague |

Adam and Chris are two junior doctors covering a medical ward. Adam works a 9 am to 5 pm shift, whilst Chris works 11 am to 7 pm. Both have a similar workload. Adam is constantly complaining that he finds the work hard to deal with. Chris seems to find the work very manageable. At the end of his shift at 5 pm, Adam tends to tell Chris that he has done as many of his tasks as possible and that Chris will need to finish his remaining tasks for him since he works until 7 pm.

How appropriate are each of the following responses by **Chris** in this situation?

23.1 Tell Adam that he will only agree to take on the urgent tasks, but that Adam will need to do the non-urgent ones himself.

| A – A very appropriate thing to do | C – Inappropriate but not awful |
| B – Appropriate, but not ideal | D – A very inappropriate thing to do |

23.2 Ask other junior colleagues to help him with some of Adam's tasks.

| A – A very appropriate thing to do | C – Inappropriate but not awful |
| B – Appropriate, but not ideal | D – A very inappropriate thing to do |

23.3 Suggest to Adam that he should arrange a meeting with his supervisor.

| A – A very appropriate thing to do | C – Inappropriate but not awful |
| B – Appropriate, but not ideal | D – A very inappropriate thing to do |

23.4 Discuss with Adam what he is finding difficult about the role.

| A – A very appropriate thing to do | C – Inappropriate but not awful |
| B – Appropriate, but not ideal | D – A very inappropriate thing to do |

23.5 Arrange a one-off meeting with Adam in his spare time to help him develop/enhance his prioritisation skills.

| A – A very appropriate thing to do | C – Inappropriate but not awful |
| B – Appropriate, but not ideal | D – A very inappropriate thing to do |

SJ 24 Practice — Scenario 24 – Drug Error

Alison, a medical student, is shadowing Mark, a junior doctor. Alison looks at a set of a patient's drug charts, which shows that Mark has prescribed a dose of penicillin for that patient. The dose is due to be administered in one hour's time. Alison remembers from a previous discussion that the patient is allergic to penicillin and that the consultant had made the allergy very clear to the whole team by placing a special warning sticker in the patient's notes. She raises her concerns with Mark who replies: "You are right. I will cancel the prescription. Make sure you don't tell anyone about this."

How important to take into account are the following considerations for **Alison** when deciding how to respond to the situation?

24.1 That Mark is usually very reliable and makes few mistakes.

A – Very important
B – Important
C – Of minor importance
D – Not important at all

24.2 That, when Mark has made mistakes in the past, he has always owned up to them freely.

A – Very important
B – Important
C – Of minor importance
D – Not important at all

24.3 That the mistake was caught in time and the patient was safe.

A – Very important
B – Important
C – Of minor importance
D – Not important at all

24.4 That the nurse who would administer the penicillin would have double-checked and would have likely spotted the error.

A – Very important
B – Important
C – Of minor importance
D – Not important at all

24.5 That the patient is unaware of the incident.

A – Very important
B – Important
C – Of minor importance
D – Not important at all

SJ 25 Practice — Scenario 25 – Tube Station Incident

Jack, a medical student, has finished a busy day. He is feeling tired and is looking forward to going out with his partner for a relaxing meal. To go home he has to catch a tube for a journey that lasts 30 minutes. The Tube station is situated 300 metres from the hospital. As he is waiting on the platform, Jack sees that a man has collapsed several metres away from him. Jack has received some basic life-saving training but has never had to apply his knowledge to a real patient before. He needs to decide whether to intervene or not.

How important to take into account are the following considerations for **Jack** when deciding how to respond to the situation?

25.1 That the patient is very close to the hospital.

A – Very important
B – Important
C – Of minor importance
D – Not important at all

25.2 That, when looking around, Jack recognises a lot of medics and nurses who are more qualified than he is.

A – Very important
B – Important
C – Of minor importance
D – Not important at all

25.3 A fellow passenger has already called 999 and an ambulance is on its way.

A – Very important
B – Important
C – Of minor importance
D – Not important at all

25.4 That his partner will be upset if he is late for the dinner.

A – Very important
B – Important
C – Of minor importance
D – Not important at all

25.5 That the Tube station staff are trained in basic lifesaving and have relevant equipment such as defibrillators.

A – Very important
B – Important
C – Of minor importance
D – Not important at all

SJ 26 Practice — Scenario 26 – Relative Enquiry

Asif is a junior doctor on a busy hospital ward. He is due to go home in 30 minutes but still has two patients to review, each of whom could take up to 20 minutes, as well as 30 minutes' worth of paperwork. His colleague Ronan is a junior doctor of equal rank covering the same ward. Ronan has completed the bulk of his work and is currently looking at his personal emails before finishing his shift. Asif is approached by a junior nurse who says that the relative of one of the ward patients is on the phone and wants to speak to someone. Both Asif and Ronan are familiar with the patient in question.

How important to take into account are the following considerations for **Asif** when deciding how to respond to the situation?

26.1 That Ronan is currently engaged in non-work-related activities.

A – Very important
B – Important
C – Of minor importance
D – Not important at all

26.2 That the vast majority of calls from relatives are for a simple update that nurses can usually give with full competence.

A – Very important
B – Important
C – Of minor importance
D – Not important at all

26.3 That the patient whose relatives are calling is constantly complaining about menial matters.

A – Very important
B – Important
C – Of minor importance
D – Not important at all

26.4 That the paperwork he is doing can wait until the next morning.

A – Very important
B – Important
C – Of minor importance
D – Not important at all

26.5 That the nurse thinks the relatives were calm, seemed to want only a general update and did not ask specifically for a doctor.

A – Very important
B – Important
C – Of minor importance
D – Not important at all

1300 UCAT Practice Questions

SJ 27 Practice — Scenario 27 – Nurse Disagreement

George, a junior doctor, has written a prescription for a strong painkiller. A staff nurse with over 20 years' experience is challenging his decision to prescribe such a painkiller to the patient and refuses to give the medication to the patient. When George asks for a reason, she simply says, "Trust me, I know this patient well".

How appropriate are each of the following responses by **George** in this situation?

27.1 Cancel the prescription on the nurse's advice and prescribe another suitable painkiller that may be more acceptable to her.

A – A very appropriate thing to do
B – Appropriate, but not ideal
C – Inappropriate but not awful
D – A very inappropriate thing to do

27.2 Ask a senior doctor for guidance and prescribe the agreed painkiller, even if it is the same one as before.

A – A very appropriate thing to do
B – Appropriate, but not ideal
C – Inappropriate but not awful
D – A very inappropriate thing to do

27.3 Ask the nurse why she disagrees with the prescription.

A – A very appropriate thing to do
B – Appropriate, but not ideal
C – Inappropriate but not awful
D – A very inappropriate thing to do

27.4 Ask the nurse which painkiller she would be prepared to administer if he prescribed it and prescribe from the list she gives.

A – A very appropriate thing to do
B – Appropriate, but not ideal
C – Inappropriate but not awful
D – A very inappropriate thing to do

27.5 Tell the nurse that, as this is his decision as a doctor, he is ordering her to administer the painkiller to the patient.

A – A very appropriate thing to do
B – Appropriate, but not ideal
C – Inappropriate but not awful
D – A very inappropriate thing to do

SJ 28 Practice
Scenario 28 – Father and Daughter

Julia is a medical student working on an elderly care ward. Her best friend Amanda, who is working as an accountant elsewhere, calls to tell her that her father is currently on the orthopaedics ward at the hospital where Julia works, recovering from a hip replacement which was performed yesterday. Amanda asks Julia to check that her father is okay and let her know if there are any issues. The surgery was uneventful, and the patient is recovering well. Julia walks by the ward and sees that Amanda's father seems okay.

How appropriate are each of the following responses by **Julia** in this situation?

28.1 Check the patient notes and update Amanda on progress.

A – A very appropriate thing to do
B – Appropriate, but not ideal
C – Inappropriate but not awful
D – A very inappropriate thing to do

28.2 Tell Amanda she is not authorised to see the notes of a patient who is in a different ward and so she can't help.

A – A very appropriate thing to do
B – Appropriate, but not ideal
C – Inappropriate but not awful
D – A very inappropriate thing to do

28.3 Tell Amanda that the orthopaedics team would be best placed to update her. She will ask them to call Amanda back.

A – A very appropriate thing to do
B – Appropriate, but not ideal
C – Inappropriate but not awful
D – A very inappropriate thing to do

28.4 Tell Amanda that this can't be done without her father's consent and therefore her hands are tied.

A – A very appropriate thing to do
B – Appropriate, but not ideal
C – Inappropriate but not awful
D – A very inappropriate thing to do

28.5 Tell Amanda that her father looked well when she saw him but that is all she can say.

A – A very appropriate thing to do
B – Appropriate, but not ideal
C – Inappropriate but not awful
D – A very inappropriate thing to do

SJ 29 Practice | Scenario 29 – Dyslexic Colleague

Sian and Kiran are two junior doctors sharing the workload on the same ward. Sian has noticed that Kiran keeps his entries in the patients' notes to the bare minimum and the notes are often confused. Kiran has also started showing reluctance at completing drug charts. Having approached Kiran directly, Sian finds out from him that he has been suffering from dyslexia since childhood and he finds it hard to deal with it in the busy ward in which they currently work. Sian has recommended several times to Kiran that he raise the issue with his educational supervisor and the consultant, but he consistently refuses to do so as he is worried that he may be misunderstood. Sian is now considering raising the issue herself with his supervisor.

How important to take into account are the following considerations for **Sian** when deciding how to respond to the situation?

29.1 That it may upset Kiran that Sian goes his supervisor.

A – Very important
B – Important
C – Of minor importance
D – Not important at all

29.2 That Kiran does not want anyone to know about his dyslexia.

A – Very important
B – Important
C – Of minor importance
D – Not important at all

29.3 That the rest of the team appears to be frustrated.

A – Very important
B – Important
C – Of minor importance
D – Not important at all

29.4 That Kiran's dyslexia may affect patient care.

A – Very important
B – Important
C – Of minor importance
D – Not important at all

29.5 That other doctors who are not dyslexic are making similar mistakes to Kiran.

A – Very important
B – Important
C – Of minor importance
D – Not important at all

SJ 30 Practice
Scenario 30 – Surgical Career

Dolores, a junior doctor very keen on a surgical career, contacted the surgical unit months ago to see if she could observe a few theatre sessions. The surgery unit has finally got back to her saying that there was only one slot left before the end of her attachment: tomorrow, 8 am to 11 am. Unfortunately, Dolores is due to run a busy clinic at that time.

How appropriate are each of the following responses by **Dolores** in this situation?

30.1 Ask her clinic manager if it is possible to cancel at least one hour of the clinic so that she can attend the surgical partially.

A – A very appropriate thing to do | C – Inappropriate but not awful
B – Appropriate, but not ideal | D – A very inappropriate thing to do

30.2 Call the clinic manager at 7 am to say she is not feeling well; then attend the surgical theatre session.

A – A very appropriate thing to do | C – Inappropriate but not awful
B – Appropriate, but not ideal | D – A very inappropriate thing to do

30.3 Call the patients who are supposed to attend the clinic the next day to see if they would be willing to rebook onto another day.

A – A very appropriate thing to do | C – Inappropriate but not awful
B – Appropriate, but not ideal | D – A very inappropriate thing to do

30.4 Swap clinic with a colleague: ask one of the other junior doctors who is supposed to be on study leave that morning to run Dolores' clinic instead so that she can attend the surgical session. Dolores can then, instead, run that junior doctor's clinic on another day.

A – A very appropriate thing to do | C – Inappropriate but not awful
B – Appropriate, but not ideal | D – A very inappropriate thing to do

30.5 Not attend the theatre session and run her clinic as originally planned. Contact her next hospital early to arrange sessions.

A – A very appropriate thing to do | C – Inappropriate but not awful
B – Appropriate, but not ideal | D – A very inappropriate thing to do

551

SJ 31 Practice — Scenario 31 – Coping with Pressure

Sara is a medical student currently on a surgical attachment. Andrea, also a medical student, finds Sara in tears one lunchtime. Sara is finding the surgical attachment very demanding, feels she may not be able to cope with it, and particularly hates the way the consultant seeks to undermine her during the ward round by asking hard questions that she can never answer.

How appropriate are each of the following responses by **Andrea** in this situation?

31.1 Tell Sara that she is sorry that she is finding it hard to cope and suggest that she may want to take some time off to recharge her batteries. This will make it easier to cope with the pressure.

A – A very appropriate thing to do
B – Appropriate, but not ideal
C – Inappropriate but not awful
D – A very inappropriate thing to do

31.2 Empathise with Sara's concerns and encourage her to discuss the issues with one of the senior trainees who has experience of dealing with the consultant.

A – A very appropriate thing to do
B – Appropriate, but not ideal
C – Inappropriate but not awful
D – A very inappropriate thing to do

31.3 Explain to Sara that she may need to address the issue directly with the consultant if she can and offer to go with her to talk to the consultant if she wants support.

A – A very appropriate thing to do
B – Appropriate, but not ideal
C – Inappropriate but not awful
D – A very inappropriate thing to do

31.4 Encourage Sara to seek counselling.

A – A very appropriate thing to do
B – Appropriate, but not ideal
C – Inappropriate but not awful
D – A very inappropriate thing to do

31.5 Offer to assist Sara with some of her workload.

A – A very appropriate thing to do
B – Appropriate, but not ideal
C – Inappropriate but not awful
D – A very inappropriate thing to do

Situational Judgement – Practice

SJ 32 Practice — Scenario 32 – Aggressive Midwife

Rosie is a medical student in an obstetrics unit and needs to have signed off on a number of deliveries on her logbook. One of the midwives, Angie, has constantly been undermining Rosie publicly, criticising her approach and thought process, and refusing to sign off her procedures for the logbook. Rosie instead approached other midwives, who were full of praise for her approach, signed off the procedures for her logbook without reservation and told her to ignore Angie. Rosie has tried to talk to Angie twice, but Angie refused to talk to her and was verbally abusive. The other medical students and most junior doctors in the unit have experienced the same hostility from Angie.

How appropriate are each of the following responses by **Rosie** in this situation?

32.1 Continue to put up with Angie's ongoing negative comments.

A – A very appropriate thing to do
B – Appropriate, but not ideal
C – Inappropriate but not awful
D – A very inappropriate thing to do

32.2 Inform the consultant about Angie's behaviour.

A – A very appropriate thing to do
B – Appropriate, but not ideal
C – Inappropriate but not awful
D – A very inappropriate thing to do

32.3 Arrange a meeting with Angie to discuss her misgivings and how they can repair the relationship.

A – A very appropriate thing to do
B – Appropriate, but not ideal
C – Inappropriate but not awful
D – A very inappropriate thing to do

32.4 Ask to be transferred to a different unit.

A – A very appropriate thing to do
B – Appropriate, but not ideal
C – Inappropriate but not awful
D – A very inappropriate thing to do

32.5 Get together with the other medical students and junior doctors and write a joint letter to the consultant.

A – A very appropriate thing to do
B – Appropriate, but not ideal
C – Inappropriate but not awful
D – A very inappropriate thing to do

SJ 33 Practice — Scenario 33 – Breaking Bad News

Christina is a medical student currently on an attachment on an oncology (cancer) ward. At a morning meeting, the team discusses the blood results of Mr Anthony, a patient who has previously been treated for prostate cancer. The blood results show that there is a strong possibility the cancer has come back, though further tests would need to be done in order to confirm it. As Christina walks by him later, Mr Anthony leans towards her and says "I presume the blood results are back by now. Is the cancer back?"

How appropriate are each of the following responses by **Christina** in this situation?

33.1 Tell the patient that she thinks the blood results are okay but that a doctor will have a chat with him soon to talk about the results.

A – A very appropriate thing to do
B – Appropriate, but not ideal
C – Inappropriate but not awful
D – A very inappropriate thing to do

33.2 Tell the patient she cannot comment because she hasn't seen the blood tests in detail and is not qualified to comment on them.

A – A very appropriate thing to do
B – Appropriate, but not ideal
C – Inappropriate but not awful
D – A very inappropriate thing to do

33.3 Tell the patient that she cannot comment because she is only a medical student and would not be able to answer his questions.

A – A very appropriate thing to do
B – Appropriate, but not ideal
C – Inappropriate but not awful
D – A very inappropriate thing to do

33.4 Tell the patient she believes the results are back, but she can't comment because she is only a medical student. She will get one of the doctors to see him shortly.

A – A very appropriate thing to do
B – Appropriate, but not ideal
C – Inappropriate but not awful
D – A very inappropriate thing to do

33.5 Tell the patient the cancer has likely come back but someone senior will talk to him at some point.

A – A very appropriate thing to do
B – Appropriate, but not ideal
C – Inappropriate but not awful
D – A very inappropriate thing to do

Situational Judgement – Practice

SJ 34 Practice — Scenario 34 – Intimate Issues

A female patient, Mrs Brookes, booked an appointment with her GP two weeks ago to discuss what she referred to as "intimate issues" without specifying which doctor she wanted to see. The appointment is at 9 am. She has just arrived at the GP practice, only to find out that all clinics are run by male GPs today, which angers her because she would much prefer to discuss her "intimate issues" with a female doctor. There is only one female GP available, but she is busy all day running an already overbooked and very busy contraception clinic and can't fit in any other patients. Mrs Brookes has asked to speak to the senior GP to ask him to intervene.

How appropriate are each of the following responses by **the senior GP** in this situation?

34.1 Apologise to the patient for the situation and tell the patient that she can see the female GP as soon as she has finished with her current patient.

A – A very appropriate thing to do
B – Appropriate, but not ideal
C – Inappropriate but not awful
D – A very inappropriate thing to do

34.2 Apologise to the patient and tell her that she should rebook the appointment for a day when she can get a slot with a female GP.

A – A very appropriate thing to do
B – Appropriate, but not ideal
C – Inappropriate but not awful
D – A very inappropriate thing to do

34.3 Apologise and explain to the patient that male doctors are very qualified and experienced in dealing with sensitive issues. Explain that the only realistic way of seeing a GP today would be to see a male doctor.

A – A very appropriate thing to do
B – Appropriate, but not ideal
C – Inappropriate but not awful
D – A very inappropriate thing to do

34.4 Apologise for the mix-up and tell the patient that, if she were to see a male doctor, the practice could ensure that a female nurse sits on the consultation so that she feels more at ease.

A – A very appropriate thing to do
B – Appropriate, but not ideal
C – Inappropriate but not awful
D – A very inappropriate thing to do

1300 UCAT Practice Questions

SJ 35 Practice — Scenario 35 – Internet Medicine

Amanda is a 35-year-old professional working in a high-powered City job. She has been suffering migraines for a long time, for which she has seen many medical specialists over the years. Despite all the tests undertaken and drugs prescribed to her, the migraines are still occurring and can sometimes be debilitating. She has gone back to her GP to discuss whether anything else can be done. She has done a lot of research on the internet and tells the GP that she has found a plant-based remedy on an American website with a lot of testimonials from clients who see this remedy as "some sort of miracle". The remedy costs only £1 per tablet; she would have to take one a day and the website claims there are no side effects.

How important to take into account are the following considerations for **Amanda's GP** when deciding how to respond to the situation?

35.1 That Amanda is enamoured with the positive testimonials.

A – Very important
B – Important
C – Of minor importance
D – Not important at all

35.2 That Amanda is very educated.

A – Very important
B – Important
C – Of minor importance
D – Not important at all

35.3 That the ingredients of the remedy are not named.

A – Very important
B – Important
C – Of minor importance
D – Not important at all

35.4 That Amanda may buy the remedy even if he recommends against taking it.

A – Very important
B – Important
C – Of minor importance
D – Not important at all

35.5 That there seem to be no side effects.

A – Very important
B – Important
C – Of minor importance
D – Not important at all

Situational Judgement – Practice

SJ 36 Practice — Scenario 36 – Educated Patient

Luis is a GP trainee. A patient, Mr Andrews, has pityriasis versicolor: a common, unsightly but harmless condition that causes small patches of skin to become discoloured. Long ago, he received treatment in the form of shampoos but none of them made much difference; as a result, he stopped seeing doctors for it and decided to simply put up with it. Luis advises Mr Andrews that new antifungal shampoos can be effective, but Mr Andrews refuses to use them as they have never worked for him in the past. He says he has read on the internet that some anti-dandruff shampoos available on prescription might work and he would like Luis to prescribe them. Luis is not aware that anti-dandruff shampoos would be helpful.

How important to take into account are the following considerations for **Luis** when deciding how to respond to the situation?

36.1 That he has never come across this as a treatment during his training.

A – Very important
B – Important
C – Of minor importance
D – Not important at all

36.2 That the patient's experience of antifungal shampoos is old.

A – Very important
B – Important
C – Of minor importance
D – Not important at all

36.3 That the anti-dandruff shampoos have no side effects and there is no harm in Mr Andrews trying them.

A – Very important
B – Important
C – Of minor importance
D – Not important at all

36.4 That Luis can seek advice from a senior colleague nearby.

A – Very important
B – Important
C – Of minor importance
D – Not important at all

36.5 That the anti-dandruff shampoos mentioned by the patient can actually be obtained without prescription.

A – Very important
B – Important
C – Of minor importance
D – Not important at all

SJ 37 Practice — Scenario 37 – Speeding

Rob is a medical student shadowing Frank, a junior GP, during a morning filled with routine home visits. The patients are spread over a wide rural area and, often, Rob sees Frank driving well over the speed limit in order to get to the house calls at their scheduled times; this is worrying him. He has already warned Frank several times that his driving is dangerous, to no avail, and is considering raising the issue with his supervisor.

How important to take into account are the following considerations for **Rob** when deciding how to respond to the situation?

37.1 That the junior GP is an experienced driver.

A – Very important
B – Important
C – Of minor importance
D – Not important at all

37.2 That Rob may get a negative report if he speaks up.

A – Very important
B – Important
C – Of minor importance
D – Not important at all

37.3 That the junior GP is endangering other road users.

A – Very important
B – Important
C – Of minor importance
D – Not important at all

37.4 That it is Frank's word against Rob's.

A – Very important
B – Important
C – Of minor importance
D – Not important at all

37.5 That some patients may become slightly anxious if the GP is late.

A – Very important
B – Important
C – Of minor importance
D – Not important at all

37.6 That emergency vehicles are allowed to go over the speed limit.

A – Very important
B – Important
C – Of minor importance
D – Not important at all

SJ 38 Practice — Scenario 38 – Rude Student

Joseph and Fatima are medical students doing a placement on a ward. Every day, they practise their medical history-taking skills on patients; a patient could be asked their medical history several times a day, a fact they are made aware of and is common practice in teaching hospitals. During a ward round run by a consultant and attended by the two medical students, a patient complains that Joseph was rude to him during a previous history-taking session.

How appropriate are each of the following responses **by the consultant** in this situation?

38.1 To tell Joseph that he cannot take any more histories from this patient.

| A – Appropriate | B – Inappropriate

38.2 To ask Fatima to help Joseph with his history-taking skills before he can see any patient again.

| A – Appropriate | B – Inappropriate

38.3 To apologise to the patient, remind him that he was told that he would be seen by medical students from whom perfection can't be expected, and allow Joseph to continue seeing him.

| A – Appropriate | B – Inappropriate

38.4 To ask the patient if Joseph could take his history again, but under the supervision of a qualified and experienced doctor.

| A – Appropriate | B – Inappropriate

38.5 To make sure that the patient is not seen by medical students again.

| A – Appropriate | B – Inappropriate

38.6 To ask Joseph to apologise to the patient for being rude.

| A – Appropriate | B – Inappropriate

SJ 39 Practice — Scenario 39 – Anger with Mistakes

Ashley, a medical student, has been asked to present the medical history of a patient during a ward round. Many members of the clinical team are present, and the process takes place in the presence of the patient.

In the past few days, Ashley gave similar presentations, during which he made a few mistakes. Those were pointed out to him by the consultant running the ward round, so that he could improve. Today, Ashley made the same mistakes again during his presentation, which the consultant pointed out to him, again, on the spot, but this time in an angry tone.

How appropriate are the following responses **by Ashley** to the situation?

39.1 To point out straight away to the consultant that he is there to learn and that the angry tone is not appropriate in this context.

| A – Appropriate | B – Inappropriate |

39.2 To ask the consultant how he could make sure that he doesn't repeat the same mistakes again.

| A – Appropriate | B – Inappropriate |

39.3 To ask a junior doctor to spare him some time so that they can go through the mistakes that he made.

| A – Appropriate | B – Inappropriate |

39.4 To ask other medical students whether they have had similar reactions from the consultant.

| A – Appropriate | B – Inappropriate |

39.5 To arrange a chat with the consultant to discuss the fact that his angry comments were made in front of a patient.

| A – Appropriate | B – Inappropriate |

SJ 40 Practice — Scenario 40 – Flirtatious Behaviour

Ashraf, a medical student, is doing an attachment at a GP practice and is observing consultations run by Dr Phelps. Dr Phelps is a newly qualified GP, who has just started permanent employment at the GP practice. Dr Phelps has often commented to Ashraf that he finds General Practice hard work and stressful and that Ashraf should stay away from a career as a GP if he can. Whilst observing Dr Phelps, Ashraf notices that Dr Phelps is communicating in a flirtatious manner with young female patients. Some patients occasionally flirt back.

How important to take into account are the following factors **for Ashraf** when deciding how to respond to the situation?

40.1 That Dr Phelps may lose his job over this behaviour.

| A – Important | B – Not important

40.2 That Dr Phelps may be sanctioned by the General Medical Council over this behaviour.

| A – Important | B – Not important

40.3 That Ashraf may be marked down for his attachment if he speaks out.

| A – Important | B – Not important

40.4 That Dr Phelps is struggling with his new responsibilities and the workload at the practice.

| A – Important | B – Not important

40.5 That Ashraf observed some of the patients flirting back.

| A – Important | B – Not important

40.6 That there is no policy in the staff manual forbidding flirtatious behaviour.

| A – Important | B – Not important

SJ 41 Practice — Scenario 41 – Rushed History Taking

Yasmina, a medical student, is working alongside Dan, a junior doctor, in an outpatient department, taking medical histories before the patient is seen by a more senior doctor. Yasmina notices that Dan seems to follow a different approach to history-taking to the one that she was taught, and, at times, he seems to rush the process. He also disappears from the room every so often between patients for a few minutes, for no apparent reason.

How appropriate are the following responses **by Yasmina** to the situation?

41.1 To let Dan know that his approach differs to what she learnt.

| A – Appropriate | B – Inappropriate

41.2 To tell Dan that if he is not following the method she was taught, he will miss important points of the patient's history.

| A – Appropriate | B – Inappropriate

41.3 To ask Dan if she could demonstrate to him during the next consultation how she would take the patient's history.

| A – Appropriate | B – Inappropriate

41.4 To ask Dan why he keeps leaving the room.

| A – Appropriate | B – Inappropriate

41.5 To tell Dan that when history taking is rushed, mistakes happen.

| A – Appropriate | B – Inappropriate

41.6 To inform Dan's supervisor that he is not staying the full duration with each patient and is rushing his history taking.

| A – Appropriate | B – Inappropriate

41.7 To ask her supervisor if she could be placed with a doctor who does history taking by the book.

| A – Appropriate | B – Inappropriate

SJ 42 Practice: Scenario 42 – Open Door

Holly is a medical student doing an attachment in a radiology department. As she walks past the waiting room, she spots a patient entering an unoccupied side room that is normally used to scan patients. The room contains scanners and sets of patient notes.

Holly enters the room and asks the patient what they are doing there. She notices that the patient is reading a set of notes, which turns out to be their own notes.

Holly politely asks the patient to stop looking at the notes and asks them to go back to the waiting room. She mentions the incident to a nurse who is passing by. The nurse replies that the door never closes properly, that it has never happened before, that patients wouldn't understand what is written in the notes anyway, and that the patients whose notes may also have been read will be none the wiser.

How important to take into account are the following factors **for Holly** when deciding how to respond to the situation?

42.1 That the patient was looking at their own notes.

A – Important   B – Not important

42.2 That the patient is unlikely to understand the notes' content.

A – Important   B – Not important

42.3 That the door does not close properly.

A – Important   B – Not important

42.4 That the patients whose notes were on the table will be unaware.

A – Important   B – Not important

42.5 That such incident has never happened before.

A – Important   B – Not important

SJ 43 Practice — Scenario 43 – Rogue Interpreter

Adele is a medical student currently sitting in clinic with a consultant who is seeing a Romanian-speaking patient. The patient's ability to speak English is limited and it has been decided that the consultation will take place with a Romanian interpreter available on the phone. The consultant will ask a question in English to the interpreter who will then ask that question in Romanian to the patient. The patient will reply in Romanian and the interpreter will translate the answer into English for the benefit of the consultant.

Adele, who can speak enough Romanian to understand what is being said by the interpreter, realises quickly that the interpreter is translating the questions in a slightly inaccurate manner, although she does not feel that the inaccuracies would have an impact on the consultant's assessment.

How appropriate are the following responses **by Adele** to the situation?

43.1 To wait and, just as the consultation is about to end, to tell the consultant that some questions may need to be asked again with a more accurate translation.

| A – Appropriate | B – Inappropriate

43.2 To interrupt the conversation and ask the consultant if she could have a quick word.

| A – Appropriate | B – Inappropriate

43.3 To pass a note discretely to the consultant to point out the issue.

| A – Appropriate | B – Inappropriate

43.4 To suggest that the interpreter be abandoned so that she can do the translation herself.

| A – Appropriate | B – Inappropriate

43.5 To do nothing because she does not feel that inaccuracies are material.

| A – Appropriate | B – Inappropriate

SJ 44 Practice — Scenario 44 – Sick Note

Teresa is a medical student doing a GP attachment with Dr Jones. One patient, Patrick, is being examined for backache and a possible neck injury that he says were sustained at work. After examining Patrick, Dr Jones concludes that the level of pain he experiences justifies giving Patrick two further weeks off work. Dr Jones gives Patrick a sick note that states clearly: "The patient is not fit to return to work until two weeks after the date of this certificate".

Two days later, whilst walking in the local park, Teresa recognises Patrick in the distance. He is playing five-a-side football with no obvious restrictions to his mobility.

How appropriate are the following responses **by Teresa** to the situation?

44.1 To approach Patrick to say she knows he feigned his symptoms.

| A – Appropriate | B – Inappropriate

44.2 To film the football match as proof.

| A – Appropriate | B – Inappropriate

44.3 To call Dr Jones on the spot to discuss the incident.

| A – Appropriate | B – Inappropriate

44.4 To relate the incident to the GP the next working day and suggest that the GP calls Patrick to review his assessment.

| A – Appropriate | B – Inappropriate

44.5 To inform the lead GP of the practice that Dr Jones misdiagnosed Patrick.

| A – Appropriate | B – Inappropriate

44.6 To call Patrick's employers to report the fraud.

| A – Appropriate | B – Inappropriate

SJ 45 Practice — Scenario 45 – Corridor Kiss

In the Ophthalmology department of a major hospital, a senior trainee doctor, George, is being resented by other senior trainees because he seems to be getting preferential treatment by the lead consultant, Mrs Wallis. George has also been tipped to be getting a job in that department as a consultant during a forthcoming recruitment process. Staff members believe the process has been fixed to favour George over other candidates.

Edward, another senior trainee applying for that consultant post, accidentally spots George and Mrs Wallis in a passionate embrace whilst working late one evening. They are not aware that they were seen. Edward knows that Mrs Wallis is married with young children but there are rumours that her marriage is going through difficulties.

How important to take into account are the following factors **for Edward** when deciding how to respond to the situation?

45.1 That Mrs Wallis is married with children.

| A – Important | B – Not important

45.2 That Mrs Wallis is on the selection panel for the consultant post.

| A – Important | B – Not important

45.3 That Mrs Wallis is the sub-dean of the medical school.

| A – Important | B – Not important

45.4 That Mrs Wallis' marriage is going through difficulties.

| A – Important | B – Not important

45.5 That Mrs Wallis' colleagues speak very highly of her.

| A – Important | B – Not important

45.6 That Mrs Wallis' is well known in the speciality, which may affect Edward's chances of getting a consultant post anywhere else.

| A – Important | B – Not important

SJ 46 Practice — Scenario 46 – Dominant Colleagues

Yin is a medical student who started a new attachment two months ago. The team has three junior doctors: Steven, Usha and Priya. When all three are around, the team seems to work harmoniously. However, whenever Priya is away, Steven and Usha behave aggressively towards Yin, and often make derogatory comments about her abilities in front of patients.

How appropriate are the following responses **by Yin** to the situation?

46.1 To discuss her concerns with the three junior doctors.

| A – Appropriate | B – Inappropriate

46.2 To seek advice from more senior colleagues on how to improve working relations with Steven and Usha.

| A – Appropriate | B – Inappropriate

46.3 To request to be assigned to a different hospital.

| A – Appropriate | B – Inappropriate

46.4 To wait a couple of weeks to see if the situation improves.

| A – Appropriate | B – Inappropriate

46.5 To stay away from Steven and Usha whenever possible.

| A – Appropriate | B – Inappropriate

SJ 47 Practice — Scenario 47 – Back Pain

Charles is a medical student. His GP has prescribed the painkiller codeine for persistent back pain that has been getting worse over the last few weeks. That back pain most likely originated from bad posture as well as handling equipment and patients at work. Charles noticed that, during his shifts, he is getting more and more tired and is finding it difficult to concentrate. His performance has started to get affected by it. Charles knows that sleepiness is a possible side effect of codeine.

How appropriate are the following responses **by Charles** to the situation?

47.1 To increase the number of breaks he takes during his next shift.

| A – Appropriate | B – Inappropriate

47.2 To stop taking the codeine immediately.

| A – Appropriate | B – Inappropriate

47.3 To make an appointment with his GP.

| A – Appropriate | B – Inappropriate

47.4 To speak with the senior doctor in charge of his next shift to make them aware of the situation.

| A – Appropriate | B – Inappropriate

47.5 To ask a colleague to help with his workload until he finishes taking the prescribed codeine.

| A – Appropriate | B – Inappropriate

47.6 To seek advice from a senior trainee in his team about the option to stop taking the codeine.

| A – Appropriate | B – Inappropriate

SJ 48 Practice — Scenario 48 – Repeated A&E Visits

Roberto is a medical student currently on an assignment in A&E. He gets talking to Mr Gatter, a 70-year-old patient, who was earlier admitted with chest pains. This is the eighth time that he has been admitted for chest pains in the past three weeks. Each time, extensive investigations were made, and a cardiologist documented that all investigations were normal and that the pain was most certainly not of cardiac origin. Today, all investigations have also come back as normal, there are no symptoms of cardiac disease or any signs of concern. Mr Gatter is asking for Roberto's help in getting him admitted to hospital.

How appropriate are the following responses **by Roberto** to the situation?

48.1 To tell Mr Gatter that he will ask one of the doctors to make sure he is admitted to the Acute Admissions Unit for further investigations.

| A – Appropriate | B – Inappropriate

48.2 To ask a senior colleague to talk to Mr Gatter.

| A – Appropriate | B – Inappropriate

48.3 To tell Mr Gatter that, given that it is the eighth time that it has been shown that he has no cardiac issues, next time he has chest pains he should phone his GP first, before coming to A&E.

| A – Appropriate | B – Inappropriate

48.4 To ask Mr Gatter if there is anything else that he may be worried about that could be causing the pain.

| A – Appropriate | B – Inappropriate

48.5 To tell the patient that there is nothing wrong with him.

| A – Appropriate | B – Inappropriate

SJ 49 Practice — Scenario 49 – Drug Interactions

Rashid is a dental student on an attachment in a community dental practice. He is currently at reception looking for paperwork and overhears a receptionist on the phone to a patient, Mr Lewis. He can only hear the receptionist's side of the conversation, which is as follows:

"If the dentist prescribed you those antibiotics, then you should take them." ... "If the dentist prescribed them, then they probably won't interfere with your other medications. I'm sure she will have checked." ... "I'm really sorry, Mr Lewis, you cannot talk to her, she is currently with a patient. Take the medication prescribed and let us know if any issues come up."

It is important that Mr Lewis starts taking the antibiotics soon, but there is no urgency.

Out of the following three options, choose the **one most appropriate** and the **one least appropriate** action that **Rashid** should take in response to the situation.

A. Knock on the dentist's door, explain the situation, and ask if she could confirm whether the medication was correctly prescribed.

B. Call the Mr Lewis back, ask the patient for details of his other medication and ask him to hold back on taking any medication for a few minutes until he can check the facts regarding possible drug interaction.

C. Ask the receptionist to call Mr Lewis back straight away and tell him not to take any medical until she has managed to talk to the dentist.

SJ 50 Practice — Scenario 50 – Retrospective Entry

Anita is a junior doctor observing Dr Reddy, a consultant in diabetes currently running an outpatient clinic. They are seeing a patient who was diagnosed with diabetes a month before.

During the consultation, Dr Reddy asks the patient how he got on with following the dietary recommendations set out in the factsheet that he was given at his first visit. The patient replies that he was not given any factsheet. Dr Reddy apologises for the omission, hands over a copy of the factsheet to the patient and recommends that he takes it home with him. Dr Reddy advises the patient to use the factsheet to decide how to best avoid foods that may worsen his diabetes.

Once the patient has left the room, Dr Reddy explains to Anita that small errors like this happen frequently and that, as long as there is no harm to the patient, they are nothing to be concerned about. Anita then observes Dr Reddy access the notes for the consultation that took place a month previously and add the comment: "Patient was given dietary factsheet". She points out to Dr Reddy that he wrote the comment in the wrong consultation record as it should be recorded in today's records. Dr Reddy replies that ultimately it makes no difference at all as this is not a significant issue.

Out of the following three options, choose the **one most appropriate** and the **one least appropriate** action that **Anita** should take in response to the situation.

A. While Dr Reddy is still logged in but busy assessing the next patient, delete the comment written by Dr Reddy in the previous month's record, and add it instead to today's consultation record.

B. Log into the system using her own login later that day, and write an addendum to today's consultation notes, recording the incident and her discussions with Dr Reddy.

C. Raise the issue with a senior consultant.

SJ 51 Practice — Scenario 51 – Sudden Absence

Anil is a medical student working alongside Christina, a very junior doctor, as part of a surgical team. This is a very busy environment and Anil is taking a blood test from a patient. Anil suddenly notices that Christina, who was supervising him at the time, has disappeared without saying a word. A nurse tells Anil that Christina was called to assist one of the surgeons in the operating theatre. She has redirected her bleep to Anil, who is now facing a very busy workload, some of which he is not equipped to deal with.

Out of the following three options, choose the **one most appropriate** and the **one least appropriate** action that **Anil** should take in response to the situation.

A. Contact the operating theatre to request that Christina returns to the ward to help him.

B. Write a list of the jobs that have arisen whilst Christina was in theatre so that she can complete them when she comes back from theatre.

C. Ask Christina, when she returns to the ward, to let him know in future when she needs to leave the ward.

SJ 52 Practice — Scenario 52 – Scan Request

Rosie is a junior doctor working on a medical ward. During the ward round, Rosie is asked by the consultant to request a CT scan for a patient called Mrs Peacock. After the ward round, Rosie overhears two senior trainees discuss Mrs Peacock's case. One of the senior trainees is adamant that there is no clinical indication for a CT scan and that this is an inappropriate request. The consultant has not heard the comment.

Out of the following three options, choose the **one most appropriate** and the **one least appropriate** action that **Rosie** should take in response to the situation.

A. Tell the consultant that the senior trainee feels that the CT scan is not needed and that the request is inappropriate.

B. Discuss with the consultant the reasons for the CT scan.

C. Discuss the case and conflict of opinion with the consultant radiologist who will conduct the scan.

SJ 53 Practice — Scenario 53 – Back and Forth

Archana and Richard are both junior doctors working on the same busy ward. One of the senior trainees told Archana and Richard that once they have completed their tasks, they can go home.

Archana has nearly completed all her tasks, when she gets called to another ward on the other side of the hospital, to which she must go without delay.

Richard tells Archana then she should call the ward when she has finished with the other ward to check if there is any more that needs doing. Richard says that there is no need for her to return to her ward if all the tasks have been completed.

When Archana has finished with the other ward, she calls her ward but gets no answer.

Out of the following three options, choose the **one most appropriate** and the **one least appropriate** action that **Archana** should take in response to the situation.

A. Text Richard asking him to call her back.

B. Continue telephoning her ward until someone answers.

C. Return to her ward.

SJ 54 Practice — Scenario 54 – Unable to Cope

Amina is a medical student. She is having lunch with a junior doctor, Michael, with whom she has been working for a few weeks on a very busy ward. As they are discussing their workload, Michael bursts into tears, and says he feels he is not coping well with the job. He finds the consultant too arrogant and demanding, and he is getting a strong feeling from the nurses' attitude towards him that they are getting annoyed at his lack of ability to cope with the workload. Several nurses have made comments of the type "This is typical of the snowflake generation".

Out of the following three options, choose the **one most appropriate** and the **one least appropriate** action that **Amina** should take in response to the situation.

A. Suggest to Michael that he discusses the issue with a senior trainee whom he can trust.

B. Encourage Michael to get help from his GP.

C. Advise Michael to take a few days of annual leave.

17 Situational Judgement Answers to Practice Questions

SJ 1 – Aesthetics

Although the senior doctor seemed to be joking when he made his comment, this is only speculative. In reality, however light-hearted the comment made was, it reflects a prejudiced attitude which may affect the dynamics of the team and the atmosphere within it. There is also, of course, a risk that such a comment may be heard by patients or relatives, causing them to lose faith in the work of the medical team (and, in some extreme cases, the work of the entire health service). The fact that the patient was out of the room is a relief, but it does not make the statement less prejudiced.

The fact that the nurse simply takes the comment for granted should also be of concern. Of concern too is that she is attempting to get Joshua to simply accept it. In healthcare, inappropriate behaviour should be challenged, regardless of whether it is exhibited by someone senior or junior.

Of course, we should also bear in mind that this still remains a fairly benign issue in that there is no immediate danger to the patient or the team. As such the response should be proportionate.

1.1 – D: A very inappropriate thing to do
The patient has not heard the comment and has not been harmed by it so there is nothing to apologise for. In fact, apologising would make him aware of the comment and might cause him to lose faith in the team.

Things would be different if the team had made a mistake in the care of the patient. In that case, an apology and an explanation would be necessary regardless of whether the patient had been harmed or was aware of it.

1.2 – B: Appropriate, but not ideal
It is very appropriate for Joshua to speak to the senior doctor about his discomfort towards the comment made and to do so when the nurse is not present. However, this will mean taking valuable clinic time and delaying the care of the remaining patients for an issue that is not so urgent and can wait a few hours to be discussed. Hence why it ranks B and not A.

1.3 – D: A very inappropriate thing to do

This is very inappropriate because it is a lie and it serves no purpose other than self-protection against an issue which does not affect Joshua directly (it would be different if, for example, Joshua felt he had to leave because he was being bullied, but that is not the case here). It will also affect Joshua's learning throughout the attachment, though that is a more minor point.

1.4 – C: Inappropriate but not awful

Although it is appropriate to speak to the nurse privately and remind her of the professionalism that each team member should demonstrate, it is inappropriate for Joshua to get her to do his dirty work for him: even more so if the nurse seems to be siding with the senior doctor. It is ranked C instead of D because it would have few negative consequences (at worst, if she doesn't do it then Joshua will have to do it himself).

SJ 2 – Personal Statement

This is one of those questions where it is crucial you remember that Situational Judgement is about what you SHOULD do and not what you WOULD do. In practice, many fellow students would just ignore it and move on, thinking "It is too late anyway" and "Why bother making life hard for myself?" However, this section is testing your understanding of basic ethical principles and therefore you need to answer in relation to the theoretical approach you are expected to take.

Any kind of cheating is frowned upon severely in medicine and so admitting to it so blatantly could prove fatal for David and for his uncle. When it comes to questions about cheating, there is no excuse; it will have to be reported. The medical school tutors can then draw their own conclusions and act according to the school's principles. Looking at it the other way, i.e. imagining that Sapna failed to report it, if it were later discovered that Sapna knew about the cheating but had not disclosed it, then she could get into trouble for failing to raise the issue at an appropriate level.

2.1 – D: Not important at all

The fact that he turned out to be a good recruit might be a relief but that does not excuse the cheating. For a start there is no indication that he is achieving a high rank by being honest and, even if he were, it is not an indication that he is not prone to cheating as a last resort when things are not going well for him. The fact he is a top-ranking student only means that he is academically able, but it means nothing about his integrity anyway. So this is irrelevant.

2.2 – D: Not important at all
David's uncle should have worried about that when he made the decision to help his nephew out by encouraging him to lie. In those circumstances it is fair that the ethics of David's uncle should be scrutinised and, as such, the effect on his career should not influence whether the information should be disclosed or not. This might actually help uncover some of his uncle's other unethical behaviours.

2.3 – D: Not important at all
No one knows if David is actually always honest, but even if that were true, it does not excuse previous bad behaviour and should be reported (in theory anyway, but that is the perspective the UCAT is asking you to take: what you SHOULD do).

2.4 – D: Not important at all
Whether this is true or not, this does not excuse David's lying. In essence, two wrongs don't make a right.

In this example you are asked to discuss how important these factors are in <u>Sapna</u>'s decision to report the matter to a supervisor. The answers would be different if we were asked to consider whether David's supervisor should expel him from medical school. In that situation, it would be important to consider whether, though David has made a mistake, he has shown remorse for it and has learnt his lesson from it. In such case, the school may show more leniency towards someone who is known for being honest and a strong performer. Those considerations, however, are not for Sapna to take into account. They are for the medical school to worry about.

SJ 3 – Staying Late

There are several issues to consider:

- As much as she can, Maryam should finish her jobs before she leaves. In other words, if she needs to stick around ten more minutes to finish a job, she should do so rather than hand it over to someone who knows little about what is going on. However, the situation is slightly complicated here by the fact that the computer system could be out of action for some time, and it would not be reasonable for Maryam to wait around for an unpredictable amount of time.

- Maryam could well decide to stick around but she will lose the chance to rest properly before the next morning's shift. Having said that, this is an exceptional circumstance, the computer system is expected to be back up and running by 7 pm and she does not have far to travel. So even if she left at 7 pm, it would leave her a decent amount of evening time.
- Rob is clearly trying to minimise the burden on himself by pushing it back on to Maryam.
- If no one ends up checking the blood test results, this may result in harm to patients.

3.1 – D: A very inappropriate thing to do
By leaving without ensuring that the blood tests are checked one way or the other, Maryam potentially places patients at risk of harm. Any action which places patients at risk HAS to be ranked as very inappropriate.

3.2 – B: Appropriate, but not ideal
Talking to Rob's supervisor would ensure that the situation is handled and that patients are safe; so it is appropriate. Note that, normally, answers which talk about involving a supervisor are ranked as C (inappropriate but not awful) if you have not talked to the problem individual first. However, in this case Rob has already been involved and has refused to help and there is a possible safety issue so this ranks higher. Maryam also hasn't really tried her hardest yet to convince Rob and, since she still has some scope to convince Rob to change his mind, this will rank as B, not A.

3.3 – A: A very appropriate thing to do
Sorting the situation out with Rob directly is the best course of action. Note that it is ranked A for that reason but also because the statement says that Maryam acknowledges his concerns.

3.4 – C: Inappropriate but not awful
This is inappropriate insofar as there is only so much time Maryam can stay after normal hours to finish her tasks, particularly if the rota allows for someone to deal with out-of-hours work. It would be reasonable for her to stay if she knew the computer system would be back up after 20 minutes; but 2 hours is a very long time (particularly if there is a risk the system may not be back online after that) and therefore the task should really be handled by whoever takes over from her. The main issue with this approach is to

determine whether staying late may affect patient safety (e.g. if that compromised her sleeping time). But we are told that she lives locally. If she leaves the hospital at 7.30 pm and her next shift is at 7 am the next morning, then she will have ample time to rest. Things would be different if she had to stay up all night. Hence why it is ranked C, and not D.

SJ 4 – Needlestick Injury

4.1 – A: A very appropriate thing to do
One of the most important reasons for ranking this answer as very appropriate is that Sartaj is recognising that he may not be fit to take the blood because he may panic. We know that this is true and therefore there is a real risk to patient safety. As such, it is very reasonable for him to refuse and ask if someone else can do it. It is all the more reasonable since he won't be required to carry out that procedure in his future career. If he had planned to work in a specialty where needles are used, then it may have been reasonable for him to refuse in this instance, but he would have had to find a way to overcome that fear soon.

A second important reason is that he is letting the senior doctor know about it in a nice way, with an apology, and in a situation where the senior doctor can actually do something about it. If Sartaj simply failed to take the blood without informing anyone then the patient would be at risk, and this would be very inappropriate.

The combination of safety and a sensible/sensitive approach makes this option rank as very appropriate.

4.2 – C: Inappropriate but not awful
The approach that Sartaj is taking here is safe because he won't be doing the procedure himself. However, he is not being upfront with the consultant. Sartaj knows that he can't do it and so he should be honest about it. If anything, it will ensure the consultant is reminded of the problem. However, he didn't actually lie, and merely said something that could be interpreted in different ways, so that ranks as C instead of D.

4.3 – C: Inappropriate but not awful
In doing so, Sartaj recognises that he may be a risk to the patient and ensures that the procedure is carried out in a safe environment, under supervision. If he did end up finding it difficult, then someone would be there to take over. However, it would not be the most reassuring solution for the patient, who may end up seeing Sartaj panic whilst having a needle in their

Situational Judgement – Practice

arm. Given that Sartaj won't be using needles very soon, he might as well ask whoever was going to observe the procedure to do it themselves. That would be both faster and safer and would keep the patient's confidence levels up. The impact on the patient is the reason the answer ranks C.

4.4 – C: Inappropriate but not awful
This is inappropriate because Sartaj is essentially having a go at a senior colleague, who may simply have forgotten about his issue. Such an approach will not help maintain goodwill between colleagues and is too confrontational. The reason it is ranked C instead of D is because it will at least ensure that the procedure is not carried out by him and so it takes care of the safety angle.

SJ 5 – Chance Encounter

5.1 – D: A very inappropriate thing to do
Admitting to his friends that the man is a patient would be a breach of confidentiality. For example, if Dr Jones were in the oncology department, his friends would automatically know the man may have cancer. If Dr Jones worked in the sexual health department, that could be even more embarrassing. Essentially just acknowledging he is a patient without revealing why would be sufficient information to constitute a breach of confidentiality.

5.2 – B: Appropriate, but not ideal
The benefit of this approach is that he is dealing with the situation away from his friends, thereby avoiding any confidentiality issues. The tone at the end is fairly amicable; however, it is a little abrupt to remind the patient of the rules when it is perfectly acceptable to have a discussion with patients outside of the professional setting as long as it is discreet and not part of an ongoing friendship or relationship. A 5-minute general discussion is hardly going to influence the care provided by the doctor to the patient.

5.3 – D: A very inappropriate thing to do
The patient will be somewhat bemused by the fact his own doctor is blanking him. This may affect the doctor-patient relationship going forward.

5.4 – A: A very appropriate thing to do
This approach has the benefit that it deals with the confidentiality side of the problem, and also enables the doctor to engage normally with the patient without allowing the situation to develop further.

5.5 – A: A very appropriate thing to do
This would obviously take place the following day once he has dealt with the patient on the spot in whatever manner he saw fit. It may sound over the top, but it would demonstrate that Dr Jones is being transparent about the situation in case there is an issue at a later stage. A verbal mention to the manager would be a good thing to do but putting it in writing would ensure an accurate contemporaneous record. Because it can only be a positive action with no flipside, it has to rank A.

SJ 6 – Career Development

6.1 – C: Of minor importance
Thomas's job is to look after patients in the psychiatric unit first and foremost. Putting pressure on other colleagues by coming and going as he pleases is unacceptable. The fact that he finds the work boring or irrelevant to his career does not mean that he shouldn't engage with it. However, though Dan should not compromise on those points (which would rank the answer as D), he also has scope to be helpful to his colleague, for example, by agreeing with him to share the work in a certain way so that Thomas can benefit more from the attachment. Therefore, to a small extent, Dan could take Thomas's career choice into consideration to be a good colleague.

6.2 – A: Very important
By not clearing his absences with senior doctors, he is creating an unsafe situation. The team will be assuming that he is fulfilling his duties and so won't necessarily cover during that time. This also demonstrates a lack of integrity and a lack of care for the impact of his actions on the team.

6.3 – D: Not important at all
This is really an issue for Thomas to worry about, rather than Dan. Raising concerns about unprofessional behaviour should not be dependent on the fact that the person in question may suffer as a consequence of their own actions. In other words, it is Thomas's choice to do what he is doing and so he is liable for the consequences of his actions. Dan does not have a duty to save Thomas from his own actions. As such, this is irrelevant.

6.4 – C: Of minor importance
If Thomas can compensate at a later stage for his absences, then that would be a good thing to consider because it would equate to an overall fair allocation of work across the whole attachment. However, this is only hypothetical and therefore is not of great value to make a decision.

Situational Judgement – Practice

SJ 7 – Venting Off

7.1 – A: Very important
It is important that patients trust the doctors who care for them. Anything which undermines that trust will be detrimental to the relationship. This consideration is therefore vital.

7.2 – D: Not important at all
The comment made by Rob is wrong, not just because it is personally targeting a specific member of the team but mostly because it is inappropriately undermining the care the team is providing as a whole. So, the fact that Dr Jones is soon to leave does not make the comment more acceptable; it is Rob's attitude that is wrong. Indeed, Rob most likely makes such comments about other colleagues too or might do so in the future.

7.3 – D: Not important at all
This is the dilemma that whistle-blowers constantly face. They need to do the right thing by reporting unacceptable behaviours, but then often end up paying the price by being vilified by their team. In this situation, the comment made by Rob will need to be reported to someone senior because it is unacceptable regardless of the consequences, simply because it is undermining the care the team is giving to patients (remember that they are testing what you SHOULD do and not necessarily what you WOULD do).

7.4 – D: Not important at all
Mrs Peacock may well lie to defend Rob but then again, she may not. Even if she did, it would not mean that the incident did not take place; it would merely make it harder to prove that it did take place. However, what matters here is that the incident is recorded and that someone senior addresses it with Rob. At best, it might make him more aware of the inadequacy of his behaviour and the incident will be addressed. At worst, nothing will happen immediately but if other colleagues start reporting similar incidents, then the unit's management will not be able to ignore the accumulating evidence. In other words, Sandra's contribution may not make an immediate impact, but it will contribute towards a resolution.

SJ 8 – Gift from Patient

8.1 – A: Very important
The doctor should not feel that their care of the patient should be influenced by the gift. If the present was of high value (e.g. a car, jewellery, or other

expensive item), the gift would be inappropriate in the context of a doctor–patient relationship. However, it is entirely sensible that doctors should be able to accept gifts of small value.

8.2 – B: Important
A gift makes sense if it bears a relation to the care received from the doctor. Thinking logically, it makes sense for a doctor to be offered a box of chocolates as a thank you present if they have made a big difference to a patient. It would make less sense to receive a gift simply for a routine one-off visit. As such, the fact that the patient is a regular does have a bearing on the decision because it provides a context of "normality". By itself, this would rank the answer as an A. Having said that, in this particular case, the gift is small and there would be no reason to upset a patient by rejecting the gift simply on the basis that they were not a regular. On balance, this should therefore be ranked as B instead of A, i.e. it is not a vital consideration.

8.3 – A: Very important
The main consideration that Jonas needs to take into account is whether the gift, by its nature or the conditions in which it is received, is likely to alter or damage the doctor-patient relationship. If the patient is looking forward to giving the gift to the doctor, then he may be offended or upset by a refusal. This may affect the doctor-patient relationship for no good reason. So, this would be a very important consideration.

8.4 – C: Of minor importance
The fact that other people do something regularly does not mean that it is the right thing to do. It can be a useful indicator, but this should not be the major driver for one's decision.

8.5 – D: Not important at all
At worst, Jonas could give the box of chocolates to someone else or, even better, share it with other members of staff in the GP practice. There is no point upsetting a patient just because he happens not to like chocolate when there are easy solutions to the problem.

SJ 9 – Preoperative Questions

9.1 – D: A very inappropriate thing to do
We are told that the patient is anxious; therefore, making him wait will only increase his stress levels. In this situation he will spend the night with no answers.

9.2 – A: A very appropriate thing to do
Since we have been told explicitly that the doctors Mr Debono saw earlier are unavailable then getting an equally qualified doctor to answer the questions is very appropriate. Had we been told that the doctors he saw earlier were just "busy for the moment" then this answer would have been ranked B because, in the end, it would be best for the patient to see the original doctors, even if that meant having to wait for 20 minutes until they became available. But the question has already ruled out this option and so we must answer by considering the new context.

9.3 – D: A very inappropriate thing to do
There are times when trying to be helpful can cause more problems. It is possible that the patient's concerns are easy to address. However, they may not be. By reassuring the patient that she should be able to answer his questions, Sian is providing a level of reassurance that she may not be able to deliver in practice. That, in turn, may affect the patient's confidence in her and/or the team's competence; this may make him more anxious. That anxiety would be reinforced by the fact that Sian is only a medical student and the patient asked to see a doctor.

9.4 – B: Appropriate, but not ideal
This is essentially a more acceptable version of 9.3 in that Sian is not promising anything she can't deliver, and the patient is reassured that he will see a suitable doctor if need be. However, the patient did specifically request to see a doctor and may not be entirely trusting of a medical student. So, this will go a long way towards proactively finding a solution to the problem but may not entirely alleviate his fears (bearing in mind there is no guarantee he will see a doctor if Sian believes she can answer his questions correctly).

SJ 10 – Busy Social Life

10.1 – C: Inappropriate but not awful
This does not address Campbell's misplaced behaviour soon enough. The reason it is ranked C instead of D is because it will help get a clearer idea of the problem. The prospect that something might be done next time is also providing a small degree of reassurance.

Some might argue that, by taking a day off, Campbell exposed the rest of the team to extra pressure and therefore impacted on patient safety. It is true to say that the team would have felt extra pressure; however, since he called in the morning to say he would be off sick then the team would have had time to adjust accordingly and organise itself to cover his shift (it would have been worse if he had informed no one or if he had turned up at work and then simply vanished). As far as the team is concerned, in terms of patient cover, it made no difference whether he was actually sick or just pretending to be sick, and as such it cannot be concluded that Campbell put patients in danger by taking the day off deceptively (that would have automatically ranked the answer D). What needs to be dealt with, however, is the deception.

10.2 – D: A very inappropriate thing to do
Saying or doing nothing is never acceptable (bear in mind you are asked to say what you SHOULD do and not what you WOULD do) unless the person's behaviour is entirely justified.

10.3 – A: A very appropriate thing to do
In approaching Campbell directly, Robert will deal with it at the appropriate level. Because patients were not at risk of harm, there is no need to raise the matter higher up unless the issue recurs.

10.4 – C: Inappropriate but not awful
Given that patients were not exposed to harm and that the goal is simply to avoid a repeat incident, it is best to raise the matter first with Campbell rather than his supervising consultant. It is thus currently inappropriate, but it may become an appropriate course of action if there was a repeat incident despite having warned Campbell the first time round.

10.5 – C: Inappropriate but not awful
Given that the secretary will be able to do nothing else other than pass on the message, it seems unfair to involve her in the process. And it might also, in passing, damage the perception that others in the team have of Campbell for no real benefit. It therefore seems pointless to introduce an intermediary into the discussion unwittingly. The answer is ranked C instead of D because it is at least an attempt, however inappropriate, to do something about the matter.

SJ 11 – No More Leaflets

11.1 – A: A very appropriate thing to do
This shows that Josie is proactive in finding a solution that will give the patient what he requires. She can't make miracles and suddenly produce a

Situational Judgement – Practice

proper leaflet but giving the patient a printout will ensure he has the information he needs in the short term until a proper leaflet materialises. The fact that Josie apologises ranks this answer as A. Without the apology it would rank B.

11.2 – C: Inappropriate but not awful
There are two things wrong with this approach:

(i) Informing the receptionist by email is very formal and could be misunderstood as emails can appear blunter than they are intended to be. It is a very impersonal way of achieving something that would be best done face to face in a two-way conversation. So, although the intention is right, the method is inappropriate.

(ii) Copying the practice manager feels a bit vindictive. If the practice manager were to be involved, then it would be far better to go and talk to him/her directly.

This approach may make team relations worse. But since the result is not hugely dramatic (i.e. no one is going to be harmed in the process) then it qualifies for a C rather than a D.

11.3 – C: Inappropriate but not awful
Ordinarily, any answer which involves talking directly to the person who has done wrong should be scored as A: A very appropriate thing to do. But here the problem is that the way it is being done may actually cause a range of issues and make things worse. Particularly, taking the receptionist away from her main duties for an issue which is really not urgent at all and can wait for the end of the day will be disruptive to the flow of the patients through the clinic. Patients will not get booked in, paperwork will not get done and other staff will have to work harder to compensate, not counting the fact that the receptionist might leave the meeting feeling upset, which risks impacting on the rest of her day. Hence it is ranked C (as opposed to D, which would only really be suitable if there were greater risks).

11.4 – C: Inappropriate but not awful
It would be best to have a word with the receptionist and only escalate to the practice manager if the receptionist persisted in her bad behaviour. Raising the matter at this stage is premature and inappropriate. Such course of action would be more appropriate if this was recurring behaviour.

SJ 12 – Poor Presentation

The best course of action in this situation would be to talk to Sandra directly (an option which is not actually in any of the proposed responses). Therefore, any other approach which is likely to help resolve the situation will be ranked B and any detrimental option will be ranked C or D.

12.1 – D: A very inappropriate thing to do
This is basically the "Sandra is responsible for her own problems" approach. This approach is wrong in many levels:

(i)   It does not actually address the problem. It merely serves to embarrass Sandra when it is discovered later that her part of the presentation was poor.

(ii) It shows poor teamwork (for example it is possible that Sandra is actually struggling as opposed to lazy).

(iii) It will likely cause problem for Ahmed who will find out late that there is an issue, at a time when possibly little can be done to remedy the problem. One might take the view that it is partially Ahmed's fault for being too remote from the two students, but the issue here is that this is a deliberate attempt by Barbara to set Sandra up.

As such, it shows very poor judgement and poor teamwork from Barbara and, essentially, a vindictive nature. The deliberate nature of the act and the impact not just on Sandra but on a quasi-innocent third party (Ahmed) is what is causing it to rank at the worst possible level.

12.2 – B: Appropriate, but not ideal
A progress meeting will have the benefit of ensuring that the issues are raised when there is still time to sort out the problem with Sandra's work. It might also provide a more objective forum to discuss the presentation as a whole and therefore highlight the deficiencies in Sandra's work. However, this is, in a way, a slightly cowardly approach; it would be more appropriate to sort the issue out with Sandra directly first.

12.3 – B: Appropriate, but not ideal
This may or may not work, but at least it is a reasonable and personal attempt at finding a way to raise the issues, though possibly a bit round the houses to be effective.

Situational Judgement – Practice

12.4 – C: Inappropriate but not awful
This would help achieve the desired result, but it would be best to talk to Sandra directly first. At the UCAT, talking to someone's superior before you have attempted to resolve the issue with the individual concerned will always rank as inappropriate but not awful.

SJ 13 – Heavy Burden

13.1 – B: Appropriate, but not ideal
Ideally this is something that Jo should be able to do herself. In normal circumstances, dumping work on to other people would be ranked C but, since it could be construed that it is part of the supervisor's responsibility to look after Jo's wellbeing and her training, this can be upgraded to B, i.e. it is not entirely unfair to ask the supervisor to get involved.

13.2 – D: A very inappropriate thing to do
Not only is it admitting defeat, but it will also lead to her failing her academic year, will likely affect her wellbeing and may even have an impact on patients. The truth is she is just a medical student, and we are told that she is being utilised well beyond normal expectations. As such, she has cause to complain and should not just take it on board without fighting her corner, which may in the end cause her to fail in her studies.

13.3 – A: A very appropriate thing to do
The issue of being overburdened on the ward could be easily resolved through discussions, but if the personal issues are lingering then it may be best to sort them out once and for all. And if all it takes to achieve that is to have a few days off then so be it, particularly if it means that her performance will improve thereafter. It might of course mean that she may miss a few lectures, but the same would happen if she had a heavy cold/flu, and she could easily catch up later on.

13.4 – B: Appropriate, but not ideal
This would go some way towards addressing the issue, although it may be difficult to predict how much is due to the ward work and how much is due to the personal problems. The main issue with this answer, however, and the reason why it is rated B rather than A, is that she is imposing it onto the consultant rather than engaging in a consultative process to come to a mutual agreement. It is possible that simply pulling out of projects and cases may impact on the work of other people. To be marked as A, the statement

should be worded: "Sit down with the consultant to discuss how she can be given a more manageable workload."

SJ 14 – Late Handover

14.1 – A: A very appropriate thing to do
This will only take a few seconds and will seek to reassure the partner if there is any delay. It also shows an ability to prioritise patient care over non-essential personal matters when the need arises.

14.2 – A: A very appropriate thing to do
This will make the handover more efficient. It will make good use of the waiting time and will ensure that the outstanding tasks are clearly laid out, thus optimising the quality of the information handed over.

14.3 – D: A very inappropriate thing to do
The lack of verbal handover means that Saud will rely on the notes to identify what needs to be done. But worse, he will need to go fishing for those notes in various places. There is a risk that issues may get missed and this may therefore pose a risk to patients.

14.4 – C: Inappropriate but not awful
This would be appropriate if the reason for leaving work was totally unavoidable, e.g. picking up a child from nursery when the nursery was about to close. Here there is no reason to burden a senior colleague with what is essentially Ron's work and if the delay is only 20 to 30 minutes. That senior colleague probably already has problems of his own to deal with without having to deal with Ron's jobs too. In other words, Ron is simply dumping his work onto another colleague without a good enough reason. But at least it ensures patients are safe, hence why it ranks C and not D.

SJ 15 – Staying Late

15.1 – D: Not important at all
Whenever patient safety is potentially compromised, nothing should be an excuse for not taking action. It is better to get a bad reference and make sure that patients are safe, than to kill a patient through tiredness (imagine what the consultant's reference would be in that case!).

Situational Judgement – Practice

15.2 – B: Important
Contracts are there to act as protection for an employee against many things, including getting overworked. As such, it is important that, as much as possible, Amy works within the hours she is contracted to do. However, at the same time, she must account for the fact that on some occasions it may be necessary to deviate when there are exceptional circumstances. This consideration downgrades an A to a B.

15.3 – A: Very important
Tiredness will lead to mistakes and therefore affect patient safety. So A is the only possible answer.

15.4 – A: Very important
Amy's wellbeing is important as she needs to be fit and healthy in order to make the right decisions about patient care. Again, this affects patient safety and therefore A is the only possible answer.

15.5 – D: Not important at all
Her friends' annoyance is irrelevant as it will never be sufficiently important compared to the safety of patients. Therefore, it should not come into consideration when making a decision about the situation. It is of course possible that Amy, in turn, may get frustrated if her friends are annoyed with her and this may indirectly slightly affect her wellbeing. But it is a very speculative and indirect proposition.

Note that, here, the question is specifically about her friends' emotions and not about her lack of social life. If the question was "That she has lost all her social life and finds it hard to relax", this would score as a B.

SJ 16 – Infection Control

In situations such as these, where patients may be compromised, anything which places patients at risk is difficult to excuse.

16.1 – D: Not important at all
Whether the patients mind or not does not stop Lauren from placing them at risk of infection. Therefore, in this case, the patients' own thoughts are irrelevant. In fact, they probably don't seem to mind because they are unaware of the risks.

16.2 – D: Not important at all
The fact a doctor is not there when a policy is explained does not mean they shouldn't adhere to it. A rule is a rule, and it is undoubtedly featured prominently in the staff handbook. Besides, we are told that John has already raised the issue with Lauren recently and so she should be aware of the new policy by now.

16.3 – A: Very important
This is probably the biggest risk associated with wearing long sleeves and so it simply cannot be ignored.

16.4 – D: Not important at all
The patients' safety is being compromised and Lauren has already been warned once that week. The fact that she has a scar she wants to hide might explain her behaviour, but it does not excuse it; and certainly it does not mean that she is entitled to put patients at risk. As such, the incident will need to be reported regardless.

16.5 – D: Not important at all
The fact that other people do the wrong thing should not stop Lauren from doing the right thing.

SJ 17 – Letter Mix-up

17.1 – B: Appropriate, but not ideal
This is the right course of action; however, without an apology it gets downgraded from A to B.

17.2 – B: Appropriate, but not ideal
This is also a good course of action and, unlike 17.1, the response does contain an apology. However, it forces patients to come back to the hospital for no reason whatsoever and therefore will cause some inconvenience. The matter could easily be dealt with over the phone and by resending a letter.

17.3 – D: A very inappropriate thing to do
Although modifying the letters in the notes would ensure that the correct information is recorded in each patient's notes, it would not document that an error has been made. If there was a subsequent investigation, or if the patient demanded to see their set of notes, it would become apparent that the notes were altered retrospectively, and this would give the illusion of a cover-up. The illusion of dishonesty can be as bad as the dishonesty itself

Situational Judgement – Practice

since it may undermine confidence in the team's ability to show integrity in the care of its patients.

An appropriate course of action would be to make a note that the wrong letter was sent out and then place a copy of the new letter in the file.

17.4 – D: A very inappropriate thing to do
This option, unlike 17.3, does record the error in the notes as it should. However, it fails for a different reason: lack of honesty and transparency towards patients. If the patients realise later that they were sent the wrong letter, it will likely affect the trust they have in the care received from the medical team. One must bear in mind here that, although the doctors know the letters are similar, the patients will not. So, as far as they are concerned, the letters they should have received might be totally different. That may make them anxious.

17.5 – A: A very appropriate thing to do
The consultant is in charge of the ward, and it is therefore right that he/she should be informed.

SJ 18 – Bad Atmosphere

18.1 – D: A very inappropriate thing to do
However tempting it is to flee a conflict for the sake of an easier life, Liz will always at some stage be working with people who are difficult. Moving on to another place to escape the difficulties she is encountering is not going to help her in the long term. Nor will it force the individual in question to adopt better behaviour. It may have ranked as B or C if this was continuous and persistent behaviour despite having made several efforts to resolve the situation (i.e. much later down the line), but here this only happens when Raquel is away and there is no hint that prior action was attempted.

18.2 – A: A very appropriate thing to do
In an exam situation where you have to describe what you SHOULD do and not what you WOULD do, the most appropriate course of action will nearly always be to discuss the issue with the individuals concerned first (the exception being if you fear for your physical safety – there is no need to confront someone who you know will be aggressive towards you). Basically, give them a chance to correct their attitude before you take it any further. It may or may not work, but Liz needs to try.

18.3 – D: A very inappropriate thing to do
It is hard to see what would be gained by waiting since it seems to be a recurring problem. The more Liz waits, the more the atmosphere will degrade, with a possible impact on patient care and team spirit. Also, hopefully Raquel will be on the team most of the time and therefore the behaviour may only be observed sporadically as and when she is not present. As such, it will not serve any purpose. It scores as D because it helps perpetuate the problem, which can then only get worse.

18.4 – C: Inappropriate but not awful
Raquel may be able to provide some useful advice and even intervene, but Liz should only resort to involving third parties in her "battles" as a second resort, if she feels she cannot deal with the problem directly. The appropriate course of action would be to address the issue with Carlos and Daniel and, only if that failed, involve other parties.

18.5 – C: Inappropriate but not awful
Similar to 18.4, this may be useful – and certainly if things got worse, it would be useful to have a record of what has been happening – but this would only be a suitable course of action if direct contact with the protagonists had failed. Documenting the behaviour by itself would rank as B but giving the log to the consultant downgrades it to a C, as this would only be appropriate after Liz has dealt with Carlos and Daniel directly.

SJ 19 – Audit Data

This question deals with confidentiality, team playing and integrity all in one.

19.1 – D: A very inappropriate thing to do
Taking the notes home is very dangerous for many reasons: (i) they could get lost in transit and picked up by strangers (many people have found official government papers and even laptops on trains recently!), (ii) someone in Joshua's home could come across the notes, thus resulting in a breach of confidentiality, (iii) he might forget to bring them back, which may then impact on patient care if for some reason they are needed. With such serious consequences, it is just simply a very bad idea.

19.2 – C: Inappropriate but not awful
The supervisor will have made time for the meeting and for going through the data. Postponing the meeting would be unfair towards the supervisor since, had the meeting not been planned, he might have planned other

Situational Judgement – Practice

things instead. This also assumes that the supervisor can find time in their schedule on Tuesday and that Joshua will actually have finished the audit by then. Essentially it is inappropriate because Joshua's lack of planning is impacting negatively on someone else. That being said, postponing the meeting would be better than leaving it as it is with nothing to talk about, hence why it is not awful. It is also not awful because the consequences are fairly minor, all things considered.

19.3 – B: Appropriate, but not ideal
The fact that no patient-identifiable data is kept makes this solution appropriate. It is not ideal because the data is still leaving the hospital unnecessarily and could potentially get lost. In such circumstances it is hard to find a solution that would rank as very appropriate other than maybe asking for the keys to the clinic so that he can come in at the weekend to finish the audit.

19.4 – D: A very inappropriate thing to do
This is essentially making data up. That would be misleading and considered a grave lapse of integrity.

SJ 20 – Exam Cheat

20.1 – B: Appropriate, but not ideal
It would indeed be essential to let the deanery know about the issue so that it can deal with the problem effectively. There is, however, no real reason to keep Ellen's name confidential. In fact, it would benefit the process to reveal her name as the deanery will inevitably need to investigate the matter and Ellen would be the obvious starting point. The only possible reason one might be tempted to keep her name quiet would be to protect her; but it is not as though she has owned up to the "fraud" in a way that showed any kind of remorse. Not only is she playing along with it, but she is also trying to make Sarah complicit.

And, even if Ellen had come to Sarah to inform her that a fraud was taking place with the aim of reporting it so that it could be dealt with, instead of trying to get her to play along, it would still be appropriate for Sarah to give Ellen's name to the deanery for the purpose of the investigation. The deanery might then decide to be more lenient on Ellen because she reported the fraud but that would not be for Sarah to decide.

20.2 – D: A very inappropriate thing to do
It would be very naïve to think that Ellen would actually throw away the paper and, even if she did, there would be plenty of other copies around. This approach will achieve very little, if anything. Besides, it does not deal with the fact this has been going on for 5 years.

20.3 – D: A very inappropriate thing to do
It would indeed be fairer; but it's still fraud. It does not actually resolve anything, and it will cheapen the degree as the exam would pretty much be useless.

20.4 – D: A very inappropriate thing to do
Sarah could actually be struck off the register for playing along.

20.5 – D: A very inappropriate thing to do
It is inappropriate for several reasons:
(i) It would only serve to scare those students but would not actually resolve anything,
(ii) It is not Sarah's job to deal with the matter and
(iii) It is asking the deanery to part with data which in itself is also confidential.

SJ 21 – Quiet Attachment

21.1 – A: A very appropriate thing to do
Since Ishtiaq already does what he is supposed to do, it is very appropriate for him to offer his help to junior doctors who may struggle on other wards. Not only will this improve the care of their patients, but it will also enhance his learning experience.

21.2 – C: Inappropriate but not awful
There is a difference between helping other teams (21.1) when you are not busy and asking to be moved out of your current team altogether. On the surface it might make sense to an extent that Ishtiaq wants to move to a more interesting post (hence why it is deemed "not awful") but at the same time the team where he currently works needs him to care for its patients. Before he can even consider changing team, there are a whole load of responses that are more appropriate.

21.3 – A: A very appropriate thing to do
This demonstrates proactivity in seeking opportunities and would also enhance the work that his team does. Since we know that, clinically speaking,

he does everything required and more already, then it is entirely appropriate for him to use his spare time on other activities which are of benefit to his current team.

21.4 – C: Inappropriate but not awful
On the surface this seems like a good, proactive and useful idea. Yet this is pretty much a hobby, however useful it seems, and should really be done in his own time. Spending time preparing those courses would also mean he is not doing activities of direct benefit to his team, which, after all, employs and pays him. The reason it is ranked C and not D is because he does have genuine spare time and, therefore, engaging in setting up those courses would not be detrimental to the care of his patients or his team.

21.5 – A: A very appropriate thing to do
This is something that can be done on top of/parallel to anything he does to occupy himself in the job. This demonstrates that he is concerned about the value of the attachment to other people who may work there in future. Because it can be done on top of other actions (such as 21.1 or 21.3) then it can be ranked A.

SJ 22 – Conflict of Opinion

22.1 – B: Important
Seniority and experience are not always an indicator of quality, but the consultant's experience must carry significant weight in Rosie's decision. The reason it is ranked B and not A is because Rosie still needs to exercise judgement; she can't accept blindly what the consultant says just because he is the most experienced member of the team.

22.2 – D: Not important at all
As a junior doctor, Rosie will not know everything there is to know about the management of the patient and, to some extent, it is correct that she will need to trust the judgement of her senior colleagues when they ask her to perform a particular task. However, at the same time, she is also responsible for her own actions and, in a situation where two senior colleagues have different opinions, she can't just follow one of them blindly and plead ignorance later. She must demonstrate she took reasonable steps to make sure she was doing the right thing.

22.3 – B: Important
Rosie will need to satisfy herself that whatever she ends up doing for the patient is what she believes is the right thing. So the fact that other trainees

agree with the senior trainee's plan will be an important, though not vital, consideration in giving her the reassurance she needs. Certainly, she will need to investigate what makes them agree with the senior trainee.

22.4 – D: Not important at all
Rosie cannot let the care and safety of a patient be dictated by whether a senior colleague will take out revenge on her. The decision must be made solely on whether a particular approach is in the best interest of the patient.

22.5 – A: Very important
This may hold the key to unlock the situation because it ensures the situation is safe for patients (at worst, they may be given a treatment that achieves nothing, but no harm will be caused). In such disagreement, it may be easy to just try one plan and then switch to the other one if the first one did not work.

SJ 23 – Struggling Colleague

23.1 – B: Appropriate, but not ideal
This will ensure that patients are safe and will demonstrate a helpful supportive approach, but it will not bring any resolution to the fact that Adam is just dumping his work on Chris and that he is probably inefficient.

23.2 – C: Inappropriate but not awful
It is bad enough that Chris agrees to take on Adam's work. It is even worse that he expects other people in the team to pay the price for his own inability to say no. However, since it will ensure that patients are cared for, then it needs to be classified as "not awful".

23.3 – A: A very appropriate thing to do
This is really Adam's problem, and he should deal with it himself. It is also related to his training and his workload and, as such, it falls under the responsibility of his supervisor. Suggesting that the two should meet is therefore more than appropriate.

23.4 – A: A very appropriate thing to do
Since both Chris and Adam have a similar workload then it makes sense for Chris to discuss the issues with Adam as he may be able to help him out with a few useful tips.

Situational Judgement – Practice

23.5 – B: Appropriate, but not ideal
If Adam is deficient in several skills, this should be addressed through the proper channels, e.g. his supervisor; otherwise it will resolve some of the short-term issues Adam is encountering in his present attachment but nothing in the long term. However, since this demonstrates care and attention towards a colleague in difficulty without any negative consequences, and it is a one-off, it can be classed as appropriate. If it had involved ongoing sessions, this would be ranked as C.

SJ 24 – Drug Error

When mistakes are made, they can't be ignored. At the end of the day, Mark has made a mistake which could have been fatal if it hadn't been spotted in time. The point of admitting to mistakes is that they can be analysed, and lessons can be learnt to provide a safer environment for patient care.

24.1 – D: Not important at all
Mark's unreliability does not excuse the fact he placed a patient at risk.

24.2 – D: Not important at all
Mark may well have been honest in the past (though to be fair we don't know if he has made mistakes that he never owned up to – maybe he just admitted to the small inconsequential ones in the past and covered the others up), but in this instance he is asking Alison to cover up, so he is clearly not inclined to own up to this one.

24.3 – D: Not important at all
The fact that the mistake was caught in time is just very fortunate. The next one might not be spotted. A mistake is still a mistake, regardless of the consequences. It could have been fatal.

24.4 – D: Not important at all
If the issue was simply about the mistake, then the fact that the nurse would have double-checked would have fallen into category C, i.e. "something that could be taken into account, but it does not matter whether it is considered or not". However, since we are also dealing with Mark's dishonesty then the fact that the nurse would have double-checked later is irrelevant.

24.5 – D: Not important at all
Most patients will not be aware of a mistake unless they are told about it or unless they suffer from its consequences. Again, this does not take away the fact that a mistake was made in the first place, whoever is aware of it.

SJ 25 – Tube Station Incident

25.1 – D: Not important at all
The fact that the hospital is nearby should not influence at all whether Jack should be intervening. Having a hospital nearby does not matter if there is no one to take the patient there. It might make a small difference in that one can reasonably speculate that the Tube station must be full of healthcare professionals but that would be pure speculation (unlike scenario 25.2 – see below).

25.2 – B: Important
The important fact here is that Jack KNOWS there are medics and nurses in proximity who are more qualified than he is. It means that Jack's intervention is not so vital. However, that should not stop Jack from getting involved as his help may be required.

25.3 – D: Not important at all
All this tells us is that an ambulance is on its way and all it means is that the patient will soon be taken care of. But we don't know how long the ambulance will take to get to the patient. As such, it is a mild reassurance that the patient will end up in hospital at some stage but will not dictate in any way whether Jack should intervene or not. Someone still needs to take care of the man now.

25.4 – D: Not important at all
The decision to help or not should be based purely on whether Jack can make a difference to the man who has collapsed and not on whether it is socially convenient for him to stop.

25.5 – D: Not important at all
All it means is that help may be around. But we don't know how immediate that help is, or whether the staff are experienced or willing to give it. If the statement said "That Jack sees station staff run towards the man with first aid equipment including a defibrillator" then the answer would rank as C because he could consider the fact that they don't need his help.

Situational Judgement – Practice

SJ 26 – Relative Enquiry

26.1 – A: Very important
Since Asif has quite a few tasks to perform, including reviewing some patients, it is perfectly normal that he should see whether the phone call could be handled by someone who is better placed than him. As such, it would be very important to consider the fact that Ronan has some spare capacity and could handle the phone call.

26.2 – B: Important
If Asif is busy doing current clinical work and still has patients to see before the end of his shift, then the knowledge that the call is very likely to be a standard request for information that a nurse could handle is important as it will help him establish that he most likely does not need to take the call himself, at least in the first instance. It is not vitally important though, hence why it ranks as B and not A.

26.3 – D: Not important at all
The fact that the patient is constantly complaining about menial matters does not imply that his relatives will do the same. The call may be related to a totally different matter. As such, it is irrelevant.

26.4 – B: Important
Direct patient-related matters will rank higher in priority than non-urgent paperwork. The reason it ranks as Important as opposed to Very important is because it is not a vital consideration, i.e. it is not going to force him to drop everything to take the phone call because he knows that Ronan is free. And besides the paperwork, he also has his own patients to see before his shift ends.

26.5 – A: Very important
This information will tell Asif that the request does not warrant his dropping everything to take the phone call and that someone else could handle it.

SJ 27 – Nurse Disagreement

27.1 – C: Inappropriate but not awful
George needs to establish that the painkiller is appropriate for the patient in its own right, whether the nurse agrees with him or not. In other words, the prescription will be written based on his own clinical experience, knowledge, and acumen. Of course, if the nurse is experienced then she

may be able to contribute to the discussion and point out some issues that George may have missed, but ultimately it will be George's decision. As such, changing a prescription because of an unexplained comment made by someone else and prescribing an alternative simply because it is more acceptable to them is inappropriate. The reason it is not awful rests on the fact that the new painkiller is described as "suitable" and so we can infer there is no harm to the patient.

27.2 – A: A very appropriate thing to do
Whenever doctors are unsure, they should recognise their limitations and seek advice from senior colleagues in order to ensure that the decisions made are appropriate and safe. As such, it would be totally right for him to consult a senior doctor and prescribe a painkiller which is compatible with the advice received. It makes no difference whether this is the same controversial painkiller or not, as long as it is appropriate. If the nurse still refuses to administer it, then George will be confident that he has now prescribed the correct painkiller and the issue of the nurse's refusal will have to be dealt with as a separate matter. George will, however, be able to ask someone else to administer the painkiller or even do it himself if need be.

27.3 – A: A very appropriate thing to do
We are told the staff nurse has 20 years' experience and so she must have her reasons for refusing to administer the painkiller. In any case, it is only too right that she should explain her reasoning. This might highlight to George that he has missed an important factor in his decision-making process.

27.4 – D: A very inappropriate thing to do
Doctors should do what they feel is the right thing to do and not what others tell them they are prepared to put up with. The fact that the best possible treatment may not be on the list and, therefore, might be excluded as an option may, in fact, result in patient harm.

27.5 – D: A very inappropriate thing to do
The nurse has the right to refuse to do something she feels is inappropriate and George has no right to force her (in fact this would be construed as bullying). If someone has raised the prospect that the drug may not be appropriate, then ignoring the warnings could lead to serious harm to the patient.

Situational Judgement – Practice

SJ 28 – Father and Daughter

28.1 – D: A very inappropriate thing to do
This is a blatant breach of confidentiality. Also, it would be highly inappropriate for Julia (and any doctor for that matter) to read the notes of a patient in whose care they play no part. To access the notes, she would really need to seek approval from a senior doctor involved in the care of the patient and, even if she managed to do so, she would not be able to reveal any of their content without approval from the patient. In addition, Julia is not a specialist in orthopaedics, and it would be dangerous for her to update someone on a matter related to a field in which she has no expertise.

28.2 – B: Appropriate, but not ideal
Julia's approach is appropriate but just a bit blunt and unfriendly. She is correct in saying that she is not authorised to see the notes of a patient on a different ward; however, that does nothing to address the concerns her friend has for her father.

28.3 – A: A very appropriate thing to do
It is entirely right that the update should come from the team which looks after the patient. They will be well versed in giving updates to relatives and handling the issues relating to confidentiality that come with those requests. Julia is sticking to the rules whilst being helpful to her friend by ensuring she gets appropriate information.

28.4 – B: Appropriate, but not ideal
Like 28.2, this is correct but a bit abrupt and unhelpful.

28.5 – B: Appropriate, but not ideal
This is mildly helpful in the sense that Julia is giving a general update based on her own non-committal observations and is not breaching any confidentiality. However, Amanda would want to know more, and Julia is not helping much. There is more she could do.

SJ 29 – Dyslexic Colleague

This question is a bit of a trap because it is designed to play on emotions. In such a question, you need to make sure you are clear as to what you are asked to do. Here we are talking about a colleague who has an impairment which has already been affecting patient care, so we are not speculating. We know that the notes are confused and that he is not always completing drug charts. In such circumstances, when patient care and safety is compromised, nothing will matter when it comes to reporting it to a supervisor, provided efforts have been made before to raise the issue directly with the colleague himself (which, in this case, has been done).

Note that this is not to say that Kiran's dyslexia is not important; it simply means it is not a consideration when making the decision to report.

29.1 – D: Not important at all
The important factor here is that Kiran has already been given opportunities to address the problem himself when he knows that this is affecting patient care. As such, Kiran's feelings have already been taken into account through a softer direct approach. The situation has now got to a stage where action needs to be taken regardless.

29.2 – D: Not important at all
Kiran's dyslexia may impact on patient safety and so the decision to discuss the issue with the supervisor should be based on its own merit and not on whether Kiran wants to be open about it. If his dyslexia is impairing patient care, then the issue has to be raised regardless.

29.3 – B: Important
The team's ability to work with Kiran is an important part of ensuring good quality care for patients. However, this is not a crucial decision-making factor as the reporting could be done based on the safety issue alone. It is important though.

29.4 – A: Very important
Anything to do with patient care will need to rank high.

29.5 – D: Not important at all
The decision to raise the issue with the supervisor should rest only on whether Kiran's behaviour warrants it on its own merit. The fact that other people are making similar mistakes is irrelevant. It only means that they too should have their behaviour raised with their supervisors and not that Kiran should be let off the hook.

SJ 30 – Surgical Career

30.1 – D: A very inappropriate thing to do
Not being able to attend a surgical session which is not essential is nothing compared to telling a number of patients that the appointment they have

probably been waiting many weeks or months for has been cancelled. Not only is this inconvenient, but it may also actually affect the care of those patients. If they have to be rebooked onto other slots on a different day (e.g. squeezed into an already busy schedule), then it will put pressure on the doctors running those clinics on those other days, and it will delay the care of those patients.

30.2 – D: A very inappropriate thing to do
Lying is very inappropriate regardless of the reason, and even more so for a matter which has no real significance.

30.3 – D: A very inappropriate thing to do
This is similar to 30.1 although a little bit better in the sense that, at least, the patients have a say, but still very inappropriate and inconvenient.

30.4 – B: Appropriate, but not ideal
This would be an entirely appropriate course of action since it ensures that the clinic is not disrupted, Dolores would get to go to the theatre session and the colleague would actually only be mildly disrupted since overall she will not lose out. That mild disruption for a matter which is not essential is what is causing it to be ranked B instead of A. Note that, if the colleague in question was going to lose out because Dolores asked her to cover her clinic without a swap then this would rank as C: Inappropriate but not awful, essentially because Dolores would be imposing her agenda without any care for the impact on her colleague.

30.5 – A: A very appropriate thing to do
This ensures the clinic is covered, that colleagues are not inconvenienced for a fairly trivial matter, and that she plans better for future sessions.

SJ 31 – Coping with Pressure

31.1 – C: Inappropriate but not awful
This will only make her feel better when she is away and maybe for a few days when she comes back. But it does nothing to address the fact that she feels undermined by the consultant. Also the anxiety will return once she goes back to work. Overall it won't help resolve the issue with the consultant or the way she copes with her work and so this solution is not appropriate. Since it won't make matters worse, it must rank C and not D.

31.2 – A: A very appropriate thing to do
Sara needs support from people who are well placed to provide it and can make a difference. Talking to a senior trainee who has experience of dealing with the consultant will help her understand the issues better and find a way to deal with them.

31.3 – A: A very appropriate thing to do
Addressing the issue with the consultant directly would be good if Sara feels that she can do it. Given that she finds the consultant difficult to handle she may benefit from support. The fact that Andrea is offering such support by volunteering to go with her ranks the answer as A.

31.4 – B: Appropriate, but not ideal
Counselling will only have an impact in the longer term. It won't help resolve the core issue which is the consultant's behaviour towards her.

31.5 – D: A very inappropriate thing to do
Though it might be seen as a nice thing to do, it is actually none of Andrea's business to take on other people's workloads just because they can't cope. It will not address any aspect of the fundamental problem. It will probably make matters worse by showing Sara as someone who can't cope and will worsen her sense of self-worth and her feeling of helplessness. Sara needs to regain control of the situation and doing things for her will not help.

SJ 32 – Aggressive Midwife

32.1 – C: Inappropriate but not awful
The scenario states that Angie has already been approached twice by Rosie and so continuing to put up with her negative comments would be, in effect, tantamount to backing down. It is not "very inappropriate" in the sense that nothing awful will result from it, but it is inappropriate in a context where Angie is just making life miserable. Something has to be done.

32.2 – A: A very appropriate thing to do
Since Rosie has already tried to sort the problem out directly, it would be perfectly acceptable for her to talk to her consultant. Had she not talked to Angie previously, this option would only rank B.

32.3 – C: Inappropriate but not awful
This would be pointless as there have been two previous unfruitful attempts. It is only ranked C instead of D because it won't make matters worse. It will just be a waste of time.

32.4 – D: A very inappropriate thing to do
Not confronting this issue and asking to be transferred when the rest of the team appears to be supportive would be very inappropriate because it would hand a victory to Angie who will then replicate and probably worsen her behaviour with future trainees. It simply wouldn't solve much.

32.5 – A: A very appropriate thing to do
If the others have been experiencing the same issues and Angie has already been approached personally before, then it would be perfectly legitimate for the group to put their concerns to the consultant.

SJ 33 – Breaking Bad News

33.1 – D: A very inappropriate thing to do
Christina knows that the results are not okay and so she is giving misleading information by telling the patient otherwise. This goes beyond the inoffensive white lie designed to stall the patient. The patient will soon find out that Christina gave the wrong information, and this will likely affect the trust he has in the team. Because it will make things worse, it has to rank as D.

33.2 – B: Appropriate, but not ideal
Christina is being upfront with the patient, but she should also reassure the patient that someone will be with him soon as he is clearly keen on knowing the results.

33.3 – B: Appropriate, but not ideal
Same as 33.2.

33.4 – A: A very appropriate thing to do
Christina is being truthful. She is also letting the patient know that he will soon be informed and is proactive in ensuring someone talks to him.

33.5 – D: A very inappropriate thing to do
Breaking the news to the patient in that way will distress him and will leave him without any means of getting the information he needs to answer his questions. If he knew that a senior doctor would be seeing him soon then this would rank as C (Inappropriate but not awful) because he would only be left in limbo for a short period of time, but the loose timescale given for a senior colleague to see him makes it a very inappropriate thing to do. The term "at some point" could mean next week as well as in the next ten minutes.

SJ 34 – Intimate Issues

There are two aspects to consider in this scenario.

1. The patient's behaviour: the patient can't expect the practice to drop everything to satisfy her needs. We are told that the patient did not specify at time of booking that she wanted to see a female GP, and, to some extent, she bears some responsibility for that. In this situation, the only female GP present is not available, and the patient's issue is not urgent. Most patients have embarrassing issue to discuss, and doctors are used to it. In this case, if the patient had a compelling reason (e.g. she had been sexually assaulted by a man in the past, which resulted in severe trust issues) then there may be a case for being more amenable because seeing a male GP may make her anxious. But here we are told she is normally comfortable with male GPs so there is no reason to suspect anything of that order.

2. The team's helpfulness: the team's responsibility is to ensure they can be as helpful as possible without inconveniencing the other patients too much. It would be important to work with the patient to find a suitable solution. The problem with such situations is that there is no ideal solution. Something or someone must give. So often the best approach is to offer a range of options for the patient to choose from.

34.1 – C: Inappropriate but not awful

Allowing Mrs Brookes to jump the queue at the contraception clinic when she is no more of an emergency than the patients who are attending that clinic would be inappropriate. She must also take some responsibility for the fact that she failed to mention at time of booking that she wanted to see a female GP specifically. However, it is also right that the GP practice tries to find a solution if there is one, and that the solution minimises the impact on everyone else.

This approach is inappropriate because it would prioritise the needs of one patient over the needs of other patients without a strong enough reason; specifically, it would make all contraception patients coming after her suffer a delay. However, since, in this instance, there is no physical harm to other patients, only an inconvenience, it ranks C and not D.

34.2 – B: Appropriate, but not ideal

That would enable the patient to get what she wants without disturbing anyone else and particularly the other patients. Since we know she booked

Situational Judgement – Practice

the appointment two weeks ago with the aim of discussing those intimate issues, it means they are not urgent. However, it might mean she has to wait a long time for an appointment when she has already waited for two weeks. If we were told that there was an appointment available the next day, then this would rank as A. However, given the uncertainty over the timescale for the next appointment (which could be weeks later), then it must rank B.

34.3 – B: Appropriate, but not ideal
This approach essentially consists of trying to get the patient to reconsider her position since there is scope for her to do so. It is not unreasonable and the communication with the patient is handled honestly. However, it does not directly address Mrs Brookes' issue; it just tries to find a way around it, and it is very possible that Mrs Brookes may prefer to see a female GP on a different day instead of seeing a male GP today, even if it means having to put up with the inconvenience. A better approach would be to give her the choice between several options rather than impose any one of them.

34.4 – C: Inappropriate but not awful
This would enable the patient's issues to be addressed in front of a female member of staff, but it wouldn't resolve the fact that she would still need to confide in a male doctor, which is what she was trying to avoid in the first instance. It would also use up the nurse's time at the expense of other jobs she could be doing and other patients she could be seeing. To the extent it impacts unnecessarily on another colleague and her patients without really resolving the main issue, then it must be considered inappropriate in a context where this is not an emergency. The reason it ranks C, and not D, is that it would not solve the problem but would not make it worse either.

SJ 35 – Internet Medicine

35.1 – B: Important
This is important to consider because it will make Amanda more determined to take the drug. As such, the GP will need to take Amanda's belief in the testimonials into account when talking to her, as this increases the risk that she is exposed to.

35.2 – B: Important
The fact that she is educated means that the doctor will need to explain his rationale to her in a way that matches her level of education and is not

patronising, so as to maintain a good relationship with her. This will therefore influence the way the GP communicates but will not sway the recommendation not to take the drug.

35.3 – A: Very important
The fact the ingredients are not known matters a lot because it means that it is impossible to assess what the remedy is. It could be a totally useless herb or a dangerous chemical compound. However, it could also be a mix of ingredients which can be found in the UK under a different name and may be available legally locally. Ultimately, the fact the ingredients are unknown means that, should Amanda take the remedy, she may expose herself to harm. As such, she will need to be told in no uncertain terms of the potential consequences of taking such a remedy.

35.4 – A: Very important
If Amanda may buy the remedy regardless, then the doctor should ensure that he follows up with her on whether she is taking the remedy or not. For example, he may want to see her again in a few weeks to make sure she is okay. Or at least make sure she knows that she can come back and see him if she experiences side effects.

35.5 – D: Not important at all
This is just an unverified claim.

SJ 36 – Educated Patient

36.1 – C: Of minor importance
Doctors, and particularly those in training, will not have heard of every single solution to every possible medical problem, and may not always know about the most up-to-date information. So, though it is important that they trust their own knowledge, it is also important that they remain open to the information available to them to the extent that it may impact on their clinical decisions.

36.2 – A: Very important
We know the patient's impression of antifungal treatments based on experience from a distant past. Luis should therefore seek to explain to him how new drugs may be different from those he tried a long time ago. This would then give the patient the option to try some of the newer treatments on offer.

Situational Judgement – Practice

36.3 – B: Important
The patient has been living without treatment for some time. The fact he has come back shows that he is bothered by the condition but there won't be an urgency in trying to sort it out. If anti-dandruff shampoos have no side effects and there is no rush, then Luis will be less hesitant in prescribing them and there will be no harm in getting the patient to just "have a go and see what happens". However, this is not the most important consideration, which should be whether the shampoo is likely to be effective.

36.4 – A: Very important
If Luis is unable to find the information he needs, he should seek advice from a colleague. This option therefore cannot be ignored.

36.5 – C: Of minor importance
The fact that the shampoos are available without prescription should not alter the way Luis advises the patient and particularly whether anti-dandruff shampoos are effective for that condition. It will simply mean that the shampoos will be easy to obtain. However, it has a small degree of importance because the patient's hopes may be raised by what he has read, and he may go on to purchase the anti-dandruff shampoo freely and waste his money on something that may be ineffective; hence why Luis should provide accurate advice as much as he can so that the patient can make the right decision for himself.

SJ 37 – Speeding

Be careful with this question. We are not trying to ascertain whether any of the facts presented could be a justification for the speeding, but whether they could play a role in the response to the incident. Here we are told about a frequent occurrence, so there are two main considerations: (i) the actual fast driving itself and (ii) what can be done to address the underlying issues.

37.1 – D: Not important at all
Speeding is dangerous whether you are experienced or not. Putting his own life in danger is bad enough but endangering that of others such as Rob and other road users is not acceptable. Besides, it is illegal. The fact he is an experienced driver will therefore not lead Rob to react any differently.

37.2 – D: Not important at all
His safety and that of others should not depend on possible revenge from Frank.

37.3 – A: Very important
There is a degree of irony about a doctor trying to improve the life of his patients whilst simultaneously endangering that of others.

37.4 – D: Not important at all
It is entirely possible that Rob may not be believed but that should not stop him from reporting the matter.

37.5 – D: Not important at all
It is tempting to say that the patient's anxiety matters; however, we are told these are routine home visits and there is no indication there will be significant physical or psychological harm. In any case this would be greatly counterbalanced by the likelihood of Frank putting himself and the public at risk, and the fact Frank may lose his driving licence, in which case he would no longer be able to make those visits. Therefore, this factor will be irrelevant in Rob's decision as to whether to report the matter to Frank's supervisor or not. It would, however, be an important factor to consider by the practice when it organises its schedule for the home visits, but that is not what we are asked to consider here.

37.6 – D: Not important at all
This is no excuse for the GP's speeding. He is not driving an emergency vehicle and is not even dealing with an emergency anyway.

SJ 38 – Rude Student

38.1 – B: Inappropriate
No discussion has yet taken place with either the patient or Joseph. Joseph may have been unacceptably rude; in which case he may need to be kept away from a patient who has lost trust in him. But it could also be a misunderstanding. Without the full facts, it is inappropriate to stop Joseph from seeing the patient, when this could be used as a learning opportunity.

38.2 – B: Inappropriate
Though there may be some value in Joseph being helped by Fatima, it is not her role to take care of his training and such support from her should not be used as a condition for him to start seeing patients again. This should be done by an experienced doctor who can offer proper support.

38.3 – B: Inappropriate
Apologising to the patient and reminding him of the fact that he was aware he would be seen by students makes sense (if mentioned sensitively). But

it is not appropriate to allow Joseph to continue seeing the patient without resolving the lack of trust the patient now has towards him.

38.4 – A: Appropriate
Allowing the patient to be seen by Joseph with an experienced chaperone is a constructive step to allow Joseph to learn and to make the patient feel more at ease. Note that this would be inappropriate if the patient had expressly stated that he didn't want to be seen by Joseph again. But he hasn't.

38.5 – B: Inappropriate
The patient knows that he can be approached and has only complained about Joseph. As such it would be inappropriate to keep all students away from him and deprive them from a learning opportunity.

38.6 – B: Inappropriate
Joseph's rudeness has not yet been ascertained. The best he can currently apologise for is the distress caused to the patient by his approach.

SJ 39 – Anger with Mistakes

39.1 – B: Inappropriate
Although it would be appropriate to point out to the consultant that their angry tone was not warranted, this should not be done in front of the patient.

39.2 – A: Appropriate
Ashley may be struggling to retain information or to understand the purpose of what he is doing. Asking the consultant for support on how to improve is entirely appropriate in the context of what is effectively a teaching environment, provided this is requested in a nice manner.

39.3 – A: Appropriate
Ashley should make full use of his seniors' expertise to improve his skills. In fact, this is even more appropriate than asking the consultant.

39.4 – B: Inappropriate
This would serve no purpose other than try to repair a bruised ego. It would only help spread gossip and bad will.

39.5 – A: Appropriate
The consultant should not have shown their frustration in front of a patient. Ashley is entitled to an explanation, most likely an apology and a discussion on his performance, all that away from the patient.

SJ 40 – Flirtatious Behaviour

40.1 – B: Not important
40.2 – B: Not important
The fact that Dr Phelps may lose his job or be sanctioned by the GMC are irrelevant for Ashraf. They are only important points <u>for Dr Phelps</u> to consider before he chooses to engage in such behaviour.

40.3 – B: Not important
Ashraf has a responsibility to deal with the behaviour out of professionalism, and the threat of a bad report should not be a deterrent. If Dr Phelps ended up giving a bad report, Ashraf would need to address this separately.

40.4 – B: Not important
It is hard to see how Dr Phelps' struggle with his job could cause him to engage in such behaviour. Dr Phelps' behaviour is unprofessional regardless of what might have caused it and should still be addressed.

40.5 – B: Not important
The fact that some patients are responding to Dr Phelps' behaviour does not make his own behaviour more appropriate. This is irrelevant.

40.6 – B: Not important
Policies do not always cover everything and the fact that a behaviour is not expressly prohibited by a piece of paper does not make it more acceptable. Dr Phelps has a general duty to behave professionally and protect his patients.

SJ 41 – Rushed History Taking

41.1 – A: Appropriate
Yasmina is training to pass medical exams and so her approach may be more "by the book" than Dan's approach. That is not to say that Dan's approach is incorrect, but at least she needs to raise the point so that she can learn from it.

Pointing out to Dan that his approach is different to the one she learnt is a good first step if it is done in a non-judgmental and respectful manner. It will start a discussion on the matter, It turn, this may help highlight issues in her own technique and may also encourage Dan to be more careful about his own approach when in presence of a medical student.

Situational Judgement – Practice

41.2 – B: Inappropriate
There is more than one way of taking medical histories and, in any case, Dan may be taking a practical approach rather than a theoretical approach to the task. He may be conscious that his time with the patient is limited, which forces him to stick to the essential. And, although he may have 'forgotten' that he was being observed by someone eager to learn, there is no evidence that he would miss important points if he didn't stick to what Yasmina was taught. The comment is patronising.

41.3 – A: Appropriate
Yasmina is there to learn, and it is not unreasonable that she should be given the chance to demonstrate how she would approach a patient if she had to do it by herself. Given that Dan is observing her, this is totally safe, and it will give them a chance to discuss the differences between their respective approaches. Asking if she 'could' is what makes the answer appropriate. If she was imposing herself, this would be inappropriate.

41.4 – B: Inappropriate
Dan probably has a good reason to leave the room and that is none of Yasmina's business. He does so between patients and so there is no reason to assume that it is impairing patient care. The fact that what he does may be of some interest to Yasmina (e.g. if he liaises with other staff on matters pertaining to his patients) does not make it appropriate for her to ask (especially if the answer to the question involves personal matters).

41.5 – B: Inappropriate
Though Yasmina may be right, it is patronising to state the obvious to someone more trained than her. Such comment will achieve nothing.

41.6 – B: Inappropriate
Yasmina knows nothing about the effectiveness of Dan's approach which, even if it is not done by the book, may still achieve the aim of caring for the patient appropriately. She also knows nothing about the reasons for Dan's absences. Talking to his supervisor is over the top unless she can identify some possible impact on patient care. This may become appropriate at some point, but not until there are evidenced concerns about patient care.

41.7 – B: Inappropriate
There is no reason why Dan cannot take histories by the book if he is being asked to do so. Asking to change to a different supervisor would only be a last resort solution. Persistence in finding common ground would be the preferred approach. This makes swapping clinic inappropriate.

SJ 42 – Open Door

42.1 – B: Not important
The fact that the patient was looking at their own notes may be reassuring but they still entered a room that was off limit, with potential access to other people's notes. One should assume that the patient has read them and the fact that they were looking at their own notes when caught is irrelevant.

42.2 – B: Not important
Regardless of the level of patient's understanding, there is a possible breach of confidentiality (just seeing the other patients' names and dates of birth is a breach). Also the patient entered a room containing equipment.

42.3 – A: Important
The fact that the door does not close properly is the main cause of problem here (compromising both confidentiality and equipment). If the door closed properly, this incident may never have happened. This is a key risk that needs to be addressed.

42.4 – B: Not important
Though the other patients may be unaware that their notes were made available, their data may have been compromised regardless. A discussion needs to take place to determine whether those patients should be contacted or not, but this does not affect Holly's response to the situation.

42.5 – B: Not important
The fact that the incident happened once is bad enough.

SJ 43 – Rogue Interpreter

43.1 – B: Inappropriate
Waiting for the end won't interrupt the flow and would be appropriate if Adele were a qualified doctor. As a student, she may not appreciate the impact of those inaccuracies. Raising them late could waste time and effort.

43.2 – A: Appropriate
43.3 – A: Appropriate
Both the option of interrupting the consultation to have a word with the consultant or passing the consultant a note would help resolve the issue there and then. The patient may not mind the interruption if he feels that it is in his best interest.

Situational Judgement – Practice

43.4 – B: Inappropriate
Adele is not fluent in Romanian, and she can't guarantee she will do a better job than the interpreter.

43.5 – B: Inappropriate
Doing nothing is not an option here because she is not a qualified doctor, and she may not be able to appreciate the extent to which the inaccuracies affect the overall picture. That judgement should be left for the consultant to make and therefore Adele needs to make her concerns known.

SJ 44 – Sick Note

44.1 – B: Inappropriate
This may make Patrick angry and would achieve nothing constructive.

44.2 – B: Inappropriate
Aside from the legal implications of filming someone specific and the fact it is bordering on stalking, Teresa's role is not to police crime. She obviously cannot ignore the issue altogether but filming someone is well beyond her remit, and she could also be in physical danger if she gets caught doing it.

44.3 – B: Inappropriate
There is nothing to be gained by calling Dr Jones on the spot. Nothing is urgent and nothing justifies interrupting Dr Jones' work or social life for a point that can be made later that day or even the next day.

44.4 – A: Appropriate
Dr Jones has issued a genuine certificate based on potentially false information. The information needs to be checked so that action can be taken about rescinding or maintaining the certificate.

44.5 – B: Inappropriate
If Patrick was misdiagnosed, this was purely because the patient lied. There is no evidence of malpractice, and all Dr Jones needs to do is to get to the truth and take relevant action. There is no reason to involve the practice's lead GP.

44.6 – B: Inappropriate
Fraud is the domain of the police. The fact that Patrick chooses to avoid work is not the GP's problem. The GP's responsibility is to make sure that the sick note is issued correctly.

SJ 45 – Corridor Kiss

45.1 – B: Not important
Mrs Wallis having an extramarital affair and children should be of no concern to Edward as far as his professional responsibilities are concerned. This would be a moral judgement, and not an ethical consideration. Morality should not come into play. Only ethics should.

45.2 – A: Important
Mrs Wallis is on the selection panel and has a conflict of interest regarding one of the candidates, which poses an ethical issue. She may look more favourably at appointing George (or, equally, decide that she doesn't want to work with George). There is a potential bias that needs to be addressed.

45.3 – B: Not important
Being the sub-dean of the medical school does not create an obvious conflict of interest with the fact she is having an affair with a soon-to-be consultant. There may be indirect conflicts (e.g. if she were to give George specific responsibilities as a favour) but nothing indicates this is the case.

45.4 – B: Not important
This would be a possible explanation of the affair but does not make any difference to the response when it comes to the conflict of interest.

45.5 – B: Not important
The fact that Mrs Wallis is well regarded means that Edward may ruffle a few feathers if action is taken against her, but this should not come into play in responding to the conflict of interest caused by the affair.

45.6 – B: Not important
The issue here is the conflict of interest. When it comes to what you SHOULD do, ethics will always prevail over personal considerations. As such, it is right for Edward to confront the issue regardless of the consequences. If there are negative consequences, they need to be addressed separately.

SJ 46 – Dominant Colleagues

46.1 – A: Appropriate
Whenever an issue arises, it is best to confront it in a civilised way with the parties involved.

46.2 – A: Appropriate
Although it would be best to address it with the junior doctors first, seeking advice from more senior colleagues may be useful too. They may have experience of dealing with the three junior doctors that could help Yin make sense of the situation and find a way forward.

46.3 – B: Inappropriate
This would allow Yin to escape the problem but would not resolve anything.

46.4 – B: Inappropriate
Waiting two weeks is unlikely to lead to a change in behaviour from the junior doctors. What it will do, however, is cause two more weeks of resentment, poor teamwork, and likely poorer patient care.

46.5 – B: Inappropriate
Running away won't solve the problem.

SJ 47 – Back Pain

47.1 – B: Inappropriate
Increasing the number of breaks will not resolve the issue of the side effects. It just means that tasks will take even longer to do, at the expense of other team members and of patient care.

47.2 – B: Inappropriate
Charles should not be making any judgement about his own medication. He should get advice from his GP before doing so. In any case, stopping the codeine may resolve the fatigue issue, but he will get the back pain instead, which is just as bad.

47.3 – A: Appropriate
Making an appointment with the GP will help discuss the impact of the side effects on his work. The GP may be able to prescribe different pain killers with fewer, or different / more manageable side effects. He may also be able to adjust the dose.

47.4 – A: Appropriate
Because the medication impacts on Charles' effectiveness, it is important that those in charge of the shift are aware of it, so that they can take appropriate measures. The senior doctor in charge may be able to allocate Charles different duties or keep an eye on him during that time. This will help ensure patient safety.

47.5 – B: Inappropriate
It is not Charles' role to allocate his duties to others. This should be done through the senior doctor in charge, who needs to stay in control of everything that is happening during the shift.

47.6 – B: Inappropriate
The senior trainee may not be a specialist in back pain, will not know much about Charles' medical history and also has a conflict of interest in addressing Charles' issue (since Charles works in that unit). Any advice given in such circumstances would only be informative and should not be used by Charles to make decisions about whether to stop taking codeine or not. This would need to be done by the GP.

SJ 48 – Repeated A&E Visits

48.1 – B: Inappropriate
As a medical student, Roberto has no right to set out a management plan for the patient or to promise anything to the patient. The decision to admit the patient will rest with one of the doctors. In this case, the situation is made worse by the fact that the patient will probably end up not being admitted at all and that Roberto's comment is therefore raising false hopes.

48.2 – A: Appropriate
Someone will need to address Mr Gatter's situation, and this cannot be Roberto. By asking a senior colleague to talk to Mr Gatter, Roberto will ensure he is seen by someone credible, who has authority to talk to him.

48.3 – B: Inappropriate
However tempting it may be to tell Mr Gatter not to come back so readily, there are several issues with this scenario.

First the patient should not be dissuaded to attend A&E and his attendance should not be delayed either if he has real concerns. At some point in the future, Mr Gatter may develop genuine cardiac problems that will require prompt intervention, and he needs to be left in a position where he doesn't feel he is an inconvenience. Any attempt to delay his attendance at A&E could cause his death. Secondly, this places an unnecessary burden on the GP. What should be done instead is to educate the patient about signs and symptoms so that he becomes more apt at recognising what may or may not be a cardiac problem. He should still be encouraged to come to A&E if he has any doubt.

Situational Judgement – Practice

48.4 – A: Appropriate
There may be other reasons for the pain that Mr Gatter is experiencing. Talking to him, even if it is informally, may help identify other issues.

48.5 – B: Inappropriate
The comment that there is nothing wrong with him poses several issues.

First the patient thinks that there is something wrong with him, so that comment will do nothing to maintain his faith in the system. It is also dismissive and could come across as patronising.

Secondly, if we look at it from a purely scientific perspective, it is likely incorrect. The patient's pain may be real. It's just that it hasn't been shown to be of cardiac origin.

A&E may not be the best place for the patient if he is not suffering from an emergency, but there may be grounds to investigate things further, a task the GP may need to take on.

SJ 49 – Drug Interactions

Most appropriate: Option B
The most important fact here is that Mr Lewis is running the risk of taking antibiotics that could interfere with other medication. We are not told of the consequences of that happening, but it is key that the patient be called back as soon as possible to ensure that the facts are ascertained before a final decision is made. That phone call is best done by someone who is able to understand the issue and deal with it, and that is Rashid.

The receptionist (Option C) has demonstrated that she is not apt at dealing with it and the comment she made "If the dentist prescribed them, then they probably won't interfere with your other medications. I'm sure she will have checked" shows that she doesn't understand that mistakes can happen. It may also be a while before she can talk to the dentist.

Least appropriate: Option A
Knocking on the dentist's door when she is currently with a patient may sound like a good idea at first but will be awkward. First it will be hard to discuss the other patient's case without breaching confidentiality. The dentist will also be occupied, may be unable to look at the situation properly and may also not have all the information she needs regarding the other

medications the patient is taking. As such this impromptu meeting may yield very little and may just delay everything unnecessarily. More importantly it does not allow for the patient to be called back to be told that he should not take the medication he was given. This could have serious consequences.

The best option is therefore for Rashid to call the patient back himself, gather relevant information from him about his medication, put him on a short hold and verify the facts by talking to any dentist in the practice or using reliable online resources.

SJ 50 – Retrospective Entry

Most appropriate: Option C
Dr Reddy is essentially falsifying records to show that he acted correctly despite not doing so. Options A and B would resolve the record keeping issue for that specific patient (a minor issue in the scale of things since it is unlikely to affect the overall care of the patient) but Option C would ensure that the more problematic issue of the unethical behaviour is reported and dealt with. This may have happened before and, if Dr Reddy sees nothing wrong with his behaviour, then the only person able to address the matter would be a senior consultant.

Least appropriate: Option A
Modifying records using someone else's login details is unethical. Option B (using her own login to make a record of her observations) would be more ethical and would give a faithful account of the situation.

SJ 51 – Sudden Absence

Most appropriate: Option A
Christina has left Anil is an extremely difficult situation that could make patient care suffer. She should not have gone without agreeing with the team how her work would be covered, and it was both unfair and dangerous to leave Anil on his own without prior agreement. Anil is therefore entitled to ask that she comes back to help.

Least appropriate: Option B
Some jobs may need to be done before she comes back. Not prioritising them could affect patient care and patient safety. So Option B is the worst. Asking Christina to let him know in future (Option C) is appropriate, but it doesn't take care of the immediate situation. Hence it ranks in between.

Situational Judgement – Practice

SJ 52 – Scan Request

Most appropriate: Option B
Doctors sometimes make mistakes or take decisions without knowing the full information required. It is possible that the senior trainee is right in thinking that the scan is not appropriate, but it makes sense first to understand the consultant's motivation for their decision.

Least appropriate: Option A
Although this option would highlight the conflict of opinion, it runs the risk of stirring up conflict instead of using the disagreement as an opportunity to learn. There are more constructive ways of addressing the issue.

Asking the consultant radiologist for their opinion (Option C) makes sense too as this is a constructive step but obviously not as strong as talking to the consultant who made the request.

SJ 53 – Back and Forth

Most appropriate: Option C
If no one answers, then Archana cannot assume that nothing needs doing. In fact, getting no answer could mean that the ward is very busy and needs support. Going back to check would be a minor inconvenience and would be the safest approach to take. Continuing to call the ward until someone answers (Option B) would be appropriate too but, if the ward is busy, she might as well go there and not waste time.

Least appropriate: Option A
Texting Richard is least appropriate because it is the least certain way of achieving the desired outcome. People will hear the ward phone ring, but a text message may stay unanswered for some time, particularly if Richard is busy.

SJ 54 – Unable to Cope

Most appropriate: Option A
Raising the issue with someone senior he can trust will help Michael reflect on the situation. He will benefit from the experience of someone who has probably encountered similar issues and will get the support he needs to make decisions regarding his coping strategies. The senior trainee may

also be able to help address the issue of the relationship with the nursing staff.

Least appropriate: Option C
Taking a few days off might offer some temporary relief but it will not solve the problem of his inability to cope, nor the issues that he is experiencing with the nurses.

Talking to the GP (Option B) won't directly deal with the relationship with the consultant or the nurses, but Michael will be able to talk things through with a professional in confidence and will give him access to resources such as counselling. Going to the GP may also highlight other issues such as anxiety or depression, which can then be addressed as part of the whole package. As such the option to go to his GP is preferable to taking just a few days off.

MOCK EXAM

MOCK EXAM INSTRUCTIONS

Over the following pages, you will find a full mock exam for the UCAT. This contains the required number of questions for each of the four main sections. At the beginning of each section, we have indicated the number of questions included and the maximum amount of time that you can spend on that section. The time shown is the time that you can spend on answering questions (i.e. it does not include the 1-minute administration time that you will be given on the day of the test to read some basic instructions).

You should allow 1 hour and 55 minutes in total for this mock exam, to be allocated as follows:

- Page 627: Quantitative Reasoning: 24 minutes
- Page 643: Abstract Reasoning: 13 minutes
- Page 657: Verbal Reasoning: 21 minutes
- Page 681: Decision Making: 31 minutes
- Page 701: Situational Judgement: 26 minutes

You will be reminded of these timings at the start of each section. When the time allotted to one section has expired, you must move on to the next section (i.e. you cannot use leftover time from one section to spend more time on another).

For the purpose of the quantitative reasoning questions, you are allowed use of a simple calculator.

You will find the answers to all questions from page 725.

Note that on the day of the exam you will actually be allocated two hours (i.e. five more minutes) as this includes one additional minute for each section to give you time to read the instructions.

Once you have taken the full mock exam, use the marking schedule on page 791 to calculate your score.

MOCK EXAM
QUANTITATIVE REASONING

(36 items – 24 minutes)

QR 1/9 Mock — Bottling It Up

A mail order wine company sells wines either as individual bottles or in cases of 12 bottles.

The prices, in pounds, are set out in the table below:

Wines	Case of 12 bottles on or after 01/01/08	Case of 12 bottles on or after 01/01/09	Case of 12 bottles on or after 01/01/10	Per bottle on or after 01/01/09
Red Gold Medal Winner 2007	57	40	49	6.67
White Gold Medal Winner 2007	52	39	44	6.50
White mixed case	36	24	40	4
Red mixed case	43	33	37	5.50
Classic White Selection	48	36	39	6
Classic Red Selection	50	33	25	4.40

MOCK EXAM QUESTIONS

Q1.1 By what percentage was the case of 12 bottles of White Gold Medal Winner 2007 discounted between 2008 and 2009?

    a. 13%   **b.** 15%   **c.** 17%   **d.** 25%   **e.** 33%

Q1.2 On Christmas Eve 2009, a customer wishes to purchase one case of each type. He has a voucher granting an 11% discount on all white wines and 13% discount on all red wines. What is the total cost?

    a. £180.33   **b.** £180.47   **c.** £181.11   **d.** £191.11   **e.** £193.04

Q1.3 In June 2009, a customer wants to buy one case of wine. Out of the five following options, he wishes to choose the one which offers the biggest saving in pounds between purchasing one case and purchasing individual bottles. Which option should he choose?

Option 1: White Gold Medal Winner 2007
Option 2: White mixed case
Option 3: Red mixed case
Option 4: Classic White Selection
Option 5: Classic Red Selection

    a. Option 1   **b.** Option 2   **c.** Option 3   **d.** Option 4   **e.** Option 5

Q1.4 In June 2009, a customer wishes to purchase wines from the Classic Red Selection. How much does the customer save by buying a case rather than 12 individual bottles, expressed as a fraction of the total "per bottle" cost?

    a. 3/8   **b.** 2/7   **c.** 4/7   **d.** 4/9   **e.** 2/3

QR 2/9 Mock — Waste Management

Average waste per individual for 1982 (in kg)

- Others, 36 kg
- Textile, 5 kg
- Metal, 15 kg
- Plastic, 24 kg
- Glass, 24 kg
- Organic elements, 71 kg
- Paper & cardboard, 125 kg

Average waste per individual for 1992 (in kg)

- Others, 45 kg
- Textile, 6 kg
- Metal, 16 kg
- Plastic, 25 kg
- Glass, 28 kg
- Organic elements, 78 kg
- Paper & cardboard, 151 kg

Mock Exam

**Profile of waste per individual for 2002
(as a % of total weight of individual waste)**

- Others, 15%
- Textile, 2%
- Metal, 6%
- Plastic, 10%
- Glass, 12%
- Organic elements, 25%
- Paper & cardboard, 30%

In 2002, the average weight of glass thrown away by inhabitants of Greentown was 54kg. In that year, Greentown, a town with 8700 inhabitants, recycled: 57.31% of cardboard and paper, 80% of organic elements, 80% of glass, 22% of plastic, 80% of metal, 40% of textile and 5% of everything else.

MOCK EXAM QUESTIONS

Q2.1 What was the average total weight of waste per individual in 2002?

a. 250 kg   b. 300 kg   c. 350 kg   d. 400 kg   e. 450 kg

Q2.2 By how much in percentage did the weight of paper and cardboard waste increase between 1982 and 1992?

a. 8.0%   b. 10.6%   c. 14.7%   d. 20.8%   e. 21.2%

Q2.3 In 2002, what percentage of the total recycled weight did recycled textile represent?

a. 0.15%   b. 1.15%   c. 1.45%   d. 2.10%   e. 2.26%

Q2.4 How many kilos of organic elements were not recycled in 2002?

a. 193,720   b. 195,750   c. 206,240   d. 213,230   e. 783,000

QR 3/9 Mock — The Big Freeze

Equivalence between different temperature scales

Unit of temperature	Formula
Kelvin [K]	= ([°F] + 459.67) x 5/9
Rankine [R]	= 9/5 x [K]
Celsius [°C]	= ([°F] − 32) x 5/9

Where [°F] = Fahrenheit

MOCK EXAM QUESTIONS

Q3.1 Two international explorers look at their own thermometers. One is graduated in Fahrenheit, the other in Celsius, but they both show the same number. What is this number?

    a. − 50   **b.** − 48   **c.** − 40   **d.** − 36   **e.** − 32

Q3.2 Water boils at 100 °C. What is this temperature in Rankine?

    a. 355.37   **b.** 373.15   **c.** 396.27   **d.** 574.26   **e.** 671.67

Q3.3 The average temperature of the human body is 309.95 Kelvin. What is this temperature in Fahrenheit?

    a. 97.97   **b.** 98.24   **c.** 98.34   **d.** 98.56   **e.** 98.60

Q3.4 Currently, the average temperature of the Earth's surface is 15 °C. With warming, scientists expect a rise of the average Celsius temperature by 16% over the next century. What will be the average Earth surface temperature in the next century, expressed in Fahrenheit?

    a. 63.21   **b.** 63.32   **c.** 65.36   **d.** 66.58   **e.** 68.44

QR 4/9 Mock — Running Wild

MOCK EXAM QUESTIONS

Q4.1 A mother rabbit and her son Skippy are at the same point in a field, preparing to move forward in the same linear direction. At 8am, Skippy moves forward at a speed of 1.2 km/h. His mother remains motionless until 8.16am, at which point Skippy stops and his mother decides to catch up with him, moving at a speed of 2.4 km/h. How long will it take for her to catch up with him?

a. 4 mins   b. 8 mins   c. 16 mins   d. 24 mins   e. 32 mins

Q4.2 Skippy and his mother are both jumping clockwise along the perimeter of the field (33 m long). In one second, Skippy jumps a ground distance of 20 cm whilst his mother jumps a ground distance of 50 cm. After 25 seconds, Skippy gets tired and stops. He remains still, waiting for his mother to catch up with him. From that moment on, how many seconds will it take his mother to reach him, assuming she carries on jumping on his clockwise circuit along the field perimeter at the same speed?

a. 24s   b. 38s   c. 41s   d. 51s   e. 76s

Q4.3 When Father rabbit hops on his right foot, he moves forward by 20 cm. When he hops on his left foot, he moves forward by 40 cm. When he jumps on both feet he moves forward by 70 cm. What is the minimum number of jumps he must do in order to travel exactly 198 m?

a. 280   b. 282   c. 284   d. 286   e. 288

Q4.4 Father rabbit is at point A and Mother rabbit is at point B, 1500 m away. They want to meet up and start their journey at the same time, travelling in a straight line. It normally takes the father 20 minutes to travel the whole distance. The mother's speed is 7/9 of the father's speed. At which distance from point B will they meet?

a. 656.25m   b. 843.75m   c. 966.75m   d. 1,057.66m   e. 1,166.66m

QR 5/9 Mock — Fruit Harvest

Years	Apricots Category A — Production (in tonnes)	Sales price per kg	Apricots Category B — Production (in tonnes)	Sales price per kg
2002	404	£ 0.75	300	£ 0.85
2003	73	£ 1.05	52	£ 1.20
2004	513	£ 0.60	354	£ 0.75
2005	417	£ 0.70	312	£ 0.80
2006	114	£ 0.95	57	£ 1.15

Years	Nectarines Category C — Production (in tonnes)	Sales price per kg	Nectarines Category D — Production (in tonnes)	Sales price per kg
2002	113	£ 0.95	80	£ 1.05
2003	64	£ 1.15	35	£ 1.25
2004	132	£ 0.85	97	£ 1.00
2005	120	£ 0.80	87	£ 1.15
2006	72	£ 1.10	37	£ 1.30

Note: 1 tonne = 1,000 kg

MOCK EXAM QUESTIONS

Q5.1 In which year was the total income from the sale of Apricots Category A the highest?

    a. 2002   **b.** 2003   **c.** 2004   **d.** 2005   **e.** 2006

Q5.2 Which category brought the highest income over the period covering 2002–2006?

    a. Apricots Category A   **b.** Apricots Category B
    c. Nectarines Category C   **d.** Nectarines Category D

Q5.3 In 2003, a hailstorm destroyed most of the production. Had the fruit grower installed anti-hail nets on his orchard, his production would have increased by 40% in each of the four categories but prices would have remained at the same level.

We know that:

- His orchard contains 110 rows of trees, each 654 feet long.
- An anti-hail net covers 2 rows.
- An anti-hail net costs £3 per foot.

Had he installed the net in 2003, what would his profit have been?

    a. £ 143,140 **b.** £ 251,050 **c.** £ 300,438 **d.** £ 358,960 **e.** £ 466,870

Q5.4 Apricot nectar is a drink made by crushing apricots and extracting the juice and pulp. Nothing else is added. We know that:

- Category A apricots produce 65% of their weight in nectar
- Category B apricots produce 72% of their weight in nectar
- 1 litre of apricot nectar weighs 1.2 kg

How many litres of nectar will be produced by using the entire 2006 apricot production?

    a. 95,950   **b.** 115,140   **c.** 138,168   **d.** 176,535   **e.** 189,732

QR 6/9 Mock — Sweet Music

Six villages with a total population of 10,276 inhabitants got together in 2004 to create a school for music and dance. The overall population does not change from year to year.

In 2005, the school spent £58,650.

In 2006, the total expenditure increased by 2.7%. In that year, Violintown and Drumtown, the two most populated villages, shared equally half of the new amount. The other villages shared the rest of the charges in proportion to the number of pupils each village had in the school in 2006.

Villages	Number of pupils 2005	Number of pupils 2006
Clarinetown	43	38
Drumtown	65	56
Flutetown	11	10
Harptown	28	37
Trumpetown	31	33
Violintown	37	43
TOTAL	215	217

Villages	Number of inhabitants
Clarinetown	1,508
Drumtown	56 more inhabitants than Violintown
Flutetown	386
Harptown	1456
Trumpetown	Three times more inhabitants than Flutetown
Violintown	Not provided

MOCK EXAM QUESTIONS

Q6.1 How many inhabitants are there in Violintown?

    a. 1,254   **b.** 1,749   **c.** 2,157   **d.** 2,380   **e.** 2,856

Q6.2 By what percentage did the average expenditure per pupil across all villages increase between 2005 and 2006?

    a. 0.93%   **b.** 1.75%   **c.** 2.70%   **d.** 3.13%   **e.** 4.06%

Q6.3 In 2005, the villages had opted to share the total costs for that year in proportion to the number of pupils in the school. By how much did Violintown's share of the costs increase between 2005 and 2006, to the nearest pound?

    a. £273   **b.** £1,529   **c.** £2,046   **d.** £3,673   **e.** £4,965

Q6.4 In 2007, Trombonetown wants to join the school. It has a population of 1,724 and 23 of its children would be interested in becoming pupils. Assuming that the number of pupils from other villages does not vary, what proportion of the total population would be pupils of the school?

    a. 1.74%   **b.** 1.83%   **c.** 1.96%   **d.** 2.00%   **e.** 2.05%

QR 7/9 Mock — Reward Scheme

A reward scheme works as follows:

- Clients can collect points from a range of retailers.
- Points are accumulated in a central account and can then be redeemed every quarter against a discount voucher. For every 250 points accumulated, the client receives a £2.50 voucher.
- Clients can decide to spend the vouchers in one of the retailers or can alternatively convert those vouchers into coach-miles vouchers which enable them to travel for free on any coach in the country up to the number of coach-miles they have accumulated.
- One voucher can be exchanged against 30 coach miles.

Retailers where points can be collected

Retailer	Points	Retailer	Points
The EC Electricity Company	1 point per £10 spent	The GS Grocery Store	1 point per £1 spent
The PS Petrol Station	4 points per £3 spent	The FS Flower Shop	1 point per £5 spent
The WS Wine Shop	1 point per £3 spent	The SS Stationery Shop	3 points per £10 spent
The CR Car Rental company	1 point per £40 spent	The JS Jewellery Shop	1 point per £35 spent

Notes

- Partial points cannot be granted. For example, a customer spending £47 on electricity will receive 4 points only and not 4.7 points.

- Only a multiple of 250 points can be converted into vouchers. For example, if a customer has accumulated 264 points, then 250 points will be converted into vouchers, whilst the remaining 14 will be carried forward to the next quarter.

MOCK EXAM QUESTIONS

Q7.1 In his first quarter with the scheme, a client spent the following:

- £45 Electricity
- £1,100 Grocery
- £423 Wine
- £50 Stationery

How many vouchers will he receive that quarter?

a. 4   b. 5   c. 6   d. 7   e. 8

Q7.2 A client wants to finance a 570-mile coach journey entirely with coach-miles obtained through the reward scheme. How much will he need to spend on electricity to acquire enough vouchers?

a. £47.50   b. £75   c. £475   d. £4,750   e. £47,500

Q7.3 What is the smallest amount that a client needs to spend in order to obtain vouchers worth £5?

a. £5   b. £375   c. £500   d. £775   e. £975

Q7.4 A customer obtained 30 coach-miles by spending £1250. Which type of products did he buy with that money?

a. Electricity   b. Flowers   c. Jewellery   d. Stationery   e. Wine

QR 8/9 Mock — Topping It Up

Mrs Peacock is looking after several cats in the neighbourhood by leaving a large bowl of water outside her front door so that they can come to relieve their thirst whenever they want to.

The bowl has a capacity of 1.5 litres and every day at midnight she tops up the level of water so that the bowl is completely full. Some of the water that disappears from the bowl during the day is being drunk by the local cats; however, since the bowl is left outdoors, some of the water evaporates. The rate of evaporation differs depending on the season.

Daily evaporation rate depending on the month:

Daily Evaporation

Month	Evaporation
Jan	10 ml
Feb	30 ml
Mar	50 ml
Apr	100 ml
May	150 ml
Jun	300 ml
Jul	500 ml
Aug	350 ml
Sep	200 ml
Oct	100 ml
Nov	50 ml
Dec	10 ml

A cat drinks 75ml of water per day.
Assume there are 28 days in February.

MOCK EXAM QUESTIONS

Q8.1 On 10 August at 23:59, Mrs Peacock notices that the level of water left in the bowl is 1,000 ml. How many cats drank from the bowl in the past 24 hours?

    a. 2   b. 3   c. 4   d. 5   e. 6

Q8.2 In February, 5 cats drank from the bowl every day. How much water in total did Mrs Peacock have to put in the bowl over the course of the month to replenish the level to the brim (in litres)?

    a. 0.375   b. 0.840   c. 1.5   d. 11.34   e. 42

Q8.3 In July, Mrs Peacock noticed that, as well as the 12 cats who normally drink from the bowl in that month, some birds were also using the bowl's water to refresh themselves.

On 15 July at 23:59, there was no water left in the bowl. Assuming that the birds in question each drank 5 ml of water from the bowl, how many birds drank from the bowl on that day?

    a. 0 birds   b. 12 birds   c. 20 birds   d. 100 birds   e. 120 birds

Q8.4 What is the average daily evaporation rate for the last three months of the year (expressed in ml/day)?

    a. 30   b. 50   c. 50.28   d. 53.33   e. 53.37

QR 9/9 Mock — League Table

A local authority published the following table of 'A' Level results for the entire region. The table shows the percentage of A grades obtained, as well as the percentage of grades A & B combined, measured in relation to the total number of 'A' Levels taken.

School	Number of candidates	Number of A Levels taken	% A	% A & B combined
Springwood	154	450	80%	94%
Rosamund	74	270	30%	70%
Tootham	95	380	80%	90%
Woodworm	137	280	80%	85%
Harringstone	105	320	50%	60%
TOTAL	**565**	**1700**		

MOCK EXAM QUESTIONS

Q9.1 How many 'A' Levels taken by Rosamund students were obtained at Grade B?

a. 30   b. 40   c. 74   d. 108   e. 270

Q9.2 When considering all 'A' Levels taken across all five schools together, what is the percentage of 'A' Levels for which non-A grades were obtained?

a. 4.59%   b. 6.09%   c. 9.79%   d. 18.59%   e. 33.59%

Q9.3 All Tootham students took the same number of 'A' Levels. The school has a boy:girl ratio of 40:60. How many 'A' Levels did the girls take in total?

a. 57   b. 152   c. 178   d. 228   e. 300

Q9.4 At Harringstone, 30 students only took 1 'A' Level. How many 'A' Levels did the rest of the students take on average?

a. 2.76   b. 3.05   c. 3.87   d. 4.01   e. 4.23

MOCK EXAM
ABSTRACT REASONING

(55 items – 13 minutes)

1300 UCAT Practice Questions

AR 1/15 Mock | **Exercises 1.1 to 1.5 (1 – 5 / 55 items)**

Set A

Set B

To which of the two sets above do the following shapes belong?

Shape 1.1   Shape 1.2   Shape 1.3   Shape 1.4   Shape 1.5

☐ Set A   ☐ Set A   ☐ Set A   ☐ Set A   ☐ Set A
☐ Set B   ☐ Set B   ☐ Set B   ☐ Set B   ☐ Set B
☐ Neither   ☐ Neither   ☐ Neither   ☐ Neither   ☐ Neither

644

Mock Exam

AR 2/15 Mock — Exercises 2.1 to 2.5 (6 – 10 / 55 items)

Set A

Set B

To which of the two sets above do the following shapes belong?

Shape 2.1 Shape 2.2 Shape 2.3 Shape 2.4 Shape 2.5

☐ Set A   ☐ Set A   ☐ Set A   ☐ Set A   ☐ Set A
☐ Set B   ☐ Set B   ☐ Set B   ☐ Set B   ☐ Set B
☐ Neither ☐ Neither ☐ Neither ☐ Neither ☐ Neither

1300 UCAT Practice Questions

AR 3/15 Mock
Exercises 3.1 to 3.5 (11 – 15 / 55 items)

Set A

Set B

To which of the two sets above do the following shapes belong?

Shape 3.1   Shape 3.2   Shape 3.3   Shape 3.4   Shape 3.5

☐ Set A   ☐ Set A   ☐ Set A   ☐ Set A   ☐ Set A

☐ Set B   ☐ Set B   ☐ Set B   ☐ Set B   ☐ Set B

☐ Neither ☐ Neither ☐ Neither ☐ Neither ☐ Neither

646

AR 4/15 Mock — Exercises 4.1 to 4.5 (16 – 20 / 55 items)

Set A

Set B

To which of the two sets above do the following shapes belong?

Shape 4.1 Shape 4.2 Shape 4.3 Shape 4.4 Shape 4.5

☐ Set A   ☐ Set A   ☐ Set A   ☐ Set A   ☐ Set A
☐ Set B   ☐ Set B   ☐ Set B   ☐ Set B   ☐ Set B
☐ Neither   ☐ Neither ☐ Neither ☐ Neither ☐ Neither

1300 UCAT Practice Questions

AR 5/15 Mock
Exercises 5.1 to 5.5 (21 – 25 / 55 items)

Set A

Set B

To which of the two sets above do the following shapes belong?

Shape 5.1   Shape 5.2   Shape 5.3   Shape 5.4   Shape 5.5

☐ Set A   ☐ Set A   ☐ Set A   ☐ Set A   ☐ Set A

☐ Set B   ☐ Set B   ☐ Set B   ☐ Set B   ☐ Set B

☐ Neither   ☐ Neither   ☐ Neither   ☐ Neither   ☐ Neither

648

Mock Exam

AR 6/15 Mock
Exercises 6.1 to 6.5 (26 – 30 / 55 items)

Set A

Set B

To which of the two sets above do the following shapes belong?

Shape 6.1 Shape 6.2 Shape 6.3 Shape 6.4 Shape 6.5

☐ Set A ☐ Set A ☐ Set A ☐ Set A ☐ Set A

☐ Set B ☐ Set B ☐ Set B ☐ Set B ☐ Set B

☐ Neither ☐ Neither ☐ Neither ☐ Neither ☐ Neither

1300 UCAT Practice Questions

AR 7/15 Mock
Exercises 7.1 to 7.5 (31 – 35 / 55 items)

Set A

Set B

To which of the two sets above do the following shapes belong?

Shape 7.1   Shape 7.2   Shape 7.3   Shape 7.4   Shape 7.5

☐ Set A   ☐ Set A   ☐ Set A   ☐ Set A   ☐ Set A
☐ Set B   ☐ Set B   ☐ Set B   ☐ Set B   ☐ Set B
☐ Neither ☐ Neither ☐ Neither ☐ Neither ☐ Neither

650

Mock Exam

AR 8/15 Mock
Exercises 8.1 to 8.5
(36 – 40 / 55 items)

Set A

Set B

To which of the two sets above do the following shapes belong?

Shape 8.1   Shape 8.2   Shape 8.3   Shape 8.4   Shape 8.5

☐ Set A   ☐ Set A   ☐ Set A   ☐ Set A   ☐ Set A
☐ Set B   ☐ Set B   ☐ Set B   ☐ Set B   ☐ Set B
☐ Neither ☐ Neither ☐ Neither ☐ Neither ☐ Neither

1300 UCAT Practice Questions

AR 9/15 Mock — Exercises 9.1 to 9.5 (41 – 45 / 55 items)

Set A

Set B

To which of the two sets above do the following shapes belong?

Shape 9.1 | **Shape 9.2** | **Shape 9.3** | **Shape 9.4** | **Shape 9.5**

☐ Set A   ☐ Set A   ☐ Set A   ☐ Set A   ☐ Set A
☐ Set B   ☐ Set B   ☐ Set B   ☐ Set B   ☐ Set B
☐ Neither   ☐ Neither   ☐ Neither   ☐ Neither   ☐ Neither

AR 10/15 Mock — Exercises 10.1 to 10.5 (46 – 50 / 55 items)

Set A

Set B

To which of the two sets above do the following shapes belong?

Shape 10.1   Shape 10.2   Shape 10.3   Shape 10.4   Shape 10.5

- [ ] Set A   - [ ] Set A   - [ ] Set A   - [ ] Set A   - [ ] Set A
- [ ] Set B   - [ ] Set B   - [ ] Set B   - [ ] Set B   - [ ] Set B
- [ ] Neither   - [ ] Neither   - [ ] Neither   - [ ] Neither   - [ ] Neither

1300 UCAT Practice Questions

AR 11/15 Mock
Exercise 11/15 (51 / 55 items)

is to

as

is to

Which figure completes the statement?

A   B   C   D

AR 12/15 Mock
Exercise 12/15 (52 / 55 items)

is to

as

is to

Which figure completes the statement?

A   B   C   D

654

Mock Exam

AR 13/15 Mock
Exercise 13/15 (53 / 55 items)

Which figure completes the above series?

A   B   C   D

AR 14/15 Mock
Exercise 14/15 (54 / 55 items)

Which figure completes the above series?

A   B   C   D

AR 15/15 Mock
Exercise 15/15
(55 / 55 items)

Which figure completes the above series?

A　　B　　C　　D

MOCK EXAM
VERBAL REASONING
(44 items – 21 minutes)

VR 1/11 Mock — Christmas Repeats

TEXT

Television viewers have grown increasingly discontent about the number of repeats in TV schedules during the Christmas period. However, despite sometimes very vocal negative publicity both from members of the public and from politicians, broadcasters have done little to modify their programme grids. The number of repeats over Christmas 2007, taking into account all channels, was 25% higher than over Christmas 2006. In a survey, Channel 5 came out worst with 60% of programmes in its grid being repeats, whilst BBC1 came out best with only 16% of its programmes being repeats. Channel 4 was the only terrestrial broadcaster that had not increased the percentage of repeats in relation to the overall number of programmes shown.

Representatives of the Liberal Democrats political party argued that an abuse of repeats would make people switch off their TV sets at Christmas. Members of family groups suggested that switching off the TV would have a positive impact on family life by encouraging children and parents to spend more time together. Broadcasters responded with their own survey, demonstrating that actually members of the public enjoyed watching old films and repeats of their favourite programmes, in part because it made them relive their own childhood and they could share their memories with their children.

In 2007, viewing share for BBC1 fell from 25.5% in 2006 to 22% in 2007, BBC2's share fell from 11.9% to 8.5%, ITV1's share fell from 20.8% to 19.3%, Channel 4's share fell by more than 11% to 8.7%, whilst Channel 5's share fell from 8.8% to 5.5%.

MOCK EXAM QUESTIONS

Q1.1 In 2007, the number of repeats on Channel 5 was higher than the number of repeats on BBC1.

☐ True

☐ False

☐ Can't tell

Q1.2 The number of repeats on Channel 4 in 2007 was the same as in 2006.

☐ True

☐ False

☐ Can't tell

Q1.3 Decreasing the proportion of repeats would make viewers go back to terrestrial channels.

☐ True

☐ False

☐ Can't tell

Q1.4 In 2006, Channel 4 was more popular than BBC2.

☐ True

☐ False

☐ Can't tell

VR 2/11 Mock — HIV Vaccine

TEXT

In a recent media interview, Professor Luc Montagnier, the French virologist who, with his team, first identified the HIV virus in 1983 and obtained the Nobel Prize in 2008, explained that he hoped to develop a therapeutic vaccine for HIV within the next four years. Whilst efforts to develop a preventative vaccine (i.e. a vaccine administered to healthy people to stop them getting infected in the first place) have proved unsuccessful so far, a therapeutic vaccine (i.e. a vaccine administered to already-infected patients designed to help them fight the consequences of the infection and therefore reduce suffering) looks far more promising.

Luc Montagnier explains: "Currently, there are many treatments available for HIV once it has been diagnosed, but they are burdensome and toxic because they have to be taken every day. As a result, intolerances can develop in the long term and some patients may develop resistance to the treatment. These treatments can also be very expensive. Therefore the aim, eventually, is to be able to do without the treatments. This could be achieved by encouraging the immune system to fight the virus. We know this is possible because there already are people who are naturally resisting against the effects of the infection and the illness, i.e. who are infected but not ill. If a therapeutic vaccine is developed, the patient will first need to start with the combination therapy to reduce the virus load. Thereafter, the risk will need to be taken to stop the therapy and to start the vaccination. If the vaccine fails, the patient will always have the option to revert to the combination therapy."

The French scientist also stated that, although some people may not have the HIV virus in their blood, they see their immune system continue to fail. "These people are still infected. However, although the virus may have disappeared from the blood, it remains hidden in organs and tissues, where it can restart as soon as treatment has been stopped. That is what we call the reservoir of the virus. The aim of our research is to analyse that reservoir and to find a treatment that will totally eliminate the virus or at least make it less harmful for the patient."

MOCK EXAM QUESTIONS

Q2.1 Which population is the therapeutic vaccine most likely to benefit?

    A.   Patients without HIV but who are at risk of catching it.
    B.   Patients with HIV, who have a low viral load.
    C.   Patients who refuse to take combination therapy.
    D.   Patients with a natural resistance to HIV.

Q2.2 Which of the following statements can be inferred from the text about the reservoir?

    A.   It is a barrier to the eradication of the virus.
    B.   No one has yet proven its existence.
    C.   It is a separate blood pool stored within certain vital organs.
    D.   It prevents the virus from re-entering the blood stream.

Q2.3 Patients who are administered the therapeutic vaccine will no longer need combination therapy.

☐ True

☐ False

☐ Can't tell

Q2.4 It is impossible to develop a preventative vaccine for HIV.

☐ True

☐ False

☐ Can't tell

VR 3/11 Mock — E-Cigarettes

TEXT

Electronic cigarettes are being sold on the internet and in a number of high-street shops to smokers wishing to avoid the dangers of smoking. Some of these "e-cigarettes" contain toxic substances. Some also contain nicotine but are not officially recognised as substitutes for the more traditional smoking-cessation methods. Since the results of a thorough investigation are still being awaited, the health authorities are encouraging potential users to remain prudent.

E-cigarettes look like real cigarettes, taste of tobacco, and even give out smoke – this makes them very appealing to smokers. Additional asset: they can be used in public places such as restaurants. But what are they exactly? In reality, the e-cigarette does not produce any real smoke but a vapour charged with aromatic essences. The device is made up of a metal tube containing an electronic circuit, a battery and a cartridge containing a liquid. When the user draws his first puff, the microprocessor activates a device which mixes the air inhaled by the user with a warm vapour. Problem: the liquid held in the cartridge contains chemicals that can be harmful such as glycol propylene (which can cause neurological effects similar to drunkenness), linalol and menthol (both of which can cause convulsions, particular in the elderly and those with epilepsy).

Beyond the toxicity of the e-cigarette, the health authorities oppose other issues with the manufacturers, specifically the fact that e-cigarettes containing nicotine are being advertised as smoking-cessation devices: a claim which is illegal under current regulations as no licence was obtained to commercialise the product. Such a licence is compulsory for all nicotine substitutes but can be lengthy and costly to obtain. "We do not have the size or the means to make such a request," says a representative of the main manufacturer. "We await the results of the studies being currently undertaken to determine whether we can continue to commercialise this product."

MOCK EXAM QUESTIONS

Q3.1 If approved, e-cigarettes will remove the dangers of passive smoking.

☐ True

☐ False

☐ Can't tell

Q3.2 For which of the following categories of people is the e-cigarette safe?

- A. Young people who are not epileptic.
- B. Elderly people who have never smoked before.
- C. Young people who do not inhale the smoke it produces.
- D. None of the above.

Q3.3 In the future, e-cigarettes could be used to encourage smokers to give up smoking.

☐ True

☐ False

☐ Can't tell

Q3.4 Which of the following statements can be deduced from the text?

- A. Nicotine-based products are not effective smoking-cessation products.
- B. It is illegal to market nicotine-based products as smoking-cessation products.
- C. The claim made by some manufacturers that nicotine-based devices can be used for smoking cessation purposes is misleading.
- D. Some manufacturers are currently selling e-cigarettes illegally.

VR 4/11 Mock — NICE

TEXT

The National Institute for Health and Clinical Excellence (NICE) has recently announced that it would increase the threshold at which drugs are deemed to be too expensive to be made available to patients. NICE's role is to decide which drugs can be prescribed to patients under the NHS based on efficacy and cost. Until recently, NICE, whose decisions are binding, would not approve any drug with an annual cost of more than £30,000 per patient. The proposed increase in this threshold will only apply in certain cases, for example when a patient has a life expectancy of 2 years or less and where it can be demonstrated that the treatment will extend life by a significant amount of time (usually taken as 3 months). This may benefit many cancer patients.

In the past, NICE has been the subject of several controversies and criticisms. The main reproach is that NICE puts a price on life and is being seen as a rationing body. NICE is a body which reviews evidence in the context of value for money. It therefore has to balance efficacy and cost. This means that some treatments which could add a lot of value to a patient are discounted because they are too expensive. Rationing is important because the budget is finite and because there are newer and more expensive treatments every day. However, patients can feel that they are being denied the best treatment. It is a dilemma which is difficult to resolve in a cost-controlled environment. It should be remembered that NICE only deals with the provision of treatment or care in the NHS. NICE decisions do not apply in the private sector and patients can access non-approved treatments if they pay for them privately. NICE has also been criticised for being slow to reach decisions (up to 2 years). Whilst a treatment or procedure is in the process of being reviewed, it is left to the initiative of each Trust to decide whether it wishes to fund the treatment being reviewed. Different Trusts make different decisions, which leads to inequalities of care. In a recent report, Lord Darzi, Health Minister, has recommended that the approval time should be reduced to 3 months, which should improve access to care.

Mock Exam

MOCK EXAM QUESTIONS

Q4.1 Which one of the following statements can be deduced from the text?

A. In future, NICE will be required to make decisions in 3 months instead of up to 2 years.

B. Some decisions take NICE longer than 2 years to make.

C. NICE's delay in making decisions is due to the extensive research it has to conduct.

D. NICE's decisions are binding only for NHS Trusts.

Q4.2 Which one of the following statements with regard to the NHS cap on costs can be deduced from the text?

A. Currently, an NHS Trust cannot spend more than £30,000 per year on any given treatment.

B. If patients opt for private care, the NHS partially funds their treatment up to a maximum of £30,000.

C. Currently, patients cannot receive treatment in the UK unless that treatment costs under £30,000.

D. The £30,000 cap will continue to apply in many cases.

Q4.3 Some NHS patients are denied the most effective treatment available simply on the basis of cost.

☐ True

☐ False

☐ Can't tell

Q4.4 NICE decisions lead to inequalities of care within the NHS.

☐ True

☐ False

☐ Can't tell

VR 5/11 Mock — Heavy Metal

TEXT

A recent English study published in the *Chemistry Central Journal* reveals that most of the wines sold around the world contain excessive doses of heavy metals. Declan Naughton and Andrea Petroczi, from Kingston University, have analysed wines produced in sixteen countries, demonstrating that only Argentinian, Brazilian, and Italian wines have low concentrations of heavy metals. French wines are not well ranked, followed in decreasing order by Austria, Spain, Germany, and Portugal. Hungarian and Slovakian wines contain the highest levels. In order to reach these conclusions, the English researchers analysed a wide range of scientific studies showing the quantities of metal present in wines. To the data they then applied a new risk evaluation index linked to the long-term exposure to chemical pollutants; this index, named Target Hazard Quotient (THQ), was originally designed in the US by the Environmental Protection Agency. Their calculations, based on an average daily consumption of a quarter of a litre of wine over a period of time from the age of 18 to the age of 82, show that the THQ index was between 50 and 200 for the majority of wines, and going up to 300 for Hungarian and Slovakian wines. The most worrying doses relate to metals such as manganese, copper, and vanadium.

Reactions to this study are very diverse. Some scientists believe that, even though the study highlights a potential risk only, it does encourage the scientific community to ask questions about the role and potential effect on health of elements which are rarely considered by studies. Others state that the presence of minerals in wine does not mean that these are being assimilated into the body. Some American studies have also shown that there exists a substance in wine – named rhamnogalacturonan – which envelops and neutralises metallic elements.

MOCK EXAM QUESTIONS

Q5.1 Which of the following statements regarding the THQ is the author most likely to agree with?

    A. It only deals with metals and no other risks.
    B. It is based on unrealistic daily alcohol consumption.
    C. It measures the concentration of heavy metals in wine.
    D. It ranks wines from 0 to 300.

Q5.2 Which of the following statements is supported by the text?

    A. Spanish wines have a higher THQ than Portuguese wines.
    B. Argentinian wines have a higher concentration of heavy metals than Italian wines.
    C. Austrian wines have a higher concentration of heavy metals than German wines.
    D. French wines have a THQ between 200 and 300.

Q5.3 Wines with high concentrations of heavy metals are dangerous for human health.

☐ True

☐ False

☐ Can't tell

Q5.4 The scientists who published the study have reached their conclusions by questioning wine drinkers in sixteen countries.

☐ True

☐ False

☐ Can't tell

VR 6/11 Mock — Women in Ancient Egypt

TEXT

The fact that Cleopatra held such a prominent position as Pharaoh is indicative of the fact that women played a prominent role in the building of Ancient Egypt from the early times. Unlike in most other ancient civilizations (including Rome and Greece), there is strong evidence that Egyptian women enjoyed the same legal and economic rights as the Egyptian man. This notion is reflected in Egyptian art and historical inscriptions. Such gender equality stems from the fact that Egyptian national identity would have derived from all people sharing a common relationship with the king. In this relationship, which all men and women shared equally, they were in a sense equal to each other. This is not to say that Egypt was an egalitarian society. Legal distinctions in Egypt were based much more upon differences in the social classes, rather than differences in gender. Rights and privileges were not uniform from one class to another but, within the given classes, it seems that equal economic and legal rights were, for the most part, accorded to both men and women.

We know that women could manage and dispose of private property (including land, slaves, servants and money); they could also inherit one-third of community property (i.e. property accrued by them and their husband during the marriage) on the death of their husband, with the remaining two-thirds being distributed amongst the children. They had the right to take others to court, and, more importantly, we know that there was no discrimination against women in the allocation of jobs; for example, there were over a hundred female doctors in Ancient Egypt. Women could and did hold male administrative positions in Egypt. However, such cases are few, and thus appear to be the exceptions to tradition. Given the relative scarcity of such cases, they might reflect extraordinary individuals in unusual circumstances. The Egyptian woman in general was free to go about in public; she worked out in the fields and in estate workshops. Certainly, she did not wear a veil, which is first documented among the ancient Assyrians (perhaps reflecting a tradition of the ancient Semitic-speaking people of the Syrian and Arabian deserts). However, it was perhaps unsafe for an Egyptian woman to venture far from her town alone.

MOCK EXAM QUESTIONS

Q6.1 It was unsafe for Egyptian women to travel away from their home town.

☐ True

☐ False

☐ Can't tell

Q6.2 In a family comprising a man, his wife and two children, on the death of the husband, what proportion of his property would be given to each child?

    A. One-sixth.
    B. One-third.
    C. One-half.
    D. It is impossible to tell.

Q6.3 Which of the following statements is the author most likely to agree with?

    A. There were more female doctors than female administrators.
    B. There were more female doctors than male doctors.
    C. High powered jobs were male-dominated.
    D. The Assyrian civilisation predates Ancient Egypt.

Q6.4 Egypt was a fair and classless society.

☐ True

☐ False

☐ Can't tell

VR 7/11 Mock — The Eye of the World

TEXT

In the past 18 years, the famous Americano–European spatial telescope in service since 24 April 1990 has revolutionised our knowledge of space. As is often the case in great epics, its beginnings were chaotic. The catastrophe of the shuttle Challenger in 1986 delayed the launch for several years. Then, once in orbit, scientists discovered with much consternation that their best instrument, which cost the meagre amount of 2 billion dollars was ... short-sighted. The blame is firmly placed on a small defect on the main mirror, which a team of astronauts on board the shuttle Endeavour would correct 3 years later. Since then, thanks to three further maintenance NASA missions, Hubble has had an almost faultless career, collecting no fewer than 800,000 exclusive images of space, some of which are of a rare beauty and have gone round the world.

Still, as astronomer Julianne Dalcanton of the University of Washington remarks in a recent article published in the journal *Nature*, "Many people would be surprised to learn that Hubble's size is relatively modest in comparison to some of the more modern telescopes." Indeed, the diameter of its mirror (2.4 metres) is four times smaller than those of the four telescopes located in the Atacama Desert in northern Chile. Furthermore, some of its instruments are over a decade old. Despite this, Hubble has gathered images which are ten times more precise than those obtained with ground-based telescopes. Hubble's success is due to the fact that it orbits nearly 350 miles above the Earth, far removed from the atmosphere and ambient light that limits the effectiveness of ground-based telescopes, and the upcoming servicing mission will likely allow Hubble to add to its already rich legacy of scientific discovery. Indeed, the renowned telescope is preparing for its final chapter, starting with the launch of the space shuttle Atlantis on 12 May 2009 for NASA's fifth and final service mission to the telescope.

MOCK EXAM QUESTIONS

Q7.1 Hubble is the fifth biggest earth-bound telescope.

☐ True

☐ False

☐ Can't tell

Q7.2 Telescopes with smaller sized mirrors provide better quality pictures.

☐ True

☐ False

☐ Can't tell

Q7.3 The images produced by Hubble before the initial repairs were of better quality than those currently produced by the telescopes in the Chilean desert.

☐ True

☐ False

☐ Can't tell

Q7.4 Some of Hubble's instruments were replaced or added during some of the service missions.

☐ True

☐ False

☐ Can't tell

VR 8/11 Mock — Green Fly

TEXT

Last week, an Air New Zealand (ANZ) Boeing 747 was the first plane to fly using a mix of kerosene and a biofuel of so-called "second generation"; during the flight, one of its four engines flew on fuel containing 50% of a diester made from jatropha oil. All airlines are aware of the limits of first generation biofuels (made from sugar cane, soya, rapeseed or corn): some have freezing temperatures which are too high; their culture is accused of interfering with fertile soils which should be reserved for food destined for human consumption; and they encourage deforestation. Consequently, ANZ is keen to reassure that it will respect three non-negotiable criteria: the culture of any biofuel used should not interfere with food cultures; the use of the fuel should not lead to any technical modifications of the planes; and it should remain competitive with kerosene and be available immediately.

The jatropha oil was collected in India, Malawi, Mozambique and Tanzania, where it is already used to make soap and lamp oil for local markets. The plant, native to South America, can be grown on very dry soil and is not edible, meaning that its culture should not compete with food cultures. Jatropha sounds a promising opportunity: its seeds can contain up to 40% of oil and it has been said that one hectare could produce 2 tons of the plant – enough to power a Boeing 747 for over 100km. However, the first trials to extract the oil have been disappointing and some growers – particularly in Ghana – have shown reluctance to start growing the plant given the high level of manpower required and the uncertainty surrounding its use, which would make them financially dependent on the fuel refineries. In addition, some researchers have expressed concerns about the toxicity of the plant, which could have an impact on human health.

Jatropha is not the only biofuel studied by the airline industry. In February 2008, Boeing and Virgin Atlantic did a trial flight with a mix of palm oil and coconut oil only. Environmentalists criticised the flight as a publicity stunt, arguing that these oils cannot be produced in sufficient quantities in the long term to support all airlines.

MOCK EXAM QUESTIONS

Q8.1 Which of the following statements regarding jatropha can be concluded from the text?

    A.   It cannot grow on soil normally used for growing food.
    B.   Its culture would require specific irrigation equipment.
    C.   Its culture has the benefit of not being labour-intensive.
    D.   It may be toxic even if not ingested.

Q8.2 No plane can fly using 100% biofuel.

☐ True

☐ False

☐ Can't tell

Q8.3 Using jatropha would not lead to deforestation.

☐ True

☐ False

☐ Can't tell

Q8.4 Which of the following statements is the author least likely to agree with?

    A.   Using an edible biofuel may increase the risk of food shortages.

    B.   First generation biofuels may lead to aviation accidents.

    C.   Selling edible plant material for fuel tends to be more financially rewarding than selling it for food.

    D.   Growing non-edible plants for biofuel would drastically reduce the risk of deforestation.

VR 9/11 Mock — Unwanted Goods

TEXT

Dear Mrs Ackroyd,

Many thanks for your cancellation email following your recent purchase on our online teapot shop. I would like to use this opportunity to emphasise that we are one of the leading providers of teapots in the country and as such we always seek to ensure that our customers are fully satisfied with the services that we offer.

I see from our records that, on 2 April, you ordered a special teapot suitable for use in a dishwasher, which you say you received on 4 April, and I understand from your email that you now wish to cancel the order as someone else has already bought this item on your behalf. The purchase of goods from online shops such as ours is regulated by the Distance Selling Regulations 2000 which state that:

- You can cancel your order within 7 full days following receipt of the item. The retailer must accept your cancellation whatever your reasons and provide a full refund. Should the item be returned in a damaged state, the retailer is entitled to make a deduction proportionate to the loss incurred as a result. Online retailers may also make a deduction for any credit card and administration fees incurred, though this is not our policy.

- Retailers have no obligation to accept an order cancellation past this 7-day period, though, in our case, we have decided to extend this right to our customers for a period of 14 full days. Our policy is that, after this extended period, we do not grant customers any refunds, whatever the reason for their request.

I would like to thank you personally for returning the teapot undamaged; however, in view of the above, we cannot accept the cancellation of your order and are therefore unable to grant you any refund whatsoever.

Best regards
Ron Donaldson, Customer Service Manager

MOCK EXAM QUESTIONS

Q9.1 The following are reasons why a retailer may grant only a partial refund if an item is returned within 7 days of receipt, except one. Which one?

    A. The customer damages the item before sending it back.
    B. The item's colour is not of the customer's liking.
    C. The retailer has incurred credit card charges.
    D. The item is damaged during the return transit.

Q9.2 When is Mrs Ackroyd likely to have sent her cancellation email?

    A. On or after 19 April.
    B. Between 16 April and 18 April.
    C. Between 9 April and 15 April.
    D. Between 4 April and 9 April.

Q9.3 Under the Distance Selling Regulations, it is never possible to receive a full refund.

☐ True

☐ False

☐ Can't tell

Q9.4 Generally speaking, if a customer orders an item from an online retailer on 1 July then, assuming that the online retailer has no special policy providing better terms than the Distance Selling Regulations 2000, the online retailer has no obligation to grant any refund if the order is cancelled after 8 July.

☐ True

☐ False

☐ Can't tell

VR 10/11 Mock — The Veggie Diet

TEXT

Contrary to common wisdom, being a vegetarian is not unhealthy. Scientists have now identified that the exclusion of animal flesh from our diet (both from meat or fish) does not lead to deficiencies, provided the right cereals are added to the diet, as these will provide most of the required protein intake.

With regard to Vitamin B12, exclusively present in foods of animal origin, eating dairy products or milk can help the vegetarian avoid any deficiency. However, vegans (i.e. vegetarians who eat neither dairy products nor eggs) risk developing a Vitamin B12 deficiency and therefore anaemia. And we are not even talking about the calcium that dairy products almost solely bring into the diet! Vegans who do not opt for vegetables and fruits rich in calcium such as cress, spinach, almond, hazelnuts or pistachio nuts may encounter problems.

Several epidemiological studies have demonstrated that vegetarians are less prone to hypertension and coronary comorbidity, not only because of the quantity and nature of the lipids they ingest, i.e. less saturated fats, but also lifestyle habits (little alcohol or tobacco and greater physical activity), which are responsible for these health benefits. In addition, fibres create short-chain fatty acids which slow down cholesterol synthesis.

Vegetarians also win on the issues of obesity; research shows that the proportion of vegetarians who are obese is less than the proportion of non-vegetarians who are obese. The prominence of fibre in vegetarian diets makes people feel full more quickly and vegetarians therefore tend to eat smaller quantities. A reduction of the incidence of some cancers in vegetarians can primarily be explained by a significant consumption of fruits and vegetables. Not counting that the presence of numerous antioxidants in plants is supposed to have anti-carcinogenic virtues, although this has never been proven.

MOCK EXAM QUESTIONS

Q10.1 Which of the following statements can be concluded from the text?

    A. A patient with anaemia will also have Vitamin B12 deficiency.
    B. Vegans are at risk of calcium-deficiency.
    C. Meat contains calcium.
    D. Anaemia causes Vitamin B12 deficiency.

Q10.2 Which of the following statements cannot be deduced from the text?

    A. Cress contains both calcium and Vitamin B12.
    B. Dairy products contain both Vitamin B12 and calcium.
    C. Some vegetables are poor in calcium.
    D. Vegans need to take Vitamin B12 supplements.

Q10.3 Vegetarians are less prone to lung cancer than non-vegetarians.

☐ True

☐ False

☐ Can't tell

Q10.4 Most obese people are non-vegetarians.

☐ True

☐ False

☐ Can't tell

VR 11/11 Mock — Pole Position

TEXT

Should we be worried if we have a mobile phone mast (or pole) above our head? Without bearing any judgement on the negative effects of radio frequencies, a new study by the French National Centre for Scientific Research (CNRS) shows that the exposure to waves is stronger at a distance than underneath or near the pole.

In the course of the study, 200 people carried personal radiation badges which recorded the exposure to radio frequencies for 24 hours at different distances from the mobile phone pole depending on personal movements during the day.

Firstly, the study showed that the exposure to radio frequencies was at its maximum at a distance of approximately 280 metres from the pole, especially in urban areas. In the areas immediately adjoining urban areas, the maximum exposure to radio frequencies was at a distance of 1 kilometre. The study also shows that the exposure varied considerably even at identical distances from the pole.

Secondly, the electric field measured remained constant below 1.5 V/m, therefore below international norms. However, those norms are judged insufficient by a number of militant groups who lobby for a reduction to 0.6 V/m.

The French Academy of Medicine published a report in March stating that it knows no mechanism by which electromagnetic fields in this range of energy and frequency could have a negative effect on health.

MOCK EXAM QUESTIONS

Q11.1 Both the report issued by the CNRS and the French Academy of Medicine state that radiofrequencies have no effect on health.

☐ True

☐ False

☐ Can't tell

Q11.2 The level of radiation received by an individual is proportionate to the distance from the pole.

☐ True

☐ False

☐ Can't tell

Q11.3 People living near mobile phone masts in rural areas are less exposed than those living in urban areas.

☐ True

☐ False

☐ Can't tell

Q11.4 The international norm for electric field exposure is above 0.6 V/m.

☐ True

☐ False

☐ Can't tell

MOCK EXAM
DECISION MAKING
(29 items – 31 minutes)

DM 1/29 Mock — DVDs

Hassan is drawing up a list of all the DVDs he owns. A DVD contains only one title, which can be either a film or a documentary. Hassan notices that:

- All foreign DVDs contain documentaries.
- All British DVDs were released after 2001.
- Titles lasting more than two hours were all documentaries.
- Only DVDs with films released after 2001 contained bonuses.

Select YES if the following titles <u>could</u> belong to Hassan's collection and NO if they could not.

Q1.1   A documentary lasting 1 h 45 min.   YES | NO

Q1.2   A British film with no bonus.   YES | NO

Q1.3   A British documentary released in 2004.   YES | NO

Q1.4   A thriller released in 1998.   YES | NO

Q1.5   A three-hour thriller with no bonus.   YES | NO

DM 2/29 Mock — Missed Appointments

Q2   Should GPs charge patients a fee for missed appointments?

A. YES. GPs can use the extra funding to compensate for governmental budget cuts.

B. YES. It will encourage patients to either attend or cancel appointments.

C. NO. People may miss appointments due to circumstances beyond their control.

D. NO. Getting an absent patient to pay may prove challenging.

DM 3/29 Mock — Comfort In Bed

- To be comfortable, a bed must have a base made of slats.
- All salesmen from "Comfort in Bed" are insomniacs.
- All the beds sold by "Comfort in Bed" are comfortable.
- All insomniacs sleep on bed bases made with springs.

Select YES if the conclusion follows and NO if it does not.

Q3.1	Beds with spring bases are uncomfortable.	YES / NO
Q3.2	Beds with spring bases make people insomniac.	YES / NO
Q2.3	Some salesmen of comfortable beds do not sleep on the products they sell.	YES / NO
Q3.4	At "Comfort In Bed", beds with spring bases are sold only by non-insomniacs.	YES / NO
Q3.5	People who sleep on a spring base are not necessarily insomniac.	YES / NO

DM 4/29 Mock — Driving Test

Q4 Should drivers be forced to retake their driving test at regular intervals (e.g. every 10 or 20 years)?

  A. YES. Up-to-date knowledge of the Highway Code is important.

  B. YES. The fees collected could be reinvested to fund new road infrastructures.

  C. NO. Most people would pretend to drive well during the test and would continue to drive as they normally do afterwards.

  D. NO. Though most people forget the details of the Highway Code, they drive safely.

DM 5/29 Mock — Golf Club

Club C is the only one of the fifty golf clubs built in Country X that admits both men and women. At Club C, a number of women can attend the club only at weekends or after 6pm on weekdays. All men attend either on weekdays before 6pm or at weekends, depending on their schedule.

Select YES if the conclusion follows and NO if it does not.

Q5.1 The other 49 clubs in Country X only admit men. | YES | NO |

Q5.2 All women attend Club C at weekends. | YES | NO |

Q5.3 A member attending Club C at 4pm on a weekday must be a man. | YES | NO |

Q5.4 There is a period of the week when only members of one gender can be found at Club C. | YES | NO |

Q5.5 Some women visit the club both at weekends and after 6pm on weekdays. | YES | NO |

DM 6/29 Mock — Five-A-Day

Q6   Should the government increase the daily intake of fruit and vegetables by subsidising their production?

   A. YES. It will encourage greater production of fruit/vegetables.

   B. YES. Fruit/vegetables contain vital vitamins and antioxidants.

   C. NO. Historically, food retailers such as supermarkets have not passed on cost savings to the consumer.

   D. NO. There is currently a huge amount of waste, which could be sold at cheaper prices to encourage consumption.

DM 7/29 Mock — Relaxing on Holiday

Natalie confides the following information to a childhood friend:

- When I am on holiday, I play sport.
- When I am not on holiday, I don't go on a diet.
- I am currently on a diet.
- When I am relaxed, I play sport. When I am not relaxed, I don't.

Select YES if the conclusion follows and NO if it does not.

Q7.1	Natalie is not on holiday.	YES / NO
Q7.2	Natalie is not relaxed.	YES / NO
Q7.3	When Natalie is on holiday, Natalie goes on a diet.	YES / NO
Q7.4	If Natalie is not relaxed, it means she isn't on holiday.	YES / NO
Q7.5	If Natalie does not play sport, then she is not relaxed.	YES / NO

DM 8/29 Mock — £1 Coin

Q8 Should the design of the £1 coin be changed to contain more types of metal and have a different shape?

A. YES. It will make it harder to copy it.

B. YES. Changing the coin design will take old dirty coins out of circulation and replace them by new clean ones.

C. NO. Some people like the old type of coins.

D. NO. Shops will be forced to upgrade their trolleys at great expense.

DM 9/29 Mock — Cats

- Ginger cats like dogs.
- Cats with a nice basket have rich owners.
- Cats which don't have a nice basket are ginger.
- Clever cats don't have rich owners.
- In my neighbourhood, none of the cats like dogs.
- Tiger is a cute cat from my neighbourhood.

Select YES if the conclusion follows and NO if it does not.

Q9.1 Tiger is a ginger cat. YES | NO

Q9.2 Cats with a nice basket are not clever. YES | NO

Q9.3 Tiger is not clever. YES | NO

Q9.4 Cats that like dogs are not from the neighbourhood. YES | NO

Q9.5 Cats with owners that are not rich are not ginger. YES | NO

DM 10/29 Mock — Dance Classes

Q10 At a dance school with 48 students, three classes are available: rock, jazz and hip-hop. Three students have registered for all classes; five chose jazz only, three chose rock only, four are taking both hip-hop and jazz classes but not a rock class. All students attend at least one class.

What additional information is sufficient to determine how many students attend both jazz and rock classes?

A. The number of students who attend rock classes.
B. The number of students who don't attend jazz classes.
C. The number of students who attend one class only.
D. The number of students who attend hip-hop classes only.

Mock Exam

DM 11/29 Mock — Medals

Q11 Eight sport personalities enter a restaurant and sit around a round table as follows. Once they have sat down, they realise that when one adds up the total number of medals won by any two personalities sitting opposite each other, it always gives 13.

They discuss their exploits:

A says: "I won three fewer medals than F."
B says: "I know that E and G won 17 medals together."
C says: "A and D also won 17 medals together."
D says: "I won two more medals than F."

How many medals has G won?

- **A.** 7 medals
- **B.** 8 medals
- **C.** 9 medals
- **D.** 10 medals

DM 12/29 Mock — Students' Devices

Q12 A teacher organises a survey of his class of 27 students to determine how many students own a TV, a smart phone and a laptop.
- 12 students own a TV.
- 15 students own a smart phone.
- 12 students own a laptop.
- None own both a TV and a laptop without also owning a smartphone.
- Three students own all three devices.
- Four students own both a smart phone and a laptop.

Which of the following diagrams represents the information given?

A

B

C

D

Mock Exam

DM 13/29 Mock — Mammals And Reptiles

Q13 Consider a group of animals consisting purely of mammals and reptiles. Assume the following statements are true:

- Some mammals and reptiles are pure vegetarian.
- Some mammals have hooves, but no reptile does.
- All animals with hooves are pure vegetarian mammals.
- No reptile is a mammal.

Which of the following diagrams is a possible representation of the information above?

A

B

C

D

689

DM 14/29 Mock — Sports Survey

Q14 A survey of 150 people into the practice of football, tennis and netball shows the following:
- 31 play netball only, 60 play football and 20 play tennis.
- Amongst those playing tennis, 25% also play football but not netball.
- 15 people play football and netball.
- 4 people who play two sports only don't play football.

Which of the following diagrams represents the information given?

A

B

C

D

Mock Exam

DM 15/29 Mock — Jetsetters

Q15 During a trip, travellers discuss their previous holiday destinations. The diagram below represents the number of people who visited each destination.

US — India — Brazil — China — Australia
(square) (oval) (cross) (parallelogram) (crescent)

Regions with counts:
5, 4, 6, 1, 2, 3, 3, 7, 2, 6, 5

How many people who didn't go to India went on two or fewer trips?

A. 29
B. 30
C. 31
D. 36

691

1300 UCAT Practice Questions

| DM 16/29 Mock | **Furniture Factory** |

Q16 A furniture factory uses a range of materials to build their products, as represented by the diagram below.

Wood   Metal   Plastic   Bamboo   Leather

15, 4, 10, 14, 1, 17, 8, 9, 24, 3, 9, 18, 4, 6, 8

What proportion of products is made of three or more materials?

    A. 25%
    B. 30%
    C. 33.3%
    D. 40%

DM 17/29 Mock — Staffing Levels

Q17 A company has 1200 employees. There are three categories of staff: apprentices, blue collars and white collars.

- 408 men are apprentices.
- 144 women are blue collars.
- White collars represent 20% of all employees.
- Apprentices represent half of all employees.

Which of the following statements is correct?

A. Over one third of women are blue collars.
B. Over one third of blue collars are women.
C. Blue collars is the least numerous category.
D. Women represent more than 50% of white collars.

DM 18/29 Mock — Holiday Itinerary

Q18 Brenda is trying to organise an itinerary for a forthcoming holiday. She has very strict requirements:

- If she does not visit Morocco, then she will visit Tenerife.
- If she visits Morocco, then she will also visit Tunisia.
- If she visits Tenerife, then she will also visit Cape Verde.
- She has decided not to visit Cape Verde.

Which of the following statements must be true?

A. She will visit exactly three places.
B. She will visit Tunisia but not Morocco.
C. She will visit both Morocco and Tunisia.
D. She will visit either Tenerife or Cape Verde.

DM 19/29 Mock — Positive Or Negative

Q19 A man has been stopped at random in the street and is being asked for his opinion on three different topics. His answers are not known but we know that:

- If the first answer is negative then the second is positive.
- If the first answer is positive then at least one of the other two is positive.
- It is not possible for only two of the answers to be positive.

Which of the following statements <u>cannot</u> be definitely concluded?

A. The second answer is positive.
B. If the first answer is positive then the third response is too.
C. All answers are positives.
D. It is not possible to know if the first answer is negative.

DM 20/29 Mock — Pets and Hobbies

Q20 Alan, Barack and Kaviraj are the top three students in a university bowling competition. They also all have separate hobbies (boxing, swimming and tennis) and own different pets (snakes, spiders and chameleon). We know the following:

- Kaviraj enjoys playing tennis.
- Alan owns a snake, and came immediately before Barack in the bowling competition.
- The student who owns spiders does not like boxing and is ranked immediately before the student who plays tennis.

Which of the following statements <u>must</u> be true?

A. Barack has a chameleon.
B. The boxer came first in the competition.
C. The boxer has a chameleon.
D. Alan enjoys swimming.

DM 21/29 Mock — Dice Game

Q21 In this game of dice, each time you play, you win a prize. Prizes fall under four categories: W, X, Y or Z. The game consists of throwing simultaneously two normal (i.e. not loaded) dice bearing the numbers 1 to 6. The two numbers obtained are then multiplied together. The following protocol is then applied:

If the result is less than 15:
- If one of the numbers is double the other: Win prize W.
- Otherwise: Win Prize X.

If the result is equal to or greater than 15:
- If the two numbers are odd: Win Prize Y.
- Otherwise: Win Prize Z.

Which of the following statements <u>cannot</u> be true?

A. If the numbers are 3 and 5 then the player wins prize Y
B. The most distributed prize is X.
C. The least distributed prize is W.
D. The probability of getting prize X is over 50%.

DM 22/29 Mock — Health Screen

Q22 A particular disease affects 0.1% of the population. A test for that disease exists, but is not entirely reliable. If an individual has the disease then the test shows a positive result in 90% of cases. If an individual does not have the disease, the test shows a negative result in 97% of cases. What is the probability that a patient with a positive test result has the disease?

A. 0.1%
B. 2.9%
C. 3%
D. 90%

DM 23/29 Mock — Sharing Tasks

Q23 A husband and wife take turns to go shopping. Every day except for Sunday one of them goes out shopping. The husband goes shopping three days a week. Both go shopping at different times of the day.

Nine times out of ten, when the wife gets to the supermarket, she can find smoked salmon on the shelves because she gets up early. Out of the last fifty trips her husband did to the supermarket, he only managed to come back home without smoked salmon five times.

Can the following statement be concluded?: "The probability that they purchase salmon during any particular week is 90%."

- **A.** Yes, because the wife does most of the shopping.
- **B.** Yes, because they both equally contribute.
- **C.** No, because the husband shops more often and is not so successful at finding smoked salmon.
- **D.** No, because we cannot determine who goes shopping on what day.

DM 24/29 Mock — Code 1234

Q24 A code is made up of the four digits 1, 2, 3 and 4, with the following conditions:
- If 1 is in first place then 2 is in third place.
- If 2 is next to the second place then 1 is in fourth place.
- 4 is in third place.

Which of the following must be true?

- **A.** Only three combinations fulfil all criteria.
- **B.** The digit 2 cannot be in second place.
- **C.** All possible answers have the same digit in fourth place.
- **D.** Two of the possible combinations have 1 in second place.

DM 25/29 Mock — Truths and Lies

Q25 Six friends are split into three groups of two. In each group, one is lying and the other one is telling the truth. We know that:
- If Andrew tells the truth then Margot lies.
- If Andrew lies then Jane and William lie.
- If Jane tells the truth then Philip lies.

Group 1
Andrew says he doesn't like fish.
William says he likes spinach.

Group 2
Margot says she likes fish.
Jane says she doesn't like apples.

Group 3
James says he likes apples.
Philip says he doesn't like spinach.

Which of the following cannot be true?

A. James is lying.
B. Margot is lying.
C. If Jane tells the truth then Andrew tells the truth.
D. If Philip tells the truth then James lies.

DM 26/29 Mock — Clothes Storage

Q26 Rasheed likes to organise his clothes properly. He has a chest of drawers with four drawers, one above another. He uses one drawer for each type of clothes: socks, shirts, jumpers and underwear. His jumpers and his shirts are not in consecutive drawers. Neither his underwear nor his socks are in the second drawer from the top. His underwear is in a drawer that is lower than the shirts' drawer. Which of the following must be true?

A. His socks are in the top drawer.
B. The third draw from the bottom is not for jumpers.
C. His underwear and socks are in consecutive drawers.
D. The jumpers' drawer is higher than the shirts' drawer.

DM 27/29 Mock — Night At The Museum

Q27 A museum is laid out as follows (North is at the top of the map), with each of the nine rooms being named after a famous painter:

```
+---------+---------+---------+
|    A    |    B    |         |
+---------+---------+---------+
|    C    |    D    | BRAQUE  |
+---------+---------+---------+
|         |         |         |
+---------+---------+---------+
```

- The Ernst room is in the north of the building.
- From the Kandinski room, you can walk directly into the Braque, Matisse and Renoir rooms.
- From the Van Gogh room, you can walk directly into the Picasso, Cézanne and Kandinski rooms.
- From the Braque room, you can walk directly into the Ernst and the Cézanne rooms.
- From the Matisse room you can walk directly into the Picasso and the Dali rooms.

Which of the following statements is correct?

A. A = Ernst and B = Renoir.
B. C = Van Gogh and D = Kandinski.
C. Dali is directly to the north of Matisse.
D. Van Gogh is to the north of Kandinski.

DM 28/29 Mock — Summer Jobs

Q28 It is common for medium and large-size organisations to employ students over the summer, though students are paid at a fixed rate which excludes usual entitlements such as paid holidays, sick pay and bonus schemes. Permanent members of staff often wish to take their own annual leave over this period; but in addition a lot of companies often experience a peak in demand and so require additional staff. A major bonus for companies is that summer jobs attract students who may return to work full time for them once they have completed their studies. Indeed, ensuring that students learn as much as possible about a company is more likely to make them want to work there in the long term.

Which of the following statements can be concluded from the text?

A. Permanent staff go on leave in the summer because they know their employer can easily fill the gap with students.

B. Many companies whose permanent staff do not take annual leave in the summer require additional support from students in the summer.

C. Employers use summer jobs to spot new talent.

D. Students on summer jobs are treated on an equal basis with permanent employees.

DM 29/29 Mock — Employment

Q29 Consider the following diagram:

Aged over 40	Are employed	Have a university degree	Have to commute over an hour to work	Take over 20 days' holiday per year
△	✚	○	D	▭

What of the following statements is true?

- **A.** There are more employed people with a degree than there are unemployed people without a degree.
- **B.** Most of those who are employed and have a degree are over the age of 40.
- **C.** Most of the graduates who commute over an hour to work go on holiday 20 or fewer days per year.
- **D.** Most of those who are over the age of 40 are unemployed.

MOCK EXAM
SITUATIONAL JUDGEMENT

(69 items – 26 minutes)

SJ 1/22 Mock — Scenario 01 – Faking It

Mrs Jones was admitted into hospital for an infected wound following a fall, after slipping on ice. She was kept overnight for observation and has been told she will be discharged from hospital once the wound has stopped weeping and her pain has subsided. Sarah, a medical student, has built a rapport with Mrs Jones. Mrs Jones confides in her that she is replacing the dressing just before the ward round so that it appears that the weeping has subsided. She also tells Sarah that she is still in some pain but has told the nurses she is fine so that they report to the doctors that she is fit to be discharged. She asks Sarah to keep this quiet. Mrs Jones lives on her own and has no friends or relatives nearby on whom she can rely. She is concerned about her two cats at home who need feeding and she will do anything to leave the hospital as soon as possible to attend to them.

How important to take into account are the following considerations for **Sarah** when deciding how to respond to the situation?

1.1 That Mrs Jones's wound may worsen if she is discharged early.

A – Very important
B – Important
C – Of minor importance
D – Not important at all

1.2 Mrs Jones's feelings towards Sarah if she betrays her confidence.

A – Very important
B – Important
C – Of minor importance
D – Not important at all

1.3 That the cats might die if Mrs Jones is not discharged.

A – Very important
B – Important
C – Of minor importance
D – Not important at all

1.4 That she is a medical student and should not get involved.

A – Very important
B – Important
C – Of minor importance
D – Not important at all

Mock Exam

SJ 2/22 Mock — Scenario 02 – Unusual Murmur

Romeo is a medical student in a teaching hospital. Fellow medical students have mentioned that Mr Singh, a patient with an unusual heart murmur, is currently on one of the wards and that several students have had a chance to listen to his murmur. Romeo is very keen to do the same. He approaches the patient, explaining that he would just need ten minutes of his time to ask him a few questions and listen to his heart as this may be of benefit to his education. The patient tells him that he has become tired of all the requests, and that, having been examined ten times by various students, he has now had enough of it. As such, he refuses to consent to Romeo's examination.

How appropriate are each of the following responses by **Romeo** in this situation?

2.1 Apologise for the inconvenience caused. Remind the patient that he was told when he was admitted that, as this is a teaching hospital, medical students may approach patients for such tasks.

A – A very appropriate thing to do
B – Appropriate, but not ideal
C – Inappropriate but not awful
D – A very inappropriate thing to do

2.2 Tell the patient that he will be as quick as he can and that he promises no one else will bother him ever again after that.

A – A very appropriate thing to do
B – Appropriate, but not ideal
C – Inappropriate but not awful
D – A very inappropriate thing to do

2.3 Ask a senior doctor to try to convince the patient to give ten minutes of his time.

A – A very appropriate thing to do
B – Appropriate, but not ideal
C – Inappropriate but not awful
D – A very inappropriate thing to do

2.4 Apologise to the patient for the inconvenience and ask the patient if he could come back at a more convenient time.

A – A very appropriate thing to do
B – Appropriate, but not ideal
C – Inappropriate but not awful
D – A very inappropriate thing to do

SJ 3/22 Mock — Scenario 03 – Delayed Scan

Andrew, an elderly patient, was recently diagnosed with a brain tumour and further tests including an MRI scan were recommended by the consultant. On the morning of the tests, Andrew arrives at the hospital with his family and is, as scheduled, admitted onto a medical ward. When Andrew arrives on the ward, Paul, a junior doctor, tells him that the tests are planned for that afternoon. A couple of hours later, the radiology department performing the tests informs Paul that, due to several emergencies, Andrew's tests will not be performed until the next morning.

How appropriate are each of the following responses by **Paul** in this situation?

3.1 Explain to the family that the responsibility for the delay rests with the radiology department and not with the medical ward.

A – A very appropriate thing to do
B – Appropriate, but not ideal
C – Inappropriate but not awful
D – A very inappropriate thing to do

3.2 Apologise to the patient and the family for the delay, listen to their concern and explain he will keep them updated on progress.

A – A very appropriate thing to do
B – Appropriate, but not ideal
C – Inappropriate but not awful
D – A very inappropriate thing to do

3.3 Explain the reasons for the delay and inform the family about the complaint procedure.

A – A very appropriate thing to do
B – Appropriate, but not ideal
C – Inappropriate but not awful
D – A very inappropriate thing to do

3.4 Explain why the other patients have been prioritised by the radiology department.

A – A very appropriate thing to do
B – Appropriate, but not ideal
C – Inappropriate but not awful
D – A very inappropriate thing to do

SJ 4/22 Mock — Scenario 04 – Acronyms

Wendy is a medical student shadowing Nirav, a senior trainee in a cardiology unit. Nirav is currently with Brenda, an elderly patient, discussing routine aspects of her management plan. In his explanations, Nirav uses a range of acronyms that Brenda does not seem to understand. Wendy herself feels equally lost during some of the explanations. Brenda looks very confused but Nirav continues regardless. At the end of his explanation, Nirav asks Brenda if she has understood what the management plan is. Brenda replies hesitantly: "This is all a bit complicated, but I trust you, doctor."

How appropriate are each of the following responses by **Wendy** in this situation?

4.1 Explain to the patient that it doesn't really matter if she didn't understand all of it because Nirav is very experienced and will take care of her.

A – A very appropriate thing to do
B – Appropriate, but not ideal
C – Inappropriate but not awful
D – A very inappropriate thing to do

4.2 Mention to Brenda that she could see Brenda did not understand all the explanations and ask whether there are particular aspects of the management plan she would like re-explained.

A – A very appropriate thing to do
B – Appropriate, but not ideal
C – Inappropriate but not awful
D – A very inappropriate thing to do

4.3 Leave the room with Nirav and tell him that she is concerned the patient may not have understood everything.

A – A very appropriate thing to do
B – Appropriate, but not ideal
C – Inappropriate but not awful
D – A very inappropriate thing to do

SJ 5/22 Mock — Scenario 05 – Overbearing colleague

A group of students has been told to prepare a presentation on how doctors could counter the increasing prevalence of childhood obesity in the UK. They have a few weeks to prepare. At several group meetings, Claire, one of the students, who acts as note-taker for the group, has noticed that one of the other students, Petros, is very vocal and is imposing his ideas without much regard for other people's ideas. The other students don't seem to mind.

How appropriate are each of the following responses by **Claire** in this situation?

5.1 Approach Petros before one of the meetings and explain that the project will not be a success unless everyone's view is taken into account.

A – A very appropriate thing to do
B – Appropriate, but not ideal
C – Inappropriate but not awful
D – A very inappropriate thing to do

5.2 Approach Petros at the end of one of the difficult meetings and ask him to stay silent for the next meeting so that the others can contribute.

A – A very appropriate thing to do
B – Appropriate, but not ideal
C – Inappropriate but not awful
D – A very inappropriate thing to do

5.3 Allocate Petros the task of taking notes at the next meeting so that he focuses on writing instead of talking, but retains the opportunity to intervene whenever he wants.

A – A very appropriate thing to do
B – Appropriate, but not ideal
C – Inappropriate but not awful
D – A very inappropriate thing to do

SJ 6/22 Mock — Scenario 06 – Training Opportunities

Paula and Martyn are two medical students attached to a surgical ward. Each day, the consultant runs a ward round where he sees half the patients, whilst a senior trainee runs another ward round where he sees the other half of the patients. Each takes one medical student with him.

The consultant is a very good trainer and explains things properly whereas the senior trainee tends to overcomplicate things and does not involve medical students as much. As such, medical students usually prefer to shadow the consultant. No rota has been set up to set out which student accompanies the consultant and Paula has recently noticed that 90% of the time Martyn is paired with the consultant whilst she ends up with the senior trainee. She feels this is unfair.

How appropriate are each of the following responses by **Paula** in this situation?

6.1 Raise her concerns with Martyn and discuss how they could share the learning opportunities more equitably.

A – A very appropriate thing to do
B – Appropriate, but not ideal
C – Inappropriate but not awful
D – A very inappropriate thing to do

6.2 Arrange a meeting with the senior trainee to discuss the lack of involvement of medical students in his ward rounds.

A – A very appropriate thing to do
B – Appropriate, but not ideal
C – Inappropriate but not awful
D – A very inappropriate thing to do

6.3 Arrange a meeting with the consultant to discuss the lack of training opportunities in the senior trainee's ward round.

A – A very appropriate thing to do
B – Appropriate, but not ideal
C – Inappropriate but not awful
D – A very inappropriate thing to do

SJ 7/22 Mock — Scenario 07 – Epileptic Colleague

Hisham is a junior doctor diagnosed with epilepsy a while ago. He still occasionally has seizures, including one very recently. Ben, a fellow junior doctor, has recently spotted Hisham drive into the hospital car park and mentions it to Liz, another junior doctor. All three junior doctors are fully aware that someone with epilepsy is not legally allowed to drive a car unless they have been free of seizures for at least a year.

How important to take into account are the following considerations for **Liz** when deciding how to respond to the situation?

7.1 That she has not seen Hisham driving for herself.

A – Very important
B – Important
C – Of minor importance
D – Not important at all

7.2 That Hisham is mature enough to decide for himself whether he is fit to drive or not.

A – Very important
B – Important
C – Of minor importance
D – Not important at all

7.3 That Hisham is selling his car tomorrow.

A – Very important
B – Important
C – Of minor importance
D – Not important at all

Mock Exam

SJ 8/22 Mock
Scenario 08 – Drug Allergy

The usual senior doctor on the ward is away on holiday and is temporarily being replaced by a locum (replacement) doctor booked through an agency. The locum doctor does not know any of the patients at all and has been observed reacting badly to anyone who dared criticise his actions.

Stefie is a medical student and sees that the locum doctor is prescribing a drug which, having read the patient's notes earlier, she knows the patient is allergic to. The drug is due to be administered by a nurse in an hour's time; the protocol used by nurses demands they check the notes for drug allergies. She has mentioned to the locum doctor already that she knew the patient was allergic to the drug but he ignored her.

How appropriate are each of the following responses by **Stefie** in this situation?

8.1 Talk to the locum doctor again and insist he reads the patient's notes to ensure he is prescribing correctly.

A – A very appropriate thing to do
B – Appropriate, but not ideal
C – Inappropriate but not awful
D – A very inappropriate thing to do

8.2 Talk to the patient and tell them to alert the nurse to their allergy when she comes to administer the drug.

A – A very appropriate thing to do
B – Appropriate, but not ideal
C – Inappropriate but not awful
D – A very inappropriate thing to do

8.3 Approach a permanent senior doctor in the team and share your concerns with them.

A – A very appropriate thing to do
B – Appropriate, but not ideal
C – Inappropriate but not awful
D – A very inappropriate thing to do

8.4 Approach the nurse who is meant to be administering the drug so that she can act accordingly.

A – A very appropriate thing to do
B – Appropriate, but not ideal
C – Inappropriate but not awful
D – A very inappropriate thing to do

SJ 9/22 Mock — Scenario 09 – Confidentiality

Jorge is a junior doctor who works closely with Yvonne, a nurse on the ward. Yvonne recently took her mother to one of the clinics run by Jorge and his consultant, because her mother showed symptoms which are commonly associated with bowel cancer. Yvonne's mother underwent some tests a few days ago and is awaiting the results.

The consultant has sent a letter to Yvonne's mother, asking her to come back to the clinic today. Yvonne has approached Jorge asking whether the fact that the consultant has recalled her mother to the clinic means that this is bad news.

How appropriate are each of the following responses by **Jorge** in this situation?

9.1 Confirm to Yvonne that the news is indeed not good, but ask her not to tell her mother before she sees the consultant in clinic.

A – A very appropriate thing to do
B – Appropriate, but not ideal
C – Inappropriate but not awful
D – A very inappropriate thing to do

9.2 Advise Yvonne politely that he cannot tell her anything as he has a duty of confidentiality towards her mother.

A – A very appropriate thing to do
B – Appropriate, but not ideal
C – Inappropriate but not awful
D – A very inappropriate thing to do

9.3 Tell Yvonne that the consultant will be able to explain everything in detail in the clinic.

A – A very appropriate thing to do
B – Appropriate, but not ideal
C – Inappropriate but not awful
D – A very inappropriate thing to do

9.4 Give Yvonne her mother's notes without saying anything.

A – A very appropriate thing to do
B – Appropriate, but not ideal
C – Inappropriate but not awful
D – A very inappropriate thing to do

Mock Exam

SJ 10/22 Mock — Scenario 10 – Hand Wash

Sean and Juliet are two medical students currently on an attachment on a respiratory ward. As part of the preparation for one of their assessments, they are going round the ward, politely asking various patients whether they would consent to a brief and simple examination. The patients have been informed that, since they are in a teaching hospital, they may be approached by medical students but they are free to accept or refuse.

As Juliet is about to examine Mr Langford, one of the patients who has consented to be examined, Sean notices that she has not cleaned her hands with the alcohol gel, contrary to the hospital's clear hygiene and infection control policy.

How important to take into account are the following considerations for **Sean** when deciding how to respond to the situation?

10.1 That Juliet is currently going through a rough time as she has just lost her grandmother.

A – Very important
B – Important
C – Of minor importance
D – Not important at all

10.2 That Juliet is only performing a brief and superficial examination which only requires physical contact with the patient for at most a minute.

A – Very important
B – Important
C – Of minor importance
D – Not important at all

10.3 That the patient has consented to the examination.

A – Very important
B – Important
C – Of minor importance
D – Not important at all

SJ 11/22 Mock — Scenario 11 – Unusual Doctor

Brad is seen by his colleagues as an eccentric senior doctor. When the hospital introduced a "no tie allowed" policy he started to wear colourful bow-ties instead. His hair is styled in a spiky, slightly messy fashion and he wears colourful shirts. He is regarded as a very nice, sociable and approachable colleague who is also extremely proactive and competent.

Josie is a medical student working with Brad. One of the elderly patients on the ward is due to have a procedure done by Brad and, choosing a moment when she is on her own with Josie, tells her that she feels Brad is "a bit strange" and she is not entirely sure if she can trust him. The patient is asking, nicely, if it would be possible to have the procedure done by another doctor instead. Josie is considering whether to approach Brad about it.

How important to take into account are the following considerations for **Josie** when deciding how to respond to the situation?

11.1 Brad's personal feelings.

A – Very important
B – Important
C – Of minor importance
D – Not important at all

11.2 That no patient has made such a comment before.

A – Very important
B – Important
C – Of minor importance
D – Not important at all

11.3 There is a risk that the patient refuses to be treated by Brad.

A – Very important
B – Important
C – Of minor importance
D – Not important at all

SJ 12/22 Mock — Scenario 12 – Public Gossip

Tim and George are two medical students currently on an attachment in different wards of the same psychiatric unit. They are both on the same bus on their way back to their halls of residence and are sharing their experiences of the attachment with each other. Their conversation is audible by other passengers, one of them being Karen, a junior doctor in a different hospital.

Tim is making fun of some of the patients with unusual conditions and symptoms which may seem amusing to a lay person. George is replying with stories about some of the nurses being a bit strange and one of the consultants being rude to those nurses. Neither of them are naming any of the staff or the patients.

How important to take into account are the following considerations for **Karen** when deciding how to respond to the situation?

12.1 That passengers other than Karen can hear them.

A – Very important
B – Important
C – Of minor importance
D – Not important at all

12.2 That they are not breaching confidentiality.

A – Very important
B – Important
C – Of minor importance
D – Not important at all

12.3 That Karen works in a different hospital.

A – Very important
B – Important
C – Of minor importance
D – Not important at all

SJ 13/22 Mock — Scenario 13 – Breaking Bad News

Rashid is a 12-year-old patient awaiting the results of a brain scan which was done yesterday. Zoe, a medical student, was at a team meeting this morning, where it was mentioned that the scan revealed a brain tumour. Rashid's parents have been informed of the diagnosis but, whenever Rashid asks them whether they know anything, his parents simply answer that they are still waiting to hear from the doctors. The whole team, including Zoe, knows that the parents are finding it difficult to tell Rashid about the tumour because they feel very fragile emotionally. They have asked the team to break the news to Rashid, and the consultant said he would do it shortly.

Rashid is growing impatient and calls Zoe over. He asks her whether she knows anything about what is going on.

How appropriate are each of the following responses by **Zoe** in this situation?

13.1 Apologise for the delay and explain that, although the scan results are back, she is not qualified to discuss them with him.

A – A very appropriate thing to do
B – Appropriate, but not ideal
C – Inappropriate but not awful
D – A very inappropriate thing to do

13.2 Explain to Rashid that she will check with someone senior and that a doctor will be with him soon to explain what the situation is.

A – A very appropriate thing to do
B – Appropriate, but not ideal
C – Inappropriate but not awful
D – A very inappropriate thing to do

13.3 Tell Rashid his parents have been discussing the results with the doctors and that they probably know more than she can tell him. He might therefore want to ask his parents for an update.

A – A very appropriate thing to do
B – Appropriate, but not ideal
C – Inappropriate but not awful
D – A very inappropriate thing to do

Mock Exam

SJ 14/22 Mock — Scenario 14 – Bad Presentation

Kim and Andy are two dental students. They have been asked to prepare a presentation which will count towards their final assessment for the year on a topic with which they are unfamiliar. The brief is that they will both be marked on the quality of the whole presentation. In addition, each must present one half of the presentation and they will be marked on their own presentation skills.

Kim and Andy shared the work required equally between each other. Two days before the presentation is due to be given, Kim realises that Andy has done very little and is coming up with a lot of bogus excuses, whereas she has finished her own section. It is also apparent he has no real grasp of the topic. The topic will be presented in front of an audience of junior doctors and nurses.

How appropriate are each of the following responses by **Kim** in this situation?

14.1 Sit down with Andy, work out a plan of action and help him do his section of the presentation.

A – A very appropriate thing to do
B – Appropriate, but not ideal
C – Inappropriate but not awful
D – A very inappropriate thing to do

14.2 Take over Andy's section and meet with him the day before the presentation to see what he needs to say on the day.

A – A very appropriate thing to do
B – Appropriate, but not ideal
C – Inappropriate but not awful
D – A very inappropriate thing to do

14.3 Apologise to the tutor for the predicted poor quality of the presentation. Inform him that Andy has not been pulling his weight and that she does not want to be penalised for his behaviour.

A – A very appropriate thing to do
B – Appropriate, but not ideal
C – Inappropriate but not awful
D – A very inappropriate thing to do

| SJ 15/22 Mock | Scenario 15 – Bruises |

Jane is a medical student, currently on an attachment in a GP practice. She is, at this time, observing a GP who is talking to a mother about her child, who is also present in the room. The mother is worried about a cough that the child has developed and that does not seem to go away. The GP listens to the child's chest with his stethoscope after the mother has removed the child's t-shirt. Jane sees what appears to be a bruise on the child's shoulder but the GP does not seem to notice it. The GP prescribes a course of antibiotics, asking the mother to come back the following week for a follow-up visit.

After the consultation, Jane mentions what she noticed on the shoulder to the GP. The GP admits that he did not see it and replies "He's probably done it through playing. You know what boys can be like, always falling over." She is concerned it may be a sign of abuse.

How important to take into account are the following considerations for **Jane** when deciding how to respond to the situation?

15.1 That the GP dismissed the bruises as accidental.

A – Very important
B – Important

C – Of minor importance
D – Not important at all

15.2 That boys tend to fall a lot when playing.

A – Very important
B – Important

C – Of minor importance
D – Not important at all

15.3 That the mother will likely come back the following week for a follow-up visit.

A – Very important
B – Important

C – Of minor importance
D – Not important at all

SJ 16/22 Mock — Scenario 16 – Dental Check-Up

Rob is a dental student currently observing a dentist in a high-street practice. The dentist is doing routine check-ups, assisted by a dental nurse.

As part of the check-up, the dentist sometimes needs to take X-rays of a number of teeth, which consists of placing a piece of film behind the tooth to be X-rayed and then placing a tube attached to the X-ray machine against the patient's cheek. Both the dentist and the nurse (and Rob) then need to get out of the room before the machine's button is pressed in order to avoid radiation.

The team is currently seeing Mr Phipps. The dentist wants to X-ray three teeth in three very different locations. After the first X-ray is taken, and as they are preparing to take the next one, Rob notices that the box of films they have been using states an expiry date which was 4 months ago.

How important to take into account are the following considerations for **Rob** when deciding how to respond to the situation?

16.1 That the patient will need to wait until in-date films are found.

A – Very important
B – Important
C – Of minor importance
D – Not important at all

16.2 That the films are only 4 months out of date and probably still working fine as the expiry date has sufficient margin built in.

A – Very important
B – Important
C – Of minor importance
D – Not important at all

16.3 That the patient should be informed of the problem.

A – Very important
B – Important
C – Of minor importance
D – Not important at all

SJ 17/22 Mock — Scenario 17 – Breast Examination

Aliana is a junior doctor on a cardiology ward. During a standard discussion with a patient, the elderly and often confused patient mentions to Aliana in passing that one of the junior doctors was a bit stroppy yesterday when he examined her breast. Aliana is a bit puzzled because there is nothing in the notes which would explain or justify why a breast examination was necessary in the first place.

How appropriate are each of the following responses by **Aliana** in this situation?

17.1 Ask the patient about the circumstances of the breast examination.

A – A very appropriate thing to do
B – Appropriate, but not ideal
C – Inappropriate but not awful
D – A very inappropriate thing to do

17.2 Ask the junior doctor about the circumstances of the breast examination and the reasons for the lack of documentation.

A – A very appropriate thing to do
B – Appropriate, but not ideal
C – Inappropriate but not awful
D – A very inappropriate thing to do

17.3 Apologise to the patient and explain the complaint procedure.

A – A very appropriate thing to do
B – Appropriate, but not ideal
C – Inappropriate but not awful
D – A very inappropriate thing to do

17.4 Discuss the patient's comments with the consultant.

A – A very appropriate thing to do
B – Appropriate, but not ideal
C – Inappropriate but not awful
D – A very inappropriate thing to do

Mock Exam

SJ 18/22 Mock — Scenario 18 – Struggling Colleague

Alan is a medical student currently on an attachment on a respiratory ward, alongside Mo, another medical student. Mo is very frustrating to work with because he can never make decisions, he needs everything explained at least twice before he understands it, and he just does the bare minimum he can get away with. Mo and Alan are both attending a ward round, during which the consultant asks if Mo has checked the blood results for the patients they are about to see. Mo hasn't. The consultant, in front of several patients and the team, tells Mo in no uncertain terms that he is totally useless at his job, that he wonders how Mo even made it to medical school and that he will write a formal report to Mo's supervisor requesting that his suitability for medical school should be reassessed.

After the ward round, Mo disappears and is found by Alan in the toilet, crying. Mo asks Alan what he should do. How appropriate are each of the following responses by **Alan** in this situation?

18.1 Tell Mo that the consultant has a point and that he should really take stock and do something about it fast before he gets expelled.

A – A very appropriate thing to do
B – Appropriate, but not ideal
C – Inappropriate but not awful
D – A very inappropriate thing to do

18.2 Tell Mo to apologise to the consultant and arrange a meeting with his own supervisor to discuss the way forward.

A – A very appropriate thing to do
B – Appropriate, but not ideal
C – Inappropriate but not awful
D – A very inappropriate thing to do

18.3 Tell Mo to apologise to the consultant for the failure to check the blood result. Reassure him that the consultant most likely did not mean to say what he said and that he should just be a bit more careful in future.

A – A very appropriate thing to do
B – Appropriate, but not ideal
C – Inappropriate but not awful
D – A very inappropriate thing to do

719

SJ 19/22 Mock — Scenario 19 – Badmouthing

Joseph is a medical student. He overhears a nurse tell a patient that the doctor looking after them is lazy and she is grateful he will be gone in two weeks' time. The conversation then moves on to other matters.

How appropriate are each of the following responses by **Joseph** in this situation?

19.1 Interrupt the nurse, ask her to follow you using a bogus pretext and, away from the patient, let her know that her comment was inappropriate.

A – A very appropriate thing to do
B – Appropriate, but not ideal
C – Inappropriate but not awful
D – A very inappropriate thing to do

19.2 Wait until the nurse has left the patient's bedside. Reassure the patient that the nurse did not mean what she said and that there is nothing to be concerned about.

A – A very appropriate thing to do
B – Appropriate, but not ideal
C – Inappropriate but not awful
D – A very inappropriate thing to do

19.3 Wait until a suitable time during the day to approach the nurse and ask her to explain her comment.

A – A very appropriate thing to do
B – Appropriate, but not ideal
C – Inappropriate but not awful
D – A very inappropriate thing to do

SJ 20/22 Mock — Scenario 20 – Body Odour

Alfred is a medical student doing an attachment with Isabella, another medical student, on a medical ward. Isabella finds that Alfred suffers from personal hygiene issues and has an unpleasant body odour. No one has ever commented upon it. Today is the last day that they will be working together before they go their separate ways onto different hospitals.

How important to take into account are the following factors **for Isabella** when deciding to respond to the situation?

20.1 That no patient or member of staff have raised the issue.

A – Important   B – Not important

20.2 That this is the last day of the attachment.

A – Important   B – Not important

SJ 21/22 Mock — Scenario 21 – Medical Finals

Raj, Heather, Tamer and Emilia are four medical students in their final year. To prepare for their clinical finals, they need to see as many patients as possible, with a particular focus on patients with interesting clinical signs.

A new patient, Mr Obike, has just been admitted with interesting clinical signs rarely seen in the hospital where they are. Inevitably, all four medical students are keen to see Mr Obike, take his medical history (a 10-minute process) and examine him (which takes another 10 minutes), but he gets tired very easily. Having been seen by Raj, Heather and Tamer, Mr Obike says to Emilia that he is too tired to continue and needs to rest for a period of time.

Emilia is concerned that he may be moved to a different ward, or discharged in the morning. Her shift ends in 20 minutes. Mr Obike tells her that he doesn't want to see anyone for the next four hours, at which point Emilia will have long gone home.

Out of the following three options, choose the **one most appropriate** and the **one least appropriate** response that **Emilia** should give to Mr Obike?

A. "I have already heard the history by listening to the other students, so I don't need to repeat it. What I am really interested in is to listen to the murmur, which should only take a few minutes. Would it be okay if I just did that?"

B. "I'll try to come back later when you are less tired. If there are other students who need your time, would you mind giving me priority?"

C. "If I don't get to examine you, I might never get another chance. I need this to be able to pass my exam. It would be very nice of you if you could stay up for another 20 minutes."

21.1 Select the MOST appropriate option: A   B   C

21.2 Select the LEAST appropriate option: A   B   C

SJ 22/22 Mock — Scenario 22 – Unfair Allocation

Michael and Talitha, two medical students, are working together on a hospital ward and are sharing various tasks. After a few weeks of working together, Michael realises that Talitha is taking on all the easier tasks, leaving Michael to deal with the longer and more complex tasks. This has enabled Talitha to spend more time on collecting data for an audit she was asked to do by her supervisor.

Out of the following three options, choose the **one most appropriate** and the **one least appropriate** action that **Michael** should take in response to the situation.

A. Speak with Talitha about his concerns regarding the distribution of work tasks.

B. Discuss the distribution of work tasks with his supervisor.

C. Discuss the distribution of work with a junior doctor.

22.1 Select the MOST appropriate option: A   B   C

22.2 Select the LEAST appropriate option: A   B   C

MOCK EXAM ANSWERS

MOCK EXAM QUANTITATIVE REASONING ANSWERS

MOCK QR 1/9 – Bottling It Up

Q1.1 – d: 25%
The ratio of the 2009 price over the 2008 price is 39/52, i.e. 75%.
The discount is therefore of 25%.

Q1.2 – a: £180.33
The undiscounted cost of all three red wine cases in 2009 is 40 + 33 + 33 = £106. Applying a discount of 13% gives 0.87 x £106 = £92.22.

The undiscounted cost of all three white wine cases in 2009 is 39 + 24 + 36 = £99. Applying a discount of 11% gives 0.89 x £99 = £88.11.

Total cost = 92.22 + 88.11 = £180.33

Q1.3 – a: Option 1
The quickest way to approach this problem is to calculate the savings made for each category (12 x bottle price MINUS case price) and then work out the savings for the different options:

	Case price (A)	Bottle price (B)	Saving (12 B – A)
White Gold Medal Winner 2007	39	6.50	39.00
White mixed case	24	4	24.00
Red mixed case	33	5.50	33.00
Classic White Selection	36	6	36.00
Classic Red Selection	33	4.40	19.80

The answer is therefore the White Gold Medal Winner 2007 i.e. Option 1.

Mock Exam

Q1.4 – a: 3/8
The cost of 12 bottles of Classic Red Selection purchased on a "per bottle" basis is 12 x 4.40 = £52.80. The saving made is therefore 52.80 – 33 = £19.80.

Expressed as a percentage of the total "per bottle" price, this gives £19.80 / £52.80 = 0.375. Since this is not easily expressed as a fraction, you can try the different solutions offered and find the appropriate one, which is 3/8.

MOCK QR 2/9 – Waste Management

Q2.1 – e: 450 kg
We are told in the text that, in 2002, the average weight of glass thrown away in 2002 was 54 kg. We also know from the 2002 pie chart that this represents 12% of the total waste per inhabitant. Therefore the total waste was 54/0.12 = 450 kg.

Q2.2 – d: 20.8%
The weight of paper and cardboard for 1982 and 1992 are 125 kg and 151 kg respectively. The ratio is 151/125 = 1.208, hence an increase of 20.8% from 1982 to 1992.

Q2.3 – c: 1.45%
There are two ways of calculating this: the long way and the quick way:

The long (but most intuitive) way
We first need to calculate the total recycled weight, which must be done category by category. We know from Question 4.1 that the total amount of waste per individual was 450 kg, therefore the total amount of waste across the whole population was 450 x 8700 = 3,915,000 kg.

Recycled weight of paper & cardboard:
30% x 3,915,000 x 57.31% = 673,105.95 kg

Recycled weight of organic elements:
25% x 3,915,000 x 80% = 783,000 kg

Recycled weight of glass:
12% x 3,915,000 x 80% = 375,840 kg

Recycled weight of plastic:
10% x 3,915,000 x 22% = 86,130 kg

Recycled weight of metal:
6% x 3,915,000 x 80% = 187,920 kg

Recycled weight of textile:
2% x 3,915,000 x 40% = 31,320 kg

Recycled weight for others:
15% x 3,915,000 x 5% = 29,362.50 kg

Total weight = 2,166,678.45 kg

Proportion of textile = 31320 / 2,166,678.45= 1.45%

The quick way
Since we are only calculating a ratio, we do not actually need to calculate individual quantities. The ratio can be calculated as follows (using percentage values instead of fractions):

(2x40) / (30x57.31 + 25x80 + 12x80 + 10x22 + 6x80 + 2x40 + 15x5)
= 80 / 5,534.3 = 1.45%

When a calculation seems complicated or long-winded, it is often worthwhile to take a step back to find ways to cut the time down. In this case, the long way may well take over 5 minutes to work out (notwithstanding the risk of error) whereas the quick way could be done in a minute or less. Given that the first two questions are relatively quick, this would enable candidates to remain well within the time limit.

Q2.4 – b: 195,750
The total amount of organic waste is 25% x 8700 inhabitants x 450 kg (see question 1) = 978,750 kg.

20% of organic elements are non-recyclable (since 80% are recyclable), i.e. 195,750 kg.

Mock Exam

MOCK QR 3/9 – The Big Freeze

Q3.1 – c: –40
We have C = (F – 32) x 5 / 9 and we want C = F.
Therefore C = (C – 32) x 5 / 9, i.e. C = –40.

You can also get to the answer simply by calculating (F – 32 x 5/9) for all the options on offer until you find the one which works, i.e.:

(– 50 – 32) x 5/9 = – 45.55 (not equal to 50 and therefore does not work)
(– 48 – 32) x 5/9 = – 44.44 (not equal to 48 and therefore does not work)
(– 40 – 32) x 5/9 = – 40 (works, since we get the same number)
This approach is just as quick.

Q3.2 – e: 671.67
We can work out the Rankine value in two stages:

1 – Convert from Celsius to Fahrenheit:
F = 9/5 C + 32, i.e. F = 212

2 – Convert from Fahrenheit to Kelvin and then from Kelvin to Rankine (note that the conversion from Kelvin to Rankine, which consists simply of multiplying by 9/5, cancels out the multiplication by 5/9 that must be done to convert from Fahrenheit to Kelvin).

Hence R = (F + 459.67) x 5/9 x 9/5, i.e. R = 212 + 459.67, i.e. 671.67.

Q3.3 – b: 98.24
The Fahrenheit value can be calculated from Kelvin as follows:
F = 9/5 x K – 459.67, i.e. F = 98.24.

Q3.4 – b: 63.32
The result can be calculated as: (15 x 1.16) x 9/5 + 32, i.e. 63.32.
Note that the wording suggests that it is the Celsius value which is to be increased by 16% and not the Fahrenheit, i.e. you should first add the increase and then convert.

1300 UCAT Practice Questions

MOCK QR 4/9 – Running Wild

Q4.1 – b: 8 mins
The quick way to get to the answer is to spot that the mother is going twice as fast as Skippy and therefore will catch up with him in half the time that it took him to get to the point where he stopped. Since it took Skippy 16 minutes to get to his destination, the mother will take 8 minutes to catch up with him.
If you used the longer approach of calculating distances, you will have calculated the following:

Distance at which Skippy stopped = 1.2 x 16/60 = 0.32 km
Time that it will take the mother to catch up = 0.32 / 2.4 = 0.1333333
Multiplying by 60 to express the result in minutes gives 8 mins.

Q4.2 – d: 51 seconds
There are two ways of working this out:

The long way
After 25 seconds, Skippy will have travelled 25x20 cm=500 cm (5 m).
At the time Skippy stops, his mother will have travelled 25x50 cm=1250 cm (12.5 m).

The distance that she has to travel to catch up with Skippy is:
33 m + 5 m – 12.5 m = 25.5 m (i.e. the total length of the circuit plus the distance Skippy has travelled minus what she has already travelled). Since she travels at a speed of 50 cm per second, the time it will take her to travel is: 25.5 / 0.50 = 51 seconds.

The shorter way
After 25 seconds, Skippy will have travelled 25x20 = 5 m.
When she catches up with him, his mother will therefore have travelled a total of 38 m (33 metres to go round + the 5 metres he has done), which, at a pace of 50 cm per second, will take her 76s. Deducting from this the first 25 seconds which we are told to ignore gives a time of 51 seconds.

Note: 76s is the total amount of time that she will have travelled from the start in order to catch up with him. The question is, however, related to the amount of time that she will take to catch up with him from the time of his immobilisation (i.e. 25 seconds less).

Mock Exam

Q4.3 – c: 284 jumps
Clearly, the fastest way to get to the end is to jump with both feet at a pace of 70 cm per jump. The maximum number of 70 cm jumps that he can do without overshooting the target is the integral part of 198/0.7, i.e. 282.

282 jumps with both feet will achieve a distance of 282 x 0.70 m = 197.4 m, leaving 60 cm still to go. The smallest number of jumps in which this can be achieved is two (one with the left foot, and one with the right foot, 40 cm and 20 cm respectively). The total minimum number of jumps is therefore 282 + 2 = 284.

Q4.4 – a: 656.25m
This question can be resolved without doing any calculation. Indeed, we know that the distance separating them is 1,500 m, which gives a half-way mark of 750 m. We know that the father goes faster than the mother; therefore, at the time they meet, he will have walked more than 750 m and she will have walked less than 750 m. We are asked to calculate the distance that the mother has walked. Since answer a. is the only answer that is lower than 750 m, then it has to be the correct answer.

If you want to calculate the result, it can be done as follows:

The father normally travels 1500 m in 20 minutes. This makes his normal speed 4.5 km/h and therefore the mother's speed 7/9 x 4.5 = 3.5 km/h.

If we call 'M' the meeting point and 'D' the distance MB that we are looking for:

```
A  ───────────────────►  M  ◄───── B
   4.5 km/h                   D
                           3.5 km/h
```

we know that when they meet they will have travelled for the same amount of time and therefore D / 3.5 = (1.5 km – D) / 4.5.

This gives:
4.5 x D = 3.5 x (1.5 – D) i.e. 8 x D = 5.35. Hence D = 0.65625 km, i.e. 656.25 m.

MOCK QR 5/9 – Fruity Harvest

Q5.1 – c: 2004
The sales figures for Apricots Category A were as follows:

2002: 404 x 0.75 = 303.00
2003: 73 x 1.05 = 76.65
2004: 513 x 0.60 = 307.80
2005: 417 x 0.70 = 291.90
2006: 114 x 0.95 = 108.30

The answer is therefore 2004.

Q5.2 – a: Apricots Category A
It is possible to reduce the amount of calculations involved by looking at the table briefly. A brief glance at the table will show that nectarines cannot be the most profitable crop since their production is much lower than the production of apricots and the sales price is not that much higher. We can therefore content ourselves with calculating the income from apricots.

Cat A: 404 x 750 + 73 x 1050 + 513 x 600 + 417 x 700 + 114 x 950 = 1.087m.

Cat B: 300 x 850 + 52 x 1200 + 354 x 750 + 312 x 800 + 57 x 1150 = 0.898m.

Hence Apricots Category A is the category with the highest income across the five years.

Q5.3 – b: £251,050
Income for 2003 = 73x1050 + 52x1200 + 64x1150 + 35x1250 = £256,400.
Projected income = 256,400 x 1.40 (40% increase) = £358,960
Cost of nets: 110 lines / 2 x 654ft x £3 = £107,910
Hence profit = £358,960 – 107,910 = £251,050

Q5.4 – a: 95,950
114 tons of Cat A apricots produce 65% x 114 = 74.1 tons of nectar.
57 tons of Cat B apricots produce 72% x 57 = 41.04 tons of nectar.
Total nectar production = 115.14 tonnes, or 115,140 kg. This occupies a volume of 115,140 / 1.2 = 95,950 litres.

Mock Exam

MOCK QR 6/9 – Sweet Music

Q6.1 – e: 2,856
If we call P the number of Violintown inhabitants, the total number of inhabitants can be calculated as follows:
1508 + (P + 56) + 386 + 1456 + 3 x 386 + P = 10,276.
This gives us 2xP + 4,564 = 10,276, i.e. P = 2,856.

Q6.2 – b: 1.75%
In 2005 the cost was £58,650 for 215 pupils, giving an average cost per pupil of £272.79.

In 2006, the costs were 2.7% higher for 217 pupils, giving an average of 58,650 x 1.027 / 217 = £277.57.
The increase in the average expenditure was therefore 277.57 / 272.79 = 1.0175, i.e. 1.75%.

Q6.3 – e: £4,965
In 2005, there were a total of 215 pupils. Violintown's share of the costs was therefore: 37 / 215 x 58,650 = £10,093.26.

In 2006, Violintown shared half the costs equally with another village and therefore was liable for a quarter of the 2006 costs. Hence, Violintown's 2006 share of the costs was 1/4 x 58,650 x 1.027 = £15,058.39.

Increase in costs = £4,965.13.

Q6.4 – d: 2.00%
The new total population would be 10,276 + 1,724 = 12,000.
The number of pupils would be 217 + 23 = 240. Hence the proportion of the population which studies at the school would be 240 / 12,000 = 0.02 i.e. 2%.

MOCK QR 7/9 – Reward Scheme

Q7.1 – b: 5 vouchers
During the course of the quarter he will have accumulated the following points:

- Electricity: 4 points

- Grocery: 1,100 points
- Wine: 141 points
- Stationery: 15 points

Total: 1,260 points. He will receive 1 voucher for every 250 points and therefore will receive a total of 5 vouchers (with 10 points leftover).

Q7.2 – e: £47,500
570 miles are equivalent to 570 / 30 = 19 vouchers. These can be acquired by gaining 19 x 250 = 4,750 points. The Electricity Company gives 1 point for each £10 spent; therefore he will need to spend £47,500.

Q7.3 – b: £375
The smallest amount needed will be obtained from the shop which provides the highest ratio of points per pound. The PS Petrol Station is the only shop which actually provides more than 1 point per pound spent (4 points per £3 spent).

To obtain a £5 discount (i.e. 2 vouchers), the client will need to acquire 500 points. At the PS Petrol Station, this would be acquired by spending: 500 / 4 x 3 = £375.

Q7.4 – b: Flowers
30 coach miles would have come from 1 voucher, which is worth 250 points. The customer spent £1,250 to acquire those 250 points, therefore the conversion rate is £5 per point, which is the rate given by the Flower Shop.

MOCK QR 8/9 – Topping It Up

Q8.1 – a: 2
The amount of water that disappeared from the bowl was 500 ml, 350 ml of which would have been due to evaporation. Therefore 150 ml were drunk by cats, which corresponds to the daily consumption of two cats.

Q8.2 – d: 11.34
The amount of water that she needed to replace every day in February is equal to the evaporation (30 ml) and the cats' consumption (5 x 75 ml = 375 ml). Total = 405 ml x 28 days = 11,340 ml or 11.34 litres.

Mock Exam

Q8.3 – c: 20 birds
The evaporation level in July is 500 ml, therefore the amount of water drunk was 1 litre. Out of that, 12 x 75 ml (= 900 ml) would have been drunk by cats, leaving 100 ml for the birds. At a rate of 5 ml per bird, this would give a total of 20 birds.

Q8.4 – e: 53.37
The average daily evaporation rate is calculated as:
(31 x 100 + 30 x 50 + 31 x 10) / (31+30+31) = 53.37 ml/day.

MOCK QR 9/9 – League Table

Q9.1 – d: 108
The percentage of 'A' Levels obtained at grade B at Rosamund was 70% – 30% = 40%. This corresponds to 0.4 x 270 = 108 'A' Levels.

Q9.2 – e: 33.59%
The percentage of non-A grades is calculated as 1–%A, i.e. 20%, 70%, 20%, 20% and 50% respectively. The average across all five schools is therefore calculated as follows:

(20%x450 + 70%x270 + 20%x380 + 20%x280 + 50%x320) / 1700
= 571 / 1700 = 33.59%

It is possible to get to the answer without any calculation as follows: the percentage of A grades is never more than 80%. Therefore the percentage of non-A grades for all schools is always more than 20%. The average will therefore be above 20%. Answer **e** (33.59%) is the only answer which is over 20%.

Q9.3 – d: 228
The girls represent 60% of 95 students, i.e. 57 students. All students took the same number of 'A' Levels, therefore everyone has taken 380 / 95 = 4 'A' Levels. This means that the girls took 4 x 57 = 228 'A' Levels.

Q9.4 – c: 3.87
If 30 students took 1 'A' Level only then the rest of the students (i.e. 105 – 30 = 75) took 320 – 30 = 290 'A' Levels between them. This gives an average of 290/75 = 3.87 'A' Levels per student.

MOCK EXAM ABSTRACT REASONING ANSWERS

MOCK AR 1/15 – Exercises 1.5 to 5.5 (1-5/55)

Set A
The number of intersections within each shape is equal to 2.

Set B
The number of intersections within each shape is equal to 4. This can be achieved in any possible way (since the shapes include one object intersecting with two others, or one object intersecting with one other, or two sets of two objects intersecting with one another).

Answers
Shape 1.1: Neither. No intersection.
Shape 1.2: Set B
Shape 1.3: Neither. 6 intersections.
Shape 1.4: Neither. No intersection.
Shape 1.5: Neither. 6 intersections.

Comments
Visually, it is relatively easy to determine that all sets have intersecting objects. It is therefore a fair bet that the number of intersections will play a role. Other questions that you should have asked yourself to check possible relationships (other than the basic ones) include:

- Are the intersections between similar objects (e.g. always a triangle intersecting with a circle)? This is not the case here.

- Is there a link with the number of some of the objects (particularly for Set B, where there are many similar objects within one shape (e.g. 2 circles, 3 squares, 2 moons, 2 pentagons))? There does not seem to be a pattern here.

MOCK AR 2/15 – Exercises 2.1 to 2.5 (6-10/55)

Set A
Each shape has two objects which are the same (e.g. 2 moons, 2 triangles, etc.). If there is one circle within the shape then the two objects in question are of the same size. If there are two circles within a shape then the two objects in question are of different sizes.

Set B
Set B is the reverse relationship, i.e. one circle means that the other two similar objects are of different sizes. The presence of two circles means that the other two similar objects are of the same size.

Answers
Shape 2.1: Neither. Three similar objects instead of the two required.
Shape 2.2: Neither. Only one other object.
Shape 2.3: Set B
Shape 2.4: Set A
Shape 2.5: Neither. Three similar objects instead of the two required.

Comments
The presence of circles in all shapes can be ascertained easily at a glance. Looking at the other non-circular objects, one can see that they are of a similar shape but sometimes vary in size. This should be sufficient to prompt you to investigate a relationship. Other possible relationships that you would need to investigate include:

- Whether there is a link with some of the objects overlapping (e.g. whether objects which have the same size overlap). This is not the case here.

- Whether the position of the objects matters. They look fairly random in this case.

Please note that the relationships could be much harder to ascertain if the sets contained some distracting features such as additional objects which would have little to do with the final outcome.

1300 UCAT Practice Questions

MOCK AR 3/15 – Exercises 3.1 to 3.5 (11-15/55)

Set A: All shapes contain 10 arrowheads.
Set B: All shapes contain 7 arrowheads.

Answers
Shape 3.1: Set A
Shape 3.2: Set A
Shape 3.3: Neither. 12 arrowheads.
Shape 3.4: Neither. 8 arrowheads.
Shape 3.5: Set A

Comments
Other relationships you would need to investigate include:

- Is there a relationship between the number of double arrows and the number of single arrows (e.g. one is a multiple of the other, or one is equal to the other plus a constant)? There is no relationship here.

- Does the location of some or all of the arrows matter? For example, in Set A, four out of the six have an arrow pointing to the right at the top of each shape. But since it only appears in four of the shapes, it cannot be taken as part of any relationship.

- Does the orientation of the double arrows matter, i.e. are they all vertical or horizontal? This is not the case here.

MOCK AR 4/15 –Exercises 4.1 to 4.5 (16-20/55)

Both sets contain diagrams that can be folded to make 3-dimensional boxes all having faces of the same shape.

Set A: contains sets that make boxes that are missing one side.
Set B: contains sets that make boxes with all sides complete.

Answer
Shape 4.1: Neither
Shape 4.2: Neither
Shape 4.3: Neither
Shape 4.4: Set A

Shape 4.5: Neither. When the object is folded it does make a pyramid with one side missing but the missing side is square, not triangular.

Comments
When an exercise contains shapes with squares presented in blocks in such a manner, the relationship usually revolves around the fact they can be folded to make a specific object (e.g. a cube, a pyramid, etc.).

MOCK AR 5/15 – Exercises 5.1 to 5.5 (21-25/55)

Set A:
The number of white circles is the square of the number of black circles (e.g. 4 whites and 2 blacks; 16 whites and 4 blacks).

Set B:
The number of white circles is the cube of the number of black circles (e.g. 8 whites and 2 blacks; 64 whites and 4 blacks).

Answers
Shape 5.1: Set A
Shape 5.2: Set A
Shape 5.3: Neither. 2 blacks, 5 whites.
Shape 5.4: Neither. 2 blacks, 6 whites.
Shape 5.5: Set B

Comments
Some of the shapes contain many circles and it could take time to count them all. Consequently, some candidates may be put off counting them. It is always worth doing a quick count on some of the less crowded shapes to see if a pattern can be established. If, after counting a sample of shapes, you detect a possible pattern, you can then move on to counting some of the more crowded shapes. The counting for the most crowded shape (first one in Set B) is made easier by the layout (7 by 7 square).

Other relationships you may want to investigate include:

- Does the position of the circles within each shape matter? Some of the shapes have the same number of white/black circles (e.g. in Set A, two shapes have 2 blacks and 4 whites), which indicates that the position of the circles within the shape is likely to be irrelevant.

- Does the relative position of black circles in relation to white circles matter? The type of relationship that you are looking for may be as follows: "if there are 2 black circles then the white squares are above the line that links them", "if there are 3 black circles, the white squares are contained within the triangle drawn by linking them", "if there are 4 black circles, the white circles are contained within the parallelogram drawn by linking them", etc. This is not the case here.

MOCK AR 6/15 – Exercises 6.1 to 6.5 (26-30/55)

Set A:
Each large object contains one <u>black</u> object only, which is of the same type, e.g. a single small black square within a large square object; a single small black triangle within a large triangle.

Set B:
Each large object contains one <u>white</u> object only, which is of the same type, e.g. a single small white square within a large square object; a single small white triangle within a large triangle.

Note that in both sets the number of small objects which are of the opposite colour is irrelevant.

Answers
Shape 6.1:   Neither. No small object is uniquely black or white.
Shape 6.2:   Neither. No small object is uniquely black or white.
Shape 6.3:   Set A
Shape 6.4:   Neither. Two objects of a unique colour but not matching the large object.
Shape 6.5:   Set A. (The uniquely coloured small object is a black circle, which matches the large circle. The fact that there is also a white circle is irrelevant.)

MOCK AR 7/15 – Exercises 7.1 to 7.5 (31-35/55)

Set A:
Within each shape the number of dots on each domino is the same, e.g. in the first shape, the two dominoes each have 7 dots (4+3 and 3+4).

Mock Exam

Set B:
Within each shape, the number of dots on each of the two diagonals adds up to the same number, i.e. the sum of the top dots on the first domino plus the bottom dots on the second domino equals the sum of bottom dots on the first domino plus the top dots on the second. In the first shape of the set, the total along the diagonals is 7 (4+3 and 2+5).

Note that the total varies between the different shapes and therefore the actual number of dots within one shape is not relevant.

Answers
Shape 7.1:   Set A
Shape 7.2:   Neither
Shape 7.3:   Neither
Shape 7.4:   Set A
Shape 7.5:   Neither

Comments
Shapes centred around dominoes will most often be related through the number of dots they contain. Try the following relationships:

- Adding or multiplying all dots in the shape.
- Adding or multiplying the dots on each independent domino.
- Adding or multiplying the dots on the diagonals.
- Adding or multiplying the dots horizontally.

MOCK AR 8/15 – Exercises 8.1 to 8.5 (36-40/55)

Set A: The number of small white objects is equal to the number of sides of the large object.

Set B: The number of small black objects is equal to the number of sides of the large object.

Answers
Shape 8.1: Set A
Shape 8.2: Set B
Shape 8.3: Set B
Shape 8.4: Neither. We would require 3 small objects of the same colour.
Shape 8.5: Neither. We would need only 1 small object of a given colour.

MOCK AR 9/15 – Exercises 9.1 to 9.5 (41-45/55)

Both sets contain at least one triangle, one circle and one square, with one of the three objects being duplicated. This creates a pair of objects and two "twins".

Set A: There is no rule about the colour of the objects. However, the twins must face each other and not lie in adjacent quarters of the shape.

Set B: Adjacent quarters must not contain objects of the same colour (i.e. we always have two black objects facing each other and two white objects facing each other). The twins must lie adjacent to each other and therefore must be of differing colour.

Answers
Shape 9.1:   Set A
Shape 9:2:   Neither. There are only 2 types of object in the shape.
Shape 9.3:   Neither. The twins follow the right relationship for Set B but we would also need to have a black square instead of a white square opposite the black circle.
Shape 9.4:   Neither. There are only 2 types of object in the shape.
Shape 9.5:   Neither. There are only 2 types of object in the shape.

Comments
The separation in four quadrants makes it easier to identify the relationships. If you identify quickly that the shapes only contain three possible objects: circle, square and triangle, then the only possible relationships are as follows:

- The object in one specific quadrant is always of the same colour (not the case here).
- Objects facing each other are either of the same type or of the same colour, or both (this is the case here for Set A).
- Objects adjacent to each other are either of the same type or of the same colour, or both (this is the case here for Set B).
- If an object of a specific type is of a certain colour, then another object of a specific type is of the same colour or the opposite colour, e.g. if the triangle is black then the circle is also black (this is not the case here).

Mock Exam

MOCK AR 10/15 – Exercises 10.1 to 10.5 (45-50/55)

The relationships are linked to the direction of the arrows and the number and type of objects within each shape. All arrows are vertical and all objects (other than the arrow) are white. The size and position of the objects do not matter.

In both sets, when the arrow points upwards, the number of objects (excluding the arrow) is even. When the arrow points downwards, the number of objects (excluding the arrow) is odd.

Set A:
- When the arrow points downwards, all other objects are different.
- When the arrow points upwards, all objects are of the same type, though not necessarily the actual same shape or the same size (e.g. 4 triangles of different natures).

Set B:
- When the arrow points upwards, all other objects are different.
- When the arrow points downwards, all objects are of the same type, though not necessarily the actual same shape or the same size (e.g. 3 different types of ovals, 5 different pentagons, or 7 diamonds).

Answers
Shape 10.1: Set A
Shape 10.2: Neither. A downward pointing arrow requires an odd number of objects to belong to either set.
Shape 10.3: Neither. 8 similar objects plus a different object.
Shape 10.4: Set B
Shape 10.5: Set A

Comments
Your eyes are naturally drawn towards large objects. Do not spend time worrying about them if you can see that only some shapes have large objects (e.g. 2nd shape, left column, Set A). You will waste valuable time. Similarly, your eye will be drawn to shapes which contain objects of a similar nature (e.g. 7 diamonds of equal size in Set B, 5 pentagons in Set B). This may well be relevant, but it may also be a sizeable distractor which will waste your time.

You may well find that you cannot take your mind away from such shapes; if it is the case, go back to basics and start counting objects and sides. Look out also for the nature of the sides (i.e. curved v. straight).

MOCK AR11/15 – Exercise 11/15 (51/55)

Answer: B
The top left frame shows a black triangle (three sides) over a white circle (one side). This becomes a black semi-circle (two sides) over a white square (four sides). Therefore we can conclude the following:

- The new shapes have one more side than the original shapes.
- The colours are swapped: the black triangle became a white square, and the white circle became a black semi-circle.
- The colour that was on top remains on top. In this case, the black object is on top in both cases.

We are therefore looking for:
- A grey pentagon (4 sides in the diamond + 1 = 5, white becomes grey).
- A white quadrilateral (3 sides in the 'Pacman' shape + 1 = 4, grey becomes white).
- A grey shape (i.e. pentagon) over a white shape (i.e. quadrilateral).

The answer is therefore Frame B.

MOCK AR12/15 – Exercise 12/15 (52/55)

Answer: C
The starting frame has one large object containing a slightly smaller object and two even smaller identical objects. The shapes in the right-hand frame have the same number of sides as those on the left; in the example: 3, 4 and 5 sides. We also have one large object containing a slightly smaller one, but the two small identical objects are on the outside.

For the right-hand shape:
- The two identical objects have the same number of sides as the largest object in the left-hand frame; in this case, they are pentagons. The two small objects remain the same colour: in this case, white.

Mock Exam

- The largest object has a number of sides equal to that of the two small objects on the left-hand side. Its colour, however, is that of the medium-sized shape on the left-hand side.
- The medium object has the same number of sides as the medium object on the left-hand side. However, it takes its colour from the largest object on the left-hand side.

So we would expect the following:
- A large black triangle.
- A white circle or ellipse contained within the large black triangle.
- Two small grey quadrilaterals sitting on the outside.

The answer is therefore Frame C.

MOCK AR13/15 – Exercise 13/15 (53/55)

Answer: D
Each arrow rotates on itself clockwise. An arrow which points upwards remains stationary for one step and then starts rotating again. So, in essence the rotation process is:

➡ ⬇ ⬅ ⬆ ⬆

MOCK AR14/15 – Exercise 14/15 (54/55)

Answer: B
The crossed lines and black dots are static. The white circle and white diamonds are rotating clockwise by an increasing number of steps (one notch between Frames 1 and 2, two notches between Frames 2 and 3, and three notches between Frames 3 and 4, skipping over the black dot if necessary (the black dot does not count as a notch). As they skip over a black dot, they switch colour (white → grey → white); if they need to skip over two black dots at once, the colour remains the same since they would switch twice simultaneously.

We are therefore expecting both shapes to move by four positions clockwise, skipping over black dots as necessary.

MOCK AR15/15 – Exercise 15/15 (55/55)

Answer: C
The black dots are moving up and down their column according to the following principle:

- Black arrow: remain stationary in the next frame.
- White arrow: Move by one space in the direction of the arrows. Therefore the arrows from the previous frame are those which matter to set the new frame. In the new frame, one of the arrows must be black and the other one white; and they must point in the current direction of travel of the black dot.

We therefore expect the new frame to have:
- A black dot in the bottom left square (stationary from Frame 4).
- A black dot in the second square from the bottom on the right-hand side (one level down from Frame 4).

Therefore the answer is Frame C.

MOCK EXAM
VERBAL REASONING
ANSWERS

MOCK VR1/11 – Christmas Repeats

Q1.1 – CAN'T TELL
We know that 16% of BBC1's programmes were repeats. We know that 60% of Channel 5's programmes were repeats. Without knowing how many programmes both broadcasters showed, it is not possible to compare the actual number of repeats.

Q1.2 – CAN'T TELL
Using the same logic as for Q1, we know that the proportion of repeats has not changed. However, without knowing the actual number of programmes in both years, we cannot comment on the actual number of repeats.

Q1.3 – CAN'T TELL
The text presents no link between the decrease in viewing share suffered by terrestrial channels and the increase in repeats. It just states the facts. In fact there is no clear evidence as to whether viewers want to see repeats or not, other than a survey by the broadcasters themselves.

Q1.4 – TRUE
We are told that Channel 4's share fell by more than 11% to 8.7%. Therefore its share in 2006 was over 19.7%. We are also told that BBC2's share in 2006 was 11.9%. Therefore Channel 4 was more popular than BBC2 in 2006.

MOCK VR2/11 – HIV Vaccine

Q2.1 – B: Patients with HIV, who have a low viral load.
The text says that if the therapeutic vaccine is invented, then patients will first need to start combination therapy to reduce the viral load and then start the vaccination. Therefore the vaccine will be most effective in HIV-positive patients with a low viral load. Looking at the other options:

- **A: Patients without HIV but who are at risk of catching it.** This would be true of the preventative vaccine. The therapeutic vaccine is clearly presented as being administered to already-infected patients.

- **C: Patients who refuse to take combination therapy.** If patients refuse combination therapy, then the text suggests their viral load would remain too high for the vaccine to be administered. Since combination therapy would need to be administered before the vaccine, this assertion cannot be correct.

- **D: Patients with a natural resistance to HIV.** All we know from the text is that the fact that some people are naturally resistant is what is providing hope that a vaccine could exist. In any case, if they are naturally resistant, they wouldn't need a vaccine.

Q2.2 – A: It is a barrier to the eradication of the virus.
According to the last paragraph, the reservoir of the virus which sits in organs and tissues can be reactivated when treatment has stopped. Therefore until that reservoir can be eliminated, it remains a clear barrier to the eradication of the virus. Looking at the other options:

- **B: No one has yet proven its existence.** The text seems to be definite about its existence and does not mention any possible doubt. So, even if that statement were true in practice, it certainly cannot be inferred from the text.

- **C: It is a separate blood pool stored within certain vital organs.** All we know from the text is that the reservoir is essentially referring to the virus "hiding" in some organs and tissues. There is no indication that it is a pool of blood (in fact the text suggests not in the blood at all).

- **D: It prevents the virus from re-entering the blood stream.** The text does not mention or infer anything of the sort. All we know is that, although the virus may have disappeared from the blood, it can still be found in tissue and organs.

Q2.3 – CAN'T TELL
If the vaccine fails, the patient will need to revert to the combination therapy. Whilst some patients may not need therapy thereafter, some may. Therefore we cannot conclusively state that the assertion is true or false.

Q2.4 – CAN'T TELL
All we know from the text is that efforts to develop a preventative vaccine have so far been unsuccessful (and that the reservoir is an obstacle). There is nothing to suggest that a preventative vaccine is impossible.

MOCK VR3/11 – E-cigarette

Q3.1 – CAN'T TELL
It is unclear as to whether the toxicity is to the user or to those around him/her, i.e. whether any of the toxic products are contained in the vapour. All we know is that the liquid in the cigarette contains toxic substances. The vapour, we are told, contains aromatic essences. There is also uncertainty about what the final approval will depend on. The text suggests that the authorities have two main issues: toxicity but also misleading advertising claims. There is no indication as to whether the authorities are aiming to make the cigarette less toxic or whether approval will mainly be linked to more honest advertising claims. If approval depended on the removal of all toxic substances, then it would be correct to say that the e-cigarette would remove the dangers of passive smoking. However, if approval depended solely on the introduction of less misleading advertising then the toxicity

Mock Exam

would remain and therefore the dangers of passive smoking may not be removed.

Q3.2 – D: None of the above.
The text gives examples of possible harm the e-cigarette can cause and names the elderly and those with epilepsy as examples. But they are only examples of the impact of some of the substances found in e-cigarettes. The fact no example is given of harm to others does not mean they are safe. As such, we are unable to conclude anything from the text with regard to how safe e-cigarettes might be to anyone.

Q3.3 – TRUE
Absolutely, we cannot say that this will happen, but the key to the answer is in the word "could". We know that e-cigarettes are currently being advertised as smoking-cessation devices, a claim which the health authorities are investigating. That claim is only illegal because proper approval was not sought, but it does not mean that it is factually incorrect. Whether or not e-cigarettes will eventually be used to encourage smokers to quit smoking is subject to final approval, but the use of the word "could" in the statement makes it a true claim (i.e. there is a viable possibility). If the statement were worded as "In the future, e-cigarettes WILL be used to encourage smokers to give up smoking", then the answer would be "Can't tell" because it would depend on whether approval is granted.

Q3.4 – D: Some manufacturers are currently selling e-cigarettes illegally.
No licence was obtained to commercialise the product (a licence is needed because of potential toxicity and possible use for smoking cessation), therefore it is illegal to commercialise the product.

Looking at the other options:

- **A: Nicotine-based products are not effective smoking-cessation products.** The text does not address their effectiveness, but merely the fact that they require a licence to be marketed as smoking-cessation devices.

- **B: It is illegal to market nicotine-based products as smoking-cessation products.** That is only true if no licence was obtained. But, with a licence, it is legal.

749

- **C: The claim made by some manufacturers that nicotine-based devices can be used for smoking cessation purposes is misleading.** The problem raised by the text is not that the claim is misleading, but simply that it needs approval via a licensing mechanism before it can be made. Without knowing more about the product, we cannot say that it is misleading.

MOCK VR4/11 – NICE

Q4.1 – D: NICE's decisions are binding only for NHS Trusts.
In the first paragraph we are told that NICE decisions are binding, though at that stage it is not entirely clear who it is binding for. The second paragraph confirms that "NICE only deals with the provision of treatment or care in the NHS" and that "NICE decisions do not apply in the private sector". Looking at the other options:

- **A: In future, NICE will be required to make decisions in 3 months instead of up to 2 years.** All we are told is that it is a recommendation, not a certainty.

- **B: Some decisions take NICE longer than 2 years to make.** All we are told is that decisions can take up to 2 years. This suggests therefore that no decision takes over 2 years to make. And though we might think intuitively that a few might take longer, this cannot be conclusively deduced from the text.

- **C: NICE's delay in making decisions is due to the extensive research it has to conduct.** Nothing in the text clarifies the reason for the delay. It could be, as the question suggests, that this is due to the need to research each drug carefully or, more likely, it could be that there is a huge backlog of cases to look into.

Q4.2 – D: The £30,000 cap will continue to apply in many cases.
All the text suggests is that the £30,000 cap will be removed for certain cases where there are very specific circumstances. There is no suggestion that it will, in fact, be removed for most cases. Looking at the other options:

- **A: Currently, an NHS Trust cannot spend more than £30,000 per year on any given treatment.** The text is clear that, in the case of pending cases of NICE approval, it is up to the Trust to decide whether to fund the treatment or not.

Mock Exam

- **B: If patients opt for private care, the NHS partially funds their treatment up to a maximum of £30,000.** Nothing in the text deals with partial funding.

- **C: Currently, patients cannot receive treatment in the UK unless that treatment costs under £30,000.** That is only true in regard to NHS treatment; however, it is clear from the text that patients can get higher-cost treatments privately.

Q4.3 – TRUE
The key sentence is "This means that some treatments which could add a lot of value to a patient are discounted because they are too expensive."

Q4.4 – FALSE
We are told that NICE decisions are binding and that NICE applies to the NHS only; therefore, within NICE, decisions will apply uniformly to all patients. Within the NHS, inequalities of care will occur when there is no NICE decision (and not as a result of NICE decisions): "Different Trusts make different decisions, which leads to inequalities of care." There may also be inequalities of care between NHS patients (who are constrained by NICE) and private patients (who can pay for unapproved treatment themselves), but such inequalities are not taking place <u>within</u> the NHS.

MOCK VR5/11 – Heavy Metal

Q5.1 – A: It only deals with metals and no other risks.
The text explains that the index was derived by looking at research into metal level. As such, this is a reasonable conclusion to draw. Looking at the other options:

- **B: It is based on unrealistic daily alcohol consumption.** It is hard to define what realistic actually means when it comes to drinking, considering it may vary between countries. So we can't conclude either way.

- **C: It measures the concentration of heavy metals in wine.** The THQ is an index measuring the level of risk to which drinkers are exposed in relation to heavy metals and not their concentration (though the text suggests there is a link between the two). Strictly speaking this assertion is actually false as, at best, it gives a likely indication of the level of concentration but does not measure it.

- **D: It ranks wines from 0 to 300.** We know that some wines have an index of 300, but that does not mean it can't go higher.

Q5.2 – C: Austrian wines have a higher concentration of heavy metals than German wines.
The list "Austria, Spain, Germany and Portugal" is in decreasing order of concentration. Therefore we can conclude that Austrian wines have a higher concentration of heavy metals than German wines. Looking at the other options:

- **A: Spanish wines have a higher THQ than Portuguese wines.** We know from the text that Spanish wines have a higher concentration of heavy metals than Portuguese wines, but we don't know for sure whether the THQ follows the same relationship. It may be, for example, that some metals are given more weight than others in computing the index.

- **B: Argentinian wines have a higher concentration of heavy metals than Italian wines.** All we know from the text is that wines from both countries have low concentrations of heavy metals, but they are not ranked in any particular order; as such we cannot ascertain which of the two has the higher concentration.

- **D: French wines have a THQ between 200 and 300.** We can probably guess that the THQ of French wine is likely to be below 300 and most likely to be around 200, but we cannot conclude that it is between those two values.

Q5.3 – CAN'T TELL
The last paragraph suggests that not all metal may be assimilated, and in particular that rhamnogalacturonan may neutralise metallic elements. However, all these aspects are introduced as part of a debate/discussion on the issue, and therefore nothing can be definitely asserted. Any risk is presented as potential only.

Q5.4 – FALSE
There were indeed sixteen countries involved but the scientists did not question any wine drinkers. They merely analysed studies which had been carried out previously by others.

Mock Exam

MOCK VR6/11 – Women in Ancient Egypt

Q6.1 – CAN'T TELL
The text states that "it was perhaps unsafe for an Egyptian woman to venture far from her town alone". The use of the word "perhaps" indicates that this a speculative statement and therefore we cannot conclude whether it is true or not.

Q6.2 – D: It is impossible to tell.
We know that two-thirds of property would be distributed between the two children. However, we are not told whether the property is being shared equally between the two children (for example, it could be that the elder gets a bigger share). There is also ambiguity about the meaning of "property". The text refers to two-thirds of the "community property" whereas the question only refers to "property" in general.

Q6.3 – C: High powered jobs were male-dominated.
The text explains that women could take up higher powered jobs (e.g. doctors, administrators) but that this was an exception to the rule. We are told also that "Given the relative scarcity of such cases, they might reflect extraordinary individuals in unusual circumstances". Looking at the other options:

- **A: There were more female doctors than female administrators.** We know that there were a hundred female doctors in Ancient Egypt (though we are not told whether these doctors lived at the same time). We also know that there were few women in administrative positions, though we are not told how many.

- **B: There were more female doctors than male doctors.** The text does not actually give the exact information we need to determine whether this is correct; however, it is pretty clear from the text that it was rare for women to hold such high-level positions and, as such, this statement is most likely false. It is therefore not a conclusion that the author would agree with.

- **D: The Assyrian civilisation predates Ancient Egypt.** The only statement in the text which relates to the Assyrians is in relation to wearing the veil. The author says that the Egyptians did not wear a veil, a tradition which was first documented amongst the Ancient Assyrians. So it could mean that the Assyrians came later, or it could mean simply that the author reached that conclusion simply on the basis there was no evidence from the Ancient Egyptians themselves (whereas the Assyrians HAD documented it).

Q6.4 – FALSE
The concept of fairness is not defined in the text but we know from the first paragraph that there were inequalities between the different classes. Therefore, although we cannot conclude from the text whether Egypt was a fair society, we do know that it was not classless. Therefore the assertion (which combines both terms with an "and") is false.

MOCK VR7/11 – The Eye of the World

Q7.1 – FALSE
Hubble is not earth-bound.

Q7.2 – CAN'T TELL
The fact that Hubble, which has a smaller mirror than the Chilean telescopes, produces pictures of better quality cannot be generalised since we are comparing telescopes that are being used in different environments. To be able to answer this question conclusively, we would need to have data which compared mirror sizes in similar circumstances (e.g. two mirrors of different sizes at the same altitude in space or in the Chilean desert).

Q7.3 – CAN'T TELL
We are not told anything about the quality of images before the repairs, when Hubble was "short-sighted". In the absence of any knowledge on the extent of the damage, we cannot conclude either way.

Q7.4 – TRUE
The text says that "some of its instruments are over a decade old", which suggests that others are less than 10 years old. In turn, this means that newer instruments were added during some of the service missions (or that older instruments were replaced).

MOCK VR8/11 – Green Fly

Q8.1 – D: It may be toxic even if not ingested.
The last sentence of the second paragraph indicates that the plant may be toxic to humans. Since we are told it is not edible and that this sentence is mentioned in the context of jatropha being used for fuel production, then we

Mock Exam

can conclude that the toxicity mentioned by the researchers is linked either to the manufacturing process or to its use as fuel (and therefore when not ingested). Looking at the other options:

- **A: It cannot grow on soil normally used for growing food.** All we are told is that it can grow in very dry soils and, as such, it won't compete with food crops. It does not mean that it can't grow on soil normally used for food: merely that it doesn't have to.

- **B: Its culture would require specific irrigation equipment.** Nothing in the text suggests that it requires specific irrigation equipment. In fact, if it can grow in very dry soils, it probably doesn't.

- **C: Its culture has the benefit of not being labour-intensive.** We are told that, in Ghana, farmers have shown reluctance to grow it because of the manpower required; so it seems that it is very labour-intensive.

Q8.2 – FALSE
Although ANZ used a mix of kerosene and biofuel, Boeing and Virgin Atlantic did a trial flight with palm oil and coconut oil only. Whether this can be done in the long term is another matter; but the text suggests that this flight actually took place and, therefore, that planes can fly on 100% biofuel.

Q8.3 – CAN'T TELL
We know from the text that the use of first generation biofuels encouraged deforestation. We conclude from this that locals would cut trees down to plant corn, soya, rapeseed or other suitable plants. If jatropha were to be used, since it can be grown on very dry soil, we can anticipate that locals would try to use naturally dry areas and would not need to cut trees down. However, unless we can be reassured that jatropha cannot be grown on the type of soil that forests occupy, there is no reason to assume that locals would not cut down trees to grow it. There is just a lesser chance that they might.

We know that it is a non-negotiable condition that the use of biofuels should not interfere with food cultures; however this is not the same as saying that it should not lead to deforestation.

Q8.4 – D: Growing non-edible plants for biofuel would drastically reduce the risk of deforestation.

The reason behind deforestation is not the fact that a plant is edible or not, but the fact that it needs fertile soil (which deforestation would provide). Therefore, growing inedible plants would not help. What would help instead is using plants which can be grown on arid soil (like jatropha). Looking at the other options:

- **A: Using an edible biofuel may increase the risk of food shortages.** Using an edible biofuel might encourage people to grow the plant for fuel purposes rather than food purposes (see first paragraph). Hence this may potentially lead to food shortages (which is why the airlines are so keen to ensure it does not interfere with food cultures).

- **B: First generation biofuels may lead to aviation accidents.** This can be inferred from the fact that we are told that some first generation fuels have a high freezing point (i.e. they will freeze too easily, with devastating consequences for a plane).

- **C: Selling edible plant material for fuel tends to be more financially rewarding than selling it for food.** If that were not true, then the growing of plants for fuel purposes would not risk interfering with food cultures. So it can reasonably be inferred from the text.

MOCK VR9/11 – Unwanted Goods

Q9.1 – B: The item's colour is not to the customer's liking.
Both bullet points make it clear that the rules apply whatever the reason for returning the teapot. Therefore the level of refund does not depend on the reason given but only on the criteria listed in the bullet points (e.g. level of admin fees, damage to the teapot, time elapsed since receipt of the teapot). The text also does not differentiate between items damaged by the customer and those damaged in transit.

Q9.2 – A: On or after 19 April.
Mrs Ackroyd did not receive any refund. This could happen only in three circumstances:
- Mrs Ackroyd cancelled within the 7 or 14-day period following receipt of the teapot and returned the teapot damaged. But she is being thanked at the end of the letter for sending the teapot back undamaged; therefore this is not a valid assumption to make.

Mock Exam

- Mrs Ackroyd cancelled within the 7 or 14-day period following receipt of the teapot and incurred a credit card and/or admin fee which was greater than the cost of the teapot; however, we are told that this is not the shop's policy.
- Mrs Ackroyd cancelled more than 14 full days after receiving the teapot. If she received the teapot on 4 April then this means she has sent her cancellation email on or after 19 April.

Q9.3 – FALSE
Based on the text, if someone cancelled an order from this shop within 7 days of receipt of a teapot and sent the teapot back undamaged, then, since they would not incur any card or administration charges, they would get a full refund.

Q9.4 – FALSE
8 July is 7 full days after the date of order (1 July). The date from which the 7 days are counted is the date the item is received, not the date of the order. Therefore it is incorrect to say that the "retailer has no obligation to grant any refund if the order is cancelled after 8 July". For example, if an item was received on 10 July then the customer would get a full refund provided they cancelled on or before 17 July.

MOCK VR10/11 – The Veggie Diet

Q10.1 – B: Vegans are at risk of calcium deficiency
Vegans do not eat dairy products, which we are told "almost solely" bring calcium into the diet. The text also states that "Vegans who do not opt for vegetables and fruits rich in calcium such as cress, spinach, almond, hazelnuts or pistachio nuts may encounter problems." Looking at the other options:

- **A: A patient with anaemia will also have Vitamin B12 deficiency.**
  The text tells us that a B12 deficiency may cause anaemia ("vegans... risk developing a Vitamin B12 deficiency and therefore anaemia"). This does not mean that all anaemia can be solely caused by a B12 deficiency. We therefore cannot conclude that a patient with anaemia will also have a Vitamin B12 deficiency. All we can conclude from this sentence is that someone who does not have anaemia cannot have a Vitamin B12 deficiency, or that someone with a Vitamin B12 deficiency will have anaemia (but not the other way round).

- **C: Meat contains calcium.** Nothing in the text actually suggests that meat contains calcium.

- **D: Anaemia causes Vitamin B12 deficiency.** All we can conclude from the text is the reverse relationship, i.e. that Vitamin B12 deficiency causes anaemia.

Q10.2 – A: Cress contains both calcium and Vitamin B12.
Vitamin B12 is exclusively present in foods of animal origin (first sentence of second paragraph). Therefore cress, which is a vegetable, cannot be a source of Vitamin B12. It is a source of calcium though. However, since the assertion asks us to comment on calcium and Vitamin B12 together, then it is false. Looking at the other options:

- **B: Dairy products contain both Vitamin B12 and calcium.** This is stated in two different places in the second paragraph.

- **C: Some vegetables are poor in calcium.** The text says that vegans need to eat vegetables that are rich in calcium. This suggests others aren't.

- **D: Vegans need to take Vitamin B12 supplements.** Since we are told that Vitamin B12 can only be found in foods of animal origin, including dairy products and milk, and that vegans eat none of that, then their only source of Vitamin B12 would need to come from food supplements.

Q10.3 – CAN'T TELL
We know that vegetarians tend to smoke less than non-vegetarians; however, we would need to understand the precise link between smoking and lung cancer to draw a conclusion (and, remember, we cannot use our external knowledge). In any case, even if we knew for certain from the text that smoking increased the risk of lung cancer, the statement would not necessarily be true. For example, it could be that vegetarians are exposed to other factors which lead to lung cancer and to which non-vegetarians may not necessarily be exposed (e.g. some pesticides, asbestos, etc.). The only way we could conclude that this statement is true would be if: (i) we were being told so; or (ii) we knew that smoking increases the risk of lung cancer and was the main cause. Finally, there is a reduction of some cancers in vegetarians but we don't know which cancers.

Q10.4 – CAN'T TELL
This question plays on the differentiation between percentages and numbers. Intuitively, one would think that, if vegetarians have a low rate of obesity compared to non-vegetarians, they would make up a minority in the obese group. However, this is not necessarily so as it depends on the relative size of the groups. For example, imagine a world where we have 1000 vegetarians, 10% of whom (i.e. 100) are obese, and 100 non-vegetarians, 50% of whom (i.e. 50) are obese. This would confirm what the text says about a lower proportion of vegetarians being obese (10% v. 50%) but when looking at the obese population, they would make up 100 out of the 150 obese people, i.e. two-thirds. So unless we know the relative sizes of the two groups, we cannot conclude either way.

MOCK VR11/11 – Pole Position

Q11.1 – FALSE
This position is correct as far as the Academy of Medicine is concerned; however, the CNRS report, we are told, does not bear judgement on the negative effects of radio frequencies. So the report does not state that there is no danger.

Q11.2 – FALSE
Since the exposure is maximal at a distance of 280 metres, it can't be linear and therefore can't be proportionate to the distance.

Q11.3 – CAN'T TELL
The text does not address the issue of rural areas, but only those relating to urban areas or areas immediately adjoining urban areas.

Q11.4 – TRUE
In fact, from the text, we can even say that it is higher than 1.5 V/m.

MOCK EXAM DECISION MAKING ANSWERS

MOCK DM 1/29 – DVDs

In this question you are asked whether the titles could belong to Hassan's collection. So, the only items which could not belong to it would be the items which are explicitly in breach of the information provided.

Therefore, if there is no explicit breach, you should answer YES.

Q1.1 – YES. We are told that if a title lasts over two hours then it has to be a documentary, but that does not mean that there can't be documentaries lasting under two hours. Hence a 1h45min documentary could feature in his collection.

Q1.2 – YES. All his DVDs were released after 2001. We also know that only the DVDs with films released after 2001 contain bonuses, but that does not mean that they HAVE to have bonuses. It is therefore perfectly possible to have a British film dating post 2001 which has no bonus.

Q1.3 – YES. All his British DVDs were released after 2001.

Q1.4 – NO. If Hassan had a thriller from 1998 in his collection, then it would have to be a foreign one since all British DVDs were released after 2001. However we are told that the foreign DVDs he has are all documentaries. Therefore he cannot have a 1998 thriller in his collection.

Q1.5 – NO. We know that all titles lasting more than two hours were documentaries.

MOCK DM 2/29 – Missed Appointments

Q2 – B: YES. It will encourage patients to either attend or cancel appointments. The reason for charging is to discourage people from missing appointments in the first place, or at least make sure that, if they cannot attend, they give notice so that they can be replaced. This answer addresses this point. Looking at the other options:

A: YES. GPs can use the extra funding to compensate for governmental budget cuts. The point of charging for missed appointments is not as a substitute for government funding but to prevent appointments being missed in the first place. In any case, this answer presents what the money could be used for and as such it is not really on topic.

C: NO. People may miss appointments due to circumstances beyond their control. This point is not unreasonable; however, it does not mean that charging cannot be implemented albeit with exceptions. And in any case, even if people have a good reason not to attend, that should not prevent them from giving some warning so that they can be replaced.

D: NO. Getting an absent patient to pay may prove challenging. That is certainly true but the fact something offers challenges does not mean that it should not be implemented.

MOCK DM 3/29 – Comfort In Bed

Q3.1 – YES. We are told that to be comfortable a bed must have a base made of slats.

Q3.2 – NO. We know that all insomniacs sleep on spring bases, but (i) it does not mean that non-insomniacs don't; and (ii) it does not mean that the springs are causing the insomnia (it could be for example that all insomniacs get up often at night and find spring bases easier to get up from than slat bases – this is what is called a link, which is not necessarily a cause).

Q3.3 – YES. All salesmen at "Comfort in Bed" sell comfortable beds (which must have a base made of slats) and they are all insomniac, which means that they sleep on a bed base made of springs. Hence they cannot be sleeping on the products they sell.

Q3.4 – NO. "Comfort in Bed" do not actually sell beds with spring bases since they only sell comfortable beds, which must have slats. And in any case, all their salesmen are insomniac; so even if they did sell beds with spring bases, they would have to be sold by insomniacs.

Q3.5 – YES. The fact that all insomniacs sleep on spring bases does not mean that others cannot.

MOCK DM 4/29 – Driving Test

Q4 – D: NO. Though most people forget the details of the Highway Code, they drive safely. Knowledge of the Highway Code is not the primary aim. Good and safe driving is. This answer argues that retesting would actually achieve little and so is a direct argument against it. Looking at the other options:

A: YES. Up-to-date knowledge of the Highway Code is important. It sure is, but knowledge of the Highway Code is not the be-all and end-all. Safe driving is. As such the scope of this answer is too narrow. Also, it assumes that people lose their knowledge of the Highway Code as they get older, which is speculative since one could argue that people become better drivers as they get older since they are getting more experienced.

B: YES: The fees collected could be reinvested to fund new road infrastructures. This only describes how the cash generated could be used, but does not in any way justify retesting.

C: NO. Most people would pretend to drive well during the test and would continue to drive as they normally do afterwards. This is entirely speculative. And even if that were true, it is possible some people may actually improve as a result of retesting.

MOCK DM 5/29 – Golf Club

Q5.1 – NO. All we are told is that Club C is the only one admitting both men and women. That means that all other clubs are not mixed, but that does not preclude some from being women-only clubs.

Q5.2 – NO. All we know is that some women can only attend after 6pm or at weekends; it is possible that they only attend on one of the two occasions. In any case, we know nothing about the other women, who could be attending at any time.

Q5.3 – NO. The women who are not restricted to evenings or weekends could actually be attending at any time, including 4pm on a weekday.

Q5.4 – YES. After 6pm on weekdays, there are no men but there could be women.

Mock Exam

Q5.5 – NO. We do not know if any of the women attend the club both after 6pm on weekdays and at weekends or whether they attend on only one of those two slots.

MOCK DM 6/29 – Five-A-Day

Q6 – C: NO. Historically, food retailers such as supermarkets have not passed on cost savings to the consumer. The text is implying that the mechanism by which consumption will increase is that subsidies will reduce costs to producers, which will then lead to lower prices and therefore higher volume of fruit and vegetables being purchased and consumed. The fact that lower costs have not historically led to those savings being passed on to the consumer indicates that this mechanism will fail.

Note: this is slightly speculative as the supermarket's past behaviour cannot be extrapolated, but historical evidence is better than pure conjecture and none of the other options are better.

Looking at the other options:

A: YES. It will encourage greater production of fruit/vegetables. The point is not necessarily to increase production but to subside prices (which may involve simply producing the same amount but for cheaper because of the subsidies).

B: YES. Fruit/vegetables contain vital vitamins and antioxidants. That reinforces the need to eat more fruit and vegetables, but not whether subsidies would be a useful mechanism to increase consumption.

D: NO. There is currently a huge amount of waste, which could be sold at cheaper prices to encourage consumption. It could, but it isn't, otherwise it would not be a counter argument. So, if the government simply left the issue alone, there is no indication that such waste would be sold at cheaper prices. The two are not incompatible anyway, but all this option offers is an alternative or a complementary solution, and not an argument against.

MOCK DM 7/29 – Relaxing On Holiday

Q7.1 – NO. When Natalie is not on holiday, she doesn't go on a diet. Since she is currently on a diet then it means she must be on holiday.

Q7.2 – NO. Since she is on holiday, then it means she plays sport. We know that when she is not relaxed she does not play sport. Since she does, she must be relaxed.

Q7.3 – NO. We know Natalie is not on a diet when she is not on holiday. But that does not tell us anything about her behaviour when she is on holiday.

Q7.4 – YES. If Natalie is not relaxed, she does not play sport. We know that when she is on holiday she plays sport. Therefore, when she does not play sport, it means that she isn't on holiday.

Q7.5 – YES. When Natalie is relaxed, she plays sport. Therefore when Natalie does not play sport, it means that she is not relaxed.

MOCK DM 8/29 – £1 Coin

Q8 – A: YES. it will make it harder to copy it. There has to be a purpose for changing the coin design. This might be purely aesthetic but in this particular case, the answer provides a valid reason which addresses a known issue: fraud.

Looking at the other options:

B: YES. Changing the coin design will take old dirty coins out of circulation and replace them by new clean ones. If offering new clean coins was the goal, there would be no need to redesign the coin in the first place. Simply offering to clean them, or to replace them with new ones, would be sufficient.

C: NO. Some people like the old type of coins. The feelings of the population are important, but (i) we know this only affects "some" people, and (ii) avoiding fraud is of larger national interest. The fact a change may displease some people is no reason to avoid it.

D: NO. Shops will be forced to upgrade their trolleys at great expense. This may well be a consequence. But the need to combat fraud is of greater and broader interest than the interest of supermarkets.

MOCK DM 9/29 – Cats

Q9.1 – NO. We know that Tiger is from the neighbourhood. Since no cats from the neighbourhood like dogs then we know that Tiger does not like dogs. We know that ginger cats like dogs. So if a cat does not like dogs then that cat cannot be ginger. Hence Tiger is not a ginger cat.

Q9.2 – YES. We know that cats with a nice basket have rich owners. We also know that clever cats don't have rich owners, which means that if a cat has a rich owner then that cat cannot be clever. Hence cats with a nice basket are not clever.

Q9.3 – YES. Tiger is from the neighbourhood and therefore does not like dogs, which means he is not ginger (see reasoning for 9.1). We know that cats which don't have a nice basket are ginger. Since Tiger is not ginger then it means he has a nice basket. We know that cats that have a nice basket are not clever. So Tiger is not clever.

Q9.4 – YES. We know that none of the cats in the neighbourhood like dogs. So if a cat likes dogs it cannot be from the neighbourhood.

Q9.5 – NO. Cats with a nice basket have rich owners so cats with non-rich owners don't have a nice basket. And therefore they must be ginger.

MOCK DM 10/29 – Dance Classes

Q10 – B: The number of students who don't attend jazz classes.
The information provided can be represented by the following Venn diagram, where X represents the number we need to know to be able to calculate the number of students who attend both jazz and rock classes (which will then be equal to X+3).

We have also labelled A and B the areas for which the numbers are unknown.

If we know the number of students who don't attend jazz classes, then the difference between the total number of students (48) and that number will be equal to the number of students who do attend jazz classes. We know that this number is also X + 3 + 4 + 5, so we will easily be able to calculate X.

Looking at the other options:

A: The number of students who attend rock classes. This number is equal to A + X + 3 + 3. So that leaves us with two variables and therefore we cannot do much with it. However, we could deduce that the number of students who do not attend rock classes (and which is equal to B + 4 + 5) is 48 minus that number. That would help us determine B, but not much more, since we do not know how many students attend rock classes or jazz classes.

C: The number of students who attend one class only. That number is equal to B + 3 + 5, so it could help us determine B. It would also help us determine A + X (since those who attend more than one class = A + X + 4 + 3). But not much more.

D: The number of students who attend hip-hop classes only. This is essentially equal to B, but without more information we cannot identify X.

MOCK DM 11/29 – Medals

D: 10 medals
A won three fewer medals than F and D won two more medals than F. So we can conclude that D won 5 more medals than A.

We know that when we add the medals won by A and D together we should get 17. Hence we can deduce that A won 6 medals and D won 11 medals (you can write equations if you want but since we are dealing with low-level integers, you could deduce it mentally more quickly).

Since A has won 6 medals, then E, who is sitting opposite, won 13 – 6 = 7 medals. And since we are told that E and G together won 17 medals, then we can conclude that G has won 17 – 7 = 10 medals

MOCK DM 12/29 – Students' Devices

Q12 – C
The first way in which we can eliminate some options is by counting how many students are in each circle. There should be 12, 15 and 12 respectively. This eliminates diagram A (12, 17 and 14) and diagram D (12, 9 and 14). This leaves diagrams B and C.

We know that no one owns both a TV and a laptop without also owning a computer. That means that the number of people who own only a TV and a laptop is 0. We also know that the number of people who own a TV is 12 and that the number of people who own a laptop is also 12. Hence the 0 should be included in both circles that add up to 12.

That is the case for diagram C (7 + 2 + 3 + 0 = 12 and 0 + 3 + 4 + 5 = 12) but that is not true of diagram B (8 + 4 + 3 + 0 = 15 and 0 + 3 + 2 + 7 = 12).

Hence diagram C is the answer.

MOCK DM 13/29 – Mammals And Reptiles

Q13 – D
There are two ways of resolving this problem. You can either just use logical reasoning to see which of the options best matches the text or, more simply, you can draw your own diagram and see which of the options it matches.

We know that mammals and reptiles are two separate entities, since no reptile is a mammal, so we can conclude that they are represented by two non-intersecting circles (because if they intersected, it would mean that there are animals which can be both reptile and mammal). So we start with this:

(Mammals) (Reptiles)

We know that some mammals and reptiles are vegetarians, which suggests that some are not. So the vegetarian circle will need to cross both circles partially. We get this:

Mammals   Veg   Reptiles

Finally, we know that some mammals have hooves and that those that do are vegetarian. This can be represented by a circle inside the mammals–vegetarian intersection.

Hooves

Mammals   Veg   Reptiles

This is essentially the same as Diagram D.

Mock Exam

MOCK DM 14/29 – Sports Survey

Q14 – B
In such an exercise, it is often best to proceed by elimination.

We know that 31 play netball only. So we can exclude diagram C since the numbers contained in the sections corresponding to one sport only are: 25, 40 and 10; and therefore none are 31.

We know that 60 play football and therefore the sum of all the numbers in one of the circles must add up to 60. We can see that this is not the case in diagram D. So we can exclude diagram D too.

This leaves us with Diagrams A and B. Using the numbers provided we can see that in both diagrams, the top left circle represents netball (31 people play netball only), the top right circle represents football (60 play football) and the bottom circle represents tennis (20 people play tennis).

However, we are told that 15 people play football and netball and therefore the intersection of the top two circles must add up to 15. That is only the case for diagram B (14 + 1). Alternatively, we are also told that 4 people who play two sports only don't play football, which essentially means that 4 people should play tennis and netball only. Diagram B is the only one of the two to have a sector with 4 people in it.

MOCK DM 15/29 – Jetsetters

Q15 – C: 31
We need to exclude anyone who is within the ellipse (India). Out of the others, all travellers have done two trips or fewer except the 7 people who visited Brazil, the US and China (in the overlapping sector for the cross, the rectangle and the parallelogram). Therefore the answer is: 5 + 4 + 6 + 3 + 2 + 6 + 5 = 31.

MOCK DM 16/29 – Furniture Factory

Q16 – C: 33.3%
The total number of products (adding all numbers on the diagram) is 150. The number of products made of three or more materials is:
10 + 8 + 9 + 17 + 6 = 50, i.e. 33.3%.

MOCK DM 17/29 – Staffing Levels

Q17 – B: Over one third of blue collars are women.
The following table shows the data presented in the text (in bold) and the numbers that can be deduced from it.

	APPRENTICES	BLUE COLLARS	WHITE COLLARS	TOTAL
MALE	**408**	216 = 360 – 144	Cannot be determined	Cannot be determined
FEMALE	192 = 600 – 408	**144**	Cannot be determined	Cannot be determined
TOTAL	**600** = 0.5 x 1200	360 = 1200 – 600 – 240	**240** = 0.2 x 1200	**1200**

We can see that the total number of blue collars is 360, of which 144 are women.

MOCK DM 18/29 – Holiday Itinerary

Q18 – C: She will visit both Morocco and Tunisia.
We know that Brenda will not visit Cape Verde, therefore it means that she will not visit Tenerife (because if she did then she would also visit Cape Verde). If she does not visit Tenerife, then it means that she will visit Morocco (we are reversing the first statement). The second statement tells us that she will therefore also visit Tunisia. So in total, she will visit Morocco and Tunisia, but not Tenerife or Cape Verde.

MOCK DM 19/29 – Positive Or Negative

Q19 – C: All answers are positives.
If Answer 1 is negative then we know that Answer 2 is positive. But since there cannot be only two positive answers, then Answer 3 has to be negative.

If Answer 1 is positive, then we know that at least one of the other two answers is positive. But since there cannot be only two positive answers then it means that the third one is also positive.

Consequently there are only two possibilities:

- 1= Negative, 2 = Positive, 3 = Negative
- 1 = Positive, 2 = Positive, 3 = Positive

Hence we can see that the second answer is always positive (option A), that if the first answer is positive then the third response is too (option B) and that nothing helps us decide whether the first answer is positive or negative (option D).

Option C states that all answers are positive. This is not correct since it is possible for 1 and 3 to be negative.

MOCK DM 20/29 – Pets and Hobbies

Q20 – B: The boxer came first in the competition.
We know from the second statement that Alan came immediately before Barack and has a snake. So we can write: Alan (snake) < Barack.

We know from the third statement that the student who owns spiders is ranked immediately before the tennis player, who we are told is Kaviraj. Therefore Kaviraj does not own spiders. Since he cannot own snakes (as we know Alan does) then we can conclude that Kaviraj owns a chameleon and that Barack owns spiders.

We can also conclude that Alan came first, Barack second and Kaviraj third. Hence the following table:

Alan	Barack	Kaviraj
1	2	3
Snake	Spiders	Chameleon
		Tennis

And since we know that the student who owns spiders (i.e. Barack) does not like boxing then he must enjoy swimming and Alan is into boxing.

Alan	Barack	Kaviraj
1	2	3
Snake	Spiders	Chameleon
Boxing	Swimming	Tennis

MOCK DM 21/29 – Dice Game

Q21 – C: The least distributed prize is W.
With two dice numbered 1 – 6 there are 6 x 6 = 36 possible combinations.

The ways in which one can obtain a score below 15 are:

Dice 1 = 1 & Dice 2 = 1, 2, 3, 4, 5, 6
Dice 1 = 2 & Dice 2 = 1, 2, 3, 4, 5, 6
Dice 1 = 3 & Dice 2 = 1, 2, 3, 4
Dice 1 = 4 & Dice 2 = 1, 2, 3
Dice 1 = 5 & Dice 2 = 1, 2
Dice 1 = 6 & Dice 2 = 1, 2

So a total of 23 possibilities. Out of those there are only four ways of getting one number which is double the other: (1,2), (2,1), (2,4) and (4,2).

Hence there are 36 – 23 = 13 ways of obtaining a score equal to or greater than 15. But only three ways in which it can be done using two odd numbers: (3,5), (5,3) and (5, 5).

Hence out of 36 possibilities, the prizes would come up as follows:

W	X	Y	Z
4	19	3	10

Hence we can see that:
- Throwing 3 and 5 would entitle the player to Prize Y (option A).
- The most often distributed prize would be X (option B).
- A player would have a probability of 19/36 of getting Prize X, hence more than 50% (option D).

Option C is incorrect since the least distributed prize is expected to be Y and not W.

Mock Exam

MOCK DM 22/29 – Health Screen

Q22 – B: 2.9%.
The easiest way to solve this problem is to draw a diagram:

```
                        10,000 people
                       /            \
         0.1% have the disease    9990 do not have the disease.
             = 10 people                 /            \
            /          \
1 negative test   9 positive tests   300 positive tests   9690 negative tests
                      (90%)                                     (97%)
```

Therefore the probability that a patient with a positive test has the disease is 9/309 = 2.9%.

You do not actually need to calculate the value to identify the correct option. 9/300 = 0.03 i.e. 3% and therefore 9/309 would be slightly lower.

MOCK DM 23/29 – Sharing Tasks

Q23 – B: Yes, because they both equally contribute.
This is one of those questions that seem to come up often and in which the same type of information is presented in different ways to make you believe that they are talking about different things when in fact they are not.

Here we are told the wife and husband take it in turns to go shopping. They shop six days a week and the husband shops three times a week, therefore the wife does too. At the same time, we are told that the wife has a 9/10 = 90% success rate at finding smoked salmon, whereas the husband only managed to come back without smoked salmon five times out of 50, i.e. a failure rate of 10% and therefore a success rate of 90% also.

Conclusion: they shop the same number of days with the same success rate of 90%, hence option B is the correct answer.

MOCK DM 24/29 – Code 1234

Q24 – A: Only three combinations fulfil all criteria.
We know that 4 is in third place. So that means that 1 cannot be in first place (otherwise 2 would be in third place). Therefore 1 is either in second or fourth place.

Possible options therefore are: __14__ and __ __41.

Starting with __14__: If 2 occupies first place then it means 2 is next to the second place and therefore 1 must be in fourth place, which contradicts the fact it is actually in second place. Hence 2 cannot be in first place and has to be in fourth place. The only possible option is therefore: 3142.

Looking at __ __41:
- If 2 occupies first place then it is next to the second place and 1 should be in fourth place, which it is. Hence option 2341 works.
- 2 could also be in second place and there is no condition that means anything should happen to the other digits if that were the case. Hence 3241 also works.

There are therefore only three possible answers: 3142, 2341 and 3241.

MOCK DM 25/29 – Truths and Lies

Q25 – A: James is lying.
We know that if Andrew lies then Jane and William lie. However since Andrew is in the same group as William, they can't both be lying at the same time. Therefore Andrew must be telling the truth otherwise we get a contradiction. Since we know that Andrew is telling the truth we know that Margot is lying. As Jane is in her group, this in turn means that Jane is telling the truth. In turn, it means that Philip is lying and that James is telling the truth.

Looking at the other options:

B: Margot is lying. We have established above that this is true.

C: If Jane tells the truth then Andrew tells the truth. We know that if Andrew lies then Jane and William lie. So if either Jane or William are in

Mock Exam

fact telling the truth then Andrew cannot be lying and hence he is telling the truth.

D: If Philip tells the truth then James lies. That is given in the text of the question, since they are in the same group.

MOCK DM 26/29 – Clothes Storage

Q26 – A: His socks are in the top drawer.
The second drawer from the top does not contain underwear or socks. Therefore it must contain either jumpers or shirts. Since jumpers and shirts are not in consecutive drawers it means that the bottom drawer also contains jumpers or shirts. It turn, it means that the first and third drawers from the top contain underwear or socks.

We know that the underwear drawer is lower than the shirts' drawer, therefore the underwear draw cannot be at the top. Hence it is in third position and the socks are at the top. That then means that the shirts are in the second drawer and the jumpers are at the bottom.

MOCK DM 27/29 – Night At The Museum

Q27 – C: Dali is directly to the north of Matisse.

A	B	W
C	D	BRAQUE
X	Y	Z

We know from the text that Kandinski is next to Braque, Matisse and Renoir, but also next to Van Gogh. The only room which has access to four other rooms is D. Hence D = KANDINSKI. In turn, it means that B, C and Y are Matisse, Renoir and Van Gogh, though not necessarily in that order.

We know that from Braque we can go directly into Ernst and Cézanne. Other than Kandinski, which is in D, the only other two rooms accessible from Braque are W and Z. And since we know that Ernst is in the north of the building, it means that W = ERNST and Z = CÉZANNE.

This then means that Y = VAN GOGH as it links to Cézanne and that X = PICASSO, since it links to Van Gogh.

Also C = MATISSE since it links to Picasso and Kandinski, and A = DALI since it links to Matisse. This leaves us with B = RENOIR.

A DALI	B RENOIR	W ERNST
C MATISSE	D KANDINSKI	BRAQUE
X PICASSO	Y VAN GOGH	Z CÉZANNE

MOCK DM 28/29 – Summer Jobs

Q28 – B: Many companies whose permanent staff do not take annual leave in the summer require additional support from students in the summer.
We are told that there are two reasons for requiring additional workforce: permanent staff's annual leave and a peak in demand. So, there will be companies that will require additional staff simply because they are experiencing a demand in their products and services, regardless of staff holidays.

Looking at the other options:

A: Permanent staff go on leave in the summer because they know their employer can easily fill the gap with students. All we know from the text is that extra resources are needed because staff go on leave. There is no evidence that they choose to go on holiday because they know their company will be able to replace them.

Mock Exam

C: Employers use summer jobs to spot new talent. This may be intuitive but the text does not present things from this angle. The text talks about attracting people who may be interested in returning later and about the fact that hands-on experience may make the company attractive to a student. In other words the text takes the angle that the purpose is to attract a sufficient pool of applicants rather than test those who are working there in the summer.

D: Students on summer jobs are treated on an equal basis with permanent employees. The text is clear that they are not entitled to the same benefits.

MOCK DM 29/29 – Employment

Q29 – C: Most of the graduates who commute over an hour to work go on holiday 20 or fewer days per year.
Graduates who commute over an hour are contained within both the circle and the D shape. There are 1 + 6 + 5 + 5 + 6 + 8 = 31 in total. Those who go on holiday 20 or fewer days per year will be outside of the rectangle. There are 5 + 6 + 8 = 19 of them. Therefore they are a majority.

Looking at the other options:

A: There are more employed people with a degree than there are unemployed people without a degree. Employed people with a degree will be inside both the cross and the circle. There are 6 + 1 + 5 = 12 of them. Unemployed people without a degree will be outside the cross and outside the circle. There are: 10 + 9 = 19 of them. Hence option A is false.

B: Most of those who are employed and have a degree are over the age of 40. We know from above there are 12 people who are employed and have a degree. Out of those 5 + 1 = 6 are inside the triangle. Hence there are as many over the age 40 as there are aged 40 or under. Hence option C is false.

D: Most of those who are over the age of 40 are unemployed. Those aged over 40 are included in the triangle. There are 42 in total. Out of those, only 9 + 6 + 3 = 18 (i.e. below 50%) are outside the cross and are therefore unemployed. Hence option D is false.

MOCK EXAM SITUATIONAL JUDGEMENT ANSWERS

MOCK SJ 1/22 – Faking It

1.1 – A: Very important
The duty of the team will be towards the patient. As such, allowing her to leave the hospital when it is not safe to do so will be something that cannot be ignored.

1.2 – C: Of minor importance
Establishing a dialogue with Mrs Jones to keep her on board will be important as it might stop her from making rash decisions. She might lose confidence in Sarah but it does not mean that she will lose confidence in the team and, if anything, it will enable the start of a dialogue during which she can openly raise the issues that concern her. In this case, her safety will be a far more important consideration than what she thinks of Sarah anyway.

1.3 – B: Important
The cats are obviously a concern for Mrs Jones since she is prepared to sacrifice her own health for them. The anxiety will harm the patient and so it is an important consideration (though still not as important as Mrs Jones's health). The cats' possible demise is also important because it means that Sarah needs to act quickly in raising the issue with her team; if the team is aware of the patient's fears, they may be able to find a solution to the problem (e.g. by making sure that the patient is cared for at home or that a neighbour is contacted to feed the cats). But, the cats' health still does not rank as highly as Mrs Jones's own health.

1.4 – D: Not important at all
Although she is a medical student, Sarah is expected to observe the same values as doctors.

MOCK SJ 2/22 – Unusual Murmur

2.1 – D: A very inappropriate thing to do
The apology is obviously welcome (though in the context it may not be genuine) but the main issue here is that Romeo is effectively telling the patient off for his attitude and is not respecting the patient's wishes. And whereas in some cases it may be true that patients are warned that medical students may approach them, it is entirely the patient's right to refuse to be subjected to unwelcome chats or investigations; the students should respect that. Lack of respect of a patient's wishes is very inappropriate, as is rudeness. It may actually make things worse by infuriating the patient further.

2.2 – C: Inappropriate but not awful
On the surface this does not look too bad; however, aside from the fact that there is no apology, the student has no right to promise the patient something he can't deliver (i.e. that the patient won't be bothered by anyone again). This is just designed to get a short gain for himself. It is misleading and inappropriate. The consequences being minor, it ranks as C.

2.3 – C: Inappropriate but not awful
If the patient has refused then it would be inappropriate to put pressure on them, especially in such a non-urgent non-essential context.

2.4 – A: A very appropriate thing to do
As well as the apology (essential to rate as A), he respects the patient and enquires about future possibilities. The patient still has the option to say no.

MOCK SJ 3/22 – Delayed Scan

3.1 – C: Inappropriate but not awful
Aside from the fact there is no apology and that it is not resolving anything, this response blames other colleagues for a clinical need which is beyond their control. This response only serves to avoid blame and does not give a constructive response. However, since the consequences do not make matters worse, it ranks as C instead of D.

Important: In this particular case, Paul is not actually to blame for the delay and so it is not unethical that he should seek to make sure that he is not blamed for it. It is just not a very professional thing to do and the consequences are not severe. Things would be very different if Paul were to blame for the delay (e.g. because he had forgotten to order the test) and then sought to blame someone else for it. In that case, the answer would rank D as it would be totally inappropriate to lie to a patient.

3.2 – A: A very appropriate thing to do
This pretty much covers as much as Paul can do.

3.3 – C: Inappropriate but not awful
The patient and the family have the right to complain and it would be appropriate to allow them to do so if they wanted to. However, it is possible that they may not actually feel that angry about things and offering them the opportunity to make a formal complaint is a bit premature. It will just waste a lot of time at this stage and won't address any of the issues anyway. In any case it does not contain an apology. And more should be done to reassure them rather than drive them down the path of expressing their anger.

3.4 – B: Appropriate, but not ideal
This would indeed help the family understand the situation better. However, an apology and an intention to update them on progress would also be needed in this situation.

MOCK SJ 4/22 – Acronyms

4.1 – D: A very inappropriate thing to do
It is inappropriate to leave the patient in the dark about the management of their condition. They will need to understand the issues before consenting to whatever the doctor is proposing. As such, although Nirav may be very experienced, he still has an obligation to make sure that the patient understands what he has said, including the risks and benefits of any intervention. Wendy should not be complicit in this and her behaviour is equally unethical.

4.2 – B: Appropriate, but not ideal
It will ensure that the patient has a chance to raise the issues she hasn't fully grasped. However, Wendy also felt a bit lost and, as such, she will not be in a position to answer all the questions Brenda may have. Wendy therefore risks just becoming a messenger between Brenda and Nirav and that conversation would be better had directly between the patient and her doctor.

4.3 – A: A very appropriate thing to do
That would ensure that Nirav is aware of the situation and goes back in at some stage to clarify some of the issues.

Mock Exam

MOCK SJ 5/22 – Overbearing Colleague

5.1 – A: A very appropriate thing to do
Talking to Petros away from the rest of the group will ensure he is not put on the spot and embarrassed in front of others. Being honest will also help resolve the issue proactively.

5.2 – C: Inappropriate but not awful
Approaching him in private is appropriate but asking him to shut up is not. Although he may be overbearing, his contribution is still valuable. It is much better to try to get him to see sense.

5.3 – B: Appropriate, but not ideal
This option is appropriate in the sense that it will achieve the desired result without undermining Petros; however, it is slightly devious, might be seen by Petros as an attempt to gag him and it would be much better if the solution came from him instead of being imposed by the others. So, though asking him to take the notes may be seen as a very appropriate thing to do, the underlying intentions and the fact it is slightly undermining downgrade the answer to a B.

MOCK SJ 6/22 – Training Opportunities

6.1 – A: A very appropriate thing to do
The best course of action will nearly always be to sort out the problem with the person concerned directly and diplomatically. Since Martyn's approach is part of the problem, this would help resolve that side of the matter.

6.2 – A: A very appropriate thing to do
The problem here is not just Martyn's behaviour in ensuring he is doing the ward round with the consultant. In fact, the root cause of the problem is the fact that the senior trainee is not performing his role well. As such, it would also be very appropriate to discuss the matter with him. Note that 6.1 and 6.2 are complementary actions and are not mutually exclusive but because they are dealing with different parts of the problem they can be considered in isolation, hence why both can be deemed to be very appropriate.

6.3 – C: Inappropriate but not awful
This course of action will deal with neither the senior trainee's behaviour, nor with Martyn's. The situation would be best dealt with directly with Martyn and with the senior trainee first. As a first line of response, this is inappropriate.

MOCK SJ 7/22 – Epileptic Colleague

7.1 – C: Of minor importance
This is a serious issue and as long as she trusts the colleague who spoke to her about Hisham's driving, she can't ignore the fact this poses a danger to the public. In this situation it would be better to act than not to act and so the fact that she has not directly observed the driving is not so relevant. The fact that she has not directly observed the driving means, however, that she will not be able to confront Hisham directly and she may want to suggest to Ben that, as a direct witness, he does it instead. As such this will be mildly relevant, hence the ranking of C.

7.2 – D: Not important at all
There are times when we can say that people are free to do what they want, e.g. everyone is free to play dangerous sports and risk injuring themselves if they wish. But when your actions may affect someone else drastically, and particularly when it comes to public and patient safety, there can be no compromise. The law preventing epileptic people from driving is there for a purpose and should apply, regardless of whether Hisham thinks he is fit to drive or not.

7.3 – D: Not important at all
The fact he is selling his car doesn't mean he won't be driving someone else's car or renting one. It is the fact he feels that he can defy the law which is worrying as it reflects a lack of integrity.

MOCK SJ 8/22 – Drug Allergy

8.1 – A: A very appropriate thing to do
The locum doctor should be made aware that he is overlooking the allergy recorded in the patient's notes. It seems odd that, when first approached about this issue, he ignored it when it could have fatal consequences. As such, one might reasonably assume he misheard or misinterpreted Stefie's original comments. The safest and most direct course of action would be to take this up with him a bit more assertively to remove any doubt about the potential danger to the patient.

8.2 – D: A very inappropriate thing to do
It is not the patient's responsibility to ensure their own clinical safety and, in any case, this would make the patient's safety rely on their ability to recall the facts and ensure they raise the issue, which is not a given. In addition, talking to the patient about the doctor's wrong prescription would surely make them very anxious and lose trust in the team's abilities.

8.3 – A: A very appropriate thing to do
In most scenarios, going above someone's head to address an issue instead of going to the person who is causing the issue would rank as C: Inappropriate but not awful. However, since Stefie has already attempted to address the issue directly with the locum doctor and the patient's safety is at risk, it makes it very appropriate to escalate the matter to a senior doctor.

8.4 – B: Appropriate, but not ideal
Since Stefie is only a medical student, the nurse will be able to help and, since she will be administering the drug herself, she also has an interest in the matter. As such, it is appropriate to involve her. She may also decide to discuss the issue with senior doctors. However, it would still be more appropriate in the first instance to raise the issue with the locum doctor himself or, if Stefie took the view she had already tried this unsuccessfully, then to approach a more senior doctor instead of the nurse. One of the problems with approaching the nurse is that it might ensure that this particular patient is safe, but it will not resolve the issue of the locum doctor's behaviour. As such, it will only have a limited impact.

MOCK SJ 9/22 – Confidentiality

9.1 – D: A very inappropriate thing to do
Breaching confidentiality is very inappropriate unless there is an extremely valid reason. One might be tempted to think that the breach of confidentiality is minimised by the fact that Yvonne will soon hear the news anyway since her mother is to attend the clinic today. However, there is no guarantee that her mother will want Yvonne to know the results or that Yvonne will keep her mouth shut. Worse, if the patient found out that Yvonne knew about the diagnosis before she did, she may lose faith in the team of doctors (which is also why this approach ranks as very inappropriate. It could make things worse, especially if Yvonne does not keep quiet about it).

9.2 – A: A very appropriate thing to do
This is a good way to handle it. Yvonne will have to wait for her mother to tell her after the clinic, or to ask her mother if she can sit in with her.

9.3 – A: A very appropriate thing to do
This is also correct and a good alternative to 9.2.

9.4 – D: A very inappropriate thing to do
This is effectively a breach of confidentiality and is very inappropriate.

MOCK SJ 10/22 – Hand Wash

10.1 – A: Very important
Some of you may have ranked this answer as D (Not important at all) on the basis that nothing can be a sufficient excuse for Juliet to place patients at risk by not washing her hands between patients, which is indeed correct. However, we are not asked to consider whether her grief makes the lack of handwashing acceptable, but how important this factor is for the purpose of the overall response to the situation. Here, Juliet's grief and state of mind may cause her to make other mistakes because she is not able to concentrate on what she is doing. Therefore, if the grief is irrelevant by itself as an excuse for the lack of handwashing, it is a very important consideration when it comes to the safety of all patients.

10.2 – D: Not important at all
Infections do not need prolonged contact to be transmitted. Obviously the risk is increased if there is prolonged contact but, if the patient becomes infected after an examination, they won't care much about the actual duration of the examination. Patient safety is a very binary thing. You either ensure it or you don't.

10.3 – D: Not important at all
The patient will have consented to the examination on the assumption it will be carried out properly and according to the correct rules and regulations. The fact that he consented does not give Juliet the right to be negligent.

MOCK SJ 11/22 – Unusual Doctor

11.1 – C: Of minor importance
Brad's priority should be to make sure he can engage with patients in a way that they feel they can have faith in him. If his manner causes concern for

Mock Exam

patients, then this will take priority over everything. His feelings are important to a small extent, in that the situation would need to be dealt with diplomatically, but he is a senior doctor and should know better. As such, it would make little difference if they were ignored.

11.2 – D: Not important at all
The fact that no patient has made a comment before does not mean that they did not have an issue with his appearance. But, more importantly, the trust every patient has in their doctor is a very individual feeling. This patient's feelings cannot be ignored on the basis that others feel differently.

11.3 – A: Very important
If the patient feels they can't trust Brad and feels that they need to refuse to be treated by him as a result, they will miss out on a procedure that is important for their care. This makes it a vital consideration in deciding whether to address the matter with Brad.

MOCK SJ 12/22 – Public Gossip

12.1 – A: Very important
Other passengers may actually be patients in the psychiatric unit or be the relatives of some of the patients there. Even if that is not the case, the conversation will paint a picture of uncaring staff and disrespectful doctors and medical students; as such, it will damage the reputation of that unit and affect the trust that the population may have in the care it provides.

12.2 – C: Of minor importance
It is obviously good that they are not naming anyone, and this point will need to be made by Karen when she talks to someone about the incident – whether it is Tim and George, or someone else at their hospital – but it does not really affect the fact that their conversation is impacting on public trust.

12.3 – D: Not important at all
Tim and George's conversation could actually affect the perception that patients have of the whole healthcare system. Regardless of where she works, she should either address the situation with the two students immediately or write to someone in their team to let them know (though the first solution would be more appropriate).

MOCK SJ 13/22 – Breaking Bad News

13.1 – B: Appropriate, but not ideal
Zoe is being fully honest with Rashid and therefore it ranks as appropriate. The reason it is ranked as not ideal (i.e. B instead of A) is because Zoe is not actually doing anything to help. She is merely stalling in a safe way. Therefore, this will not resolve the issue of Rashid's impatience (bearing in mind he doesn't know that an explanation will be given soon).

13.2 – A: A very appropriate thing to do
It is the truth and will be reassuring to Rashid.

13.3 – C: Inappropriate but not awful
Rashid's parents have said that they can't face telling him about the diagnosis, so encouraging Rashid to talk to them is pointless as they will most likely just stall him until the consultant comes along to break the news. Because it won't really make things worse, it can't be ranked as very inappropriate; therefore C is the correct answer.

MOCK SJ 14/22 – Bad Presentation

14.1 – A: A very appropriate thing to do
Both will be judged on the whole presentation and therefore this approach will ensure that both can actually be successful. This is the most proactive and positive approach.

14.2 – B: Appropriate, but not ideal
This will ensure that the work gets done and Kim will be demonstrating some teamwork in the process to make sure that their team achieves the common goal. However, obviously, it would be better if Andy invested more of his time. Kim will no doubt be reassured by the fact that Andy will have little choice but to invest some of his time into it anyway since he will have to deliver his half of the presentation.

14.3 – D: A very inappropriate thing to do
The presentation is supposed to be a team effort and therefore both should take equal responsibility for the failure. The fact that Kim is publicly trying to blame Andy means that she is refusing to acknowledge she equally failed to make the team work functionally.

MOCK SJ 15/22 – Bruises

15.1 – D: Not important at all
The GP's opinion in this case is pure supposition and not based on any kind of evidence since he has not seen the bruise. As such, it has no weight.

15.2 – C: Of minor importance
Bruises are indeed likely to be common in boys if they often fall and, as such, may be a consideration. But there is always a risk that they may not be accidental and, if Jane feels there may be abuse, then the fact that boys tend to fall a lot will not play a big role in the decision to speak up or act.

15.3 – B: Important
The fact the mother is coming back the following week means that there will be another chance to examine the child and see if the bruises are still there. It may also be an opportunity to ask relevant questions. This makes the situation a lot safer for the child than if the mother simply vanished after this consultation. The reason it scores B rather than A is because it will provide good additional information but it is only one piece of the puzzle and, as such, is not a vital element of the decision-making process, and Jane may take the view that this is too serious to wait another week.

MOCK SJ 16/22 – Dental Check-Up

16.1 – C: Of minor importance
Using out-of-date films means that the X-rays may not be of optimal quality and therefore that they may need to be redone. That means more radiation being received by the patient and therefore a risk to his health. Since we are told it is a routine check-up then the fact he will need to wait is of minor importance as it will simply be an inconvenience.

16.2 – D: Not important at all
There is a reason for the expiry date and, though it is possibly true that the films may still be perfectly fine after four months, the dentist has no right to harm a patient by exposing them to unnecessary radiation just on the off-chance that the films might be okay.

16.3 – A: Very important
Doctors should be honest with their patients, and particularly so in the event of mistakes. In this case, either the film worked, in which case the patient should be told there was an issue with the film but reassured that everything

worked out fine, or the film has failed, in which case this should be explained to the patient since he will need to consent to another X-ray being taken.

MOCK SJ 17/22 – Breast Examination

17.1 – A: A very appropriate thing to do
Enquiring without judging the situation would enable Aliana to get an idea of the facts and therefore the gravity of the situation before acting.

17.2 – A: A very appropriate thing to do
It is possible that the patient misunderstood the purpose of the examination, and the fact that it was not documented may be a simple omission or it may in fact never have taken place. Therefore, getting the other side of the story would be useful.

17.3 – D: A very inappropriate thing to do
The patient has not actually complained about anything. She simply stated what she regards as a fact. Until more information is identified there is no need to apologise. Encouraging the patient to complain would give her the impression that something wrong happened when there may be a perfectly simple explanation. This would be appropriate thing if there was evidence of malpractice but it is a premature, and could make things worse.

17.4 – C: Inappropriate but not awful
It would only be appropriate to mention the issue to the consultant if Aliana actually knew that there was an issue. That would require first talking to the patient and to the junior doctor.

MOCK SJ 18/22 – Struggling Colleague

18.1 – C: Inappropriate but not awful
This just reiterates what the consultant said and offers no comfort or solution. It will achieve nothing other than continue to make Mo miserable. The reason it is not deemed very inappropriate is because it is not making matters worse. What would be very inappropriate would be for Alan to start having a go at Mo in a similar tone.

18.2 – A: A very appropriate thing to do
Mo has clearly messed up and also clearly has issues he needs to sort out. Talking to both the consultant and the supervisor will enable him to clear the air and get support to improve going forward.

Mock Exam

18.3 – B: Appropriate, but not ideal
Getting him to apologise would be a good thing to do; however, the reassurance that the consultant did not mean what he said only serves to comfort Mo without really offering anything constructive.

MOCK SJ 19/22 – Badmouthing

19.1 – D: A very inappropriate thing to do
The nurse might be wrong but her comment has now gone and there is no urgency in dealing with it. There is certainly no reason to call her away from the patient as the conversation has moved on and the nurse has a job to do. This can be handled later when it won't interfere with patient care.

19.2 – D: A very inappropriate thing to do
It was bad enough that the nurse said what she said. Telling the patient that the nurse spoke out of turn will only make the patient more anxious about the team's abilities to care for them, as it will increase the impression of chaos.

19.3 – A: A very appropriate thing to do
There is no urgency and therefore finding a quiet moment later on is most ideal. Allowing the nurse to explain her comment will also lead to some sort of resolution.

MOCK SJ 20/22 – Body Odour

20.1 – B: Not important
Isabella has already noticed the issue before, and the problem should really be addressed regardless of whether a patient or a member of staff has already commented on it or not. People may not have mentioned anything but will inevitably have noticed the issue. This should be addressed to avoid future issues with teamwork or interaction with patients.

20.2 – B: Not important
From tomorrow, the issue may no longer be relevant to Isabella or the rest of the team, but it will be an issue for others going forward. Problems that are perpetually passed on run the risk of never being addressed.

MOCK SJ 21/22 – Medical Finals

21.1 – Most appropriate: Option B
The patient comes first. Options A and C both insist on the patient making an effort despite having already declared he was too tired to continue. Option B, however, requires only a very minimal effort from the patient (which is to give Emilia priority when he eventually feels better) and therefore is respectful of his health status. In real life, Option A (which is to reduce the time taken to just a few minutes) may be acceptable and may in fact be what most students would do. However for the purpose of the UCAT, you need to provide answers relating to what you SHOULD do and not what you WOULD do. Strictly speaking, despite being a request rather than a demand, Option A is still slightly coercive and therefore less appropriate that Option B.

The fact that Emilia is off duty at that time is not relevant. In many ways, it is better if she trains for her examination skills when she is off duty than when she is on duty (and therefore expected to do some work).

21.2 – Least appropriate: Option C
Not only is this emotional blackmail and coercion, but it is also ignoring the patient's request. It is disrespectful.

MOCK SJ 22/22 – Unfair Allocation

22.1 – Most appropriate: Option A
Raising issues with the person involved is always the best approach.

22.2 – Least appropriate: Option C
Discussing the issue with a junior doctor would be of benefit but they would not have the same level of experience and insight as Michael's supervisor.

MOCK EXAM MARKING SCHEDULES

The marking schedule below calculates an approximate score out of 600, to which you must add 300 in order to transform it into a score on a 300-to-900 scale, which is the scale used for the UCAT.

For each of the questions, write your score in reference to the maximum mark in the box provided. You should score your answers as follows:
- Zero if you gave the wrong answer or failed to answer at all.
- Max mark if you answered correctly.

QUANTITATIVE REASONING

Question	Answer	Max Mark	Your Mark
1.1	d	16	
1.2	a	16	
1.3	a	17	
1.4	a	17	
2.1	e	16	
2.2	d	16	
2.3	c	17	
2.4	b	17	
3.1	c	16	
3.2	e	16	
3.3	b	17	
3.4	b	17	
4.1	b	16	
4.2	d	16	
4.3	c	17	
4.4	a	17	
5.1	c	16	
5.2	a	16	
5.3	b	17	
5.4	a	17	
6.1	e	16	
6.2	b	16	
6.3	e	17	

6.4	d	17	
7.1	b	17	
7.2	e	17	
7.3	b	17	
7.4	b	17	
8.1	a	17	
8.2	d	17	
8.3	c	17	
8.4	e	17	
9.1	d	17	
9.2	e	17	
9.3	d	17	
9.4	c	17	
TOTAL		600 +300 = 900	/600 + 300 = /900

ABSTRACT REASONING

Shape	Answer	Max Mark	Your Mark
1.1	Neither	10	
1.2	B	10	
1.3	Neither	10	
1.4	Neither	10	
1.5	Neither	10	
2.1	Neither	10	
2.2	Neither	10	
2.3	B	10	
2.4	A	10	
2.5	Neither	10	
3.1	A	10	
3.2	A	10	
3.3	Neither	10	
3.4	Neither	10	
3.5	A	10	
4.1	Neither	10	
4.2	Neither	10	
4.3	Neither	10	
4.4	A	10	
4.5	Neither	10	

Mock Exam

5.1	A	10	
5.2	A	10	
5.3	Neither	10	
5.4	Neither	10	
5.5	B	10	
6.1	Neither	10	
6.2	Neither	10	
6.3	A	10	
6.4	Neither	10	
6.5	A	10	
7.1	A	10	
7.2	Neither	10	
7.3	Neither	10	
7.4	A	10	
7.5	Neither	10	
8.1	A	10	
8.2	B	10	
8.3	B	10	
8.4	Neither	10	
8.5	Neither	10	
9.1	A	10	
9.2	Neither	10	
9.3	Neither	10	
9.4	Neither	10	
9.5	Neither	10	
10.1	A	10	
10.2	Neither	10	
10.3	Neither	10	
10.4	B	10	
10.5	A	10	
11	B	20	
12	C	20	
13	D	20	
14	B	20	
15	C	20	
TOTAL		600 +300 = 900	/600 + 300 = /900

1300 UCAT Practice Questions

VERBAL REASONING

Question	Answer	Max Mark	Your Mark
1.1	Can't tell	14	
1.2	Can't tell	14	
1.3	Can't tell	14	
1.4	True	14	
2.1	B	14	
2.2	A	14	
2.3	Can't tell	14	
2.4	Can't tell	14	
3.1	Can't tell	14	
3.2	D	14	
3.3	True	14	
3.4	D	14	
4.1	D	14	
4.2	D	14	
4.3	True	14	
4.4	False	14	
5.1	A	14	
5.2	C	14	
5.3	Can't tell	14	
5.4	False	14	
6.1	Can't tell	14	
6.2	D	14	
6.3	C	14	
6.4	False	14	
7.1	False	14	
7.2	Can't tell	14	
7.3	Can't tell	14	
7.4	True	14	
8.1	D	13	
8.2	False	13	
8.3	Can't tell	13	
8.4	D	13	
9.1	B	13	
9.2	A	13	
9.3	False	13	
9.4	False	13	
10.1	B	13	

Question	Answer	Max Mark	Your Mark
10.2	A	13	
10.3	Can't tell	13	
10.4	Can't tell	13	
11.1	False	13	
11.2	False	13	
11.3	Can't tell	13	
11.4	True	13	
TOTAL		600 +300 = 900	/600 + 300 = /900

DECISION MAKING

Question	Answer	Max Mark	Your Mark
1.1	YES	4.8	
1.2	YES	4.8	
1.3	YES	4.8	
1.4	NO	4.8	
1.5	NO	4.8	
2	B	20	
3.1	YES	4.8	
3.2	NO	4.8	
3.3	YES	4.8	
3.4	NO	4.8	
3.5	YES	4.8	
4	D	20	
5.1	NO	4.8	
5.2	NO	4.8	
5.3	NO	4.8	
5.4	YES	4.8	
5.5	NO	4.8	
6	C	20	
7.1	NO	4.8	
7.2	NO	4.8	
7.3	NO	4.8	
7.4	YES	4.8	
7.5	YES	4.8	
8	A	20	

9.1	NO	4.8	
9.2	YES	4.8	
9.3	YES	4.8	
9.4	YES	4.8	
9.5	NO	4.8	
10	B	20	
11	D	20	
12	C	20	
13	D	20	
14	B	20	
15	C	20	
16	C	20	
17	B	20	
18	C	20	
19	C	20	
20	B	20	
21	C	20	
22	B	20	
23	B	20	
24	A	20	
25	A	20	
26	A	20	
27	C	20	
28	B	20	
29	C	20	
TOTAL		600 +300 = 900	/600 + 300 = /900

SUMMARY TABLE

QUANTITATIVE REASONING SCORE	/ 900
ABSTRACT REASONING SCORE	/ 900
VERBAL REASONING SCORE	/ 900
DECISION MAKING	/ 900

SITUATIONAL JUDGEMENT MARKING SCHEDULE

The Situational Judgement section of the UCAT is marked slightly differently to the other sections. Rather than being given an absolute score, you are simply given a band, as follows:

Band 1	Those in Band 1 demonstrated an excellent level of performance, showing similar judgement in most cases to the panel of experts.
Band 2	Those in Band 2 demonstrated a good, solid level of performance, showing appropriate judgement frequently, with many responses matching model answers.
Band 3	Those in Band 3 demonstrated a modest level of performance, with appropriate judgement shown for some questions and substantial differences from ideal responses for others.
Band 4	The performance of those in Band 4 was low, with judgement tending to differ substantially from ideal responses in many cases.

Although the UCAT marking system is a closely guarded secret, similar type questions are used throughout medicine and tend to be marked as follows:

- Each question is marked 1, 2, 3 or 4. The CORRECT answer will get a score of 4. All other answers will have a point deducted for each step that it is out. So for example:
  → If the correct answer is A, then those who answered A will score 4, those who answered B will score 3, those who answered C will score 2 and those who answered D will score 1.
  → If the correct answer is C, then those who answered C will score 4, those who answered B or D will score 3 and those who answered A will score 2.

So in essence it will follow the following matrix:

Your answer	Correct answer A	B	C	D
A	4	3	2	1
B	3	4	3	2
C	2	3	4	3
D	1	2	3	4

Using this matrix, you can now score your answers:

SITUATIONAL JUDGEMENT

Shape	Answer	Max Mark	Your Mark
1.1	A	4	A=4, B=3, C=2, D=1
1.2	C	4	A=2, B=3, C=4, D=3
1.3	B	4	A=3, B=4, C=3, D=2
1.4	D	4	A=1, B=2, C=3, D=4
2.1	D	4	A=1, B=2, C=3, D=4
2.2	C	4	A=2, B=3, C=4, D=3
2.3	C	4	A=2, B=3, C=4, D=3
2.4	A	4	A=4, B=3, C=2, D=1
3.1	C	4	A=2, B=3, C=4, D=3
3.2	A	4	A=4, B=3, C=2, D=1
3.3	C	4	A=2, B=3, C=4, D=3
3.4	B	4	A=3, B=4, C=3, D=2
4.1	D	4	A=1, B=2, C=3, D=4
4.2	B	4	A=3, B=4, C=3, D=2
4.3	A	4	A=4, B=3, C=2, D=1
5.1	A	4	A=4, B=3, C=2, D=1
5.2	C	4	A=2, B=3, C=4, D=3
5.3	B	4	A=3, B=4, C=3, D=2
6.1	A	4	A=4, B=3, C=2, D=1
6.2	A	4	A=4, B=3, C=2, D=1
6.3	C	4	A=2, B=3, C=4, D=3
7.1	C	4	A=2, B=3, C=4, D=3
7.2	D	4	A=1, B=2, C=3, D=4
7.3	D	4	A=1, B=2, C=3, D=4
8.1	A	4	A=4, B=3, C=2, D=1
8.2	D	4	A=1, B=2, C=3, D=4
8.3	A	4	A=4, B=3, C=2, D=1
8.4	B	4	A=3, B=4, C=3, D=2
9.1	D	4	A=1, B=2, C=3, D=4
9.2	A	4	A=4, B=3, C=2, D=1
9.3	A	4	A=4, B=3, C=2, D=1
9.4	D	4	A=1, B=2, C=3, D=4
10.1	A	4	A=4, B=3, C=2, D=1
10.2	D	4	A=1, B=2, C=3, D=4
10.3	D	4	A=1, B=2, C=3, D=4
11.1	C	4	A=2, B=3, C=4, D=3
11.2	D	4	A=1, B=2, C=3, D=4

Mock Exam

11.3	A	4	A=4, B=3, C=2, D=1
12.1	A	4	A=4, B=3, C=2, D=1
12.2	C	4	A=2, B=3, C=4, D=3
12.3	D	4	A=1, B=2, C=3, D=4
13.1	B	4	A=3, B=4, C=3, D=2
13.2	A	4	A=4, B=3, C=2, D=1
13.3	C	4	A=2, B=3, C=4, D=3
14.1	A	4	A=4, B=3, C=2, D=1
14.2	B	4	A=3, B=4, C=3, D=2
14.3	D	4	A=1, B=2, C=3, D=4
15.1	D	4	A=1, B=2, C=3, D=4
15.2	C	4	A=2, B=3, C=4, D=3
15.3	B	4	A=3, B=4, C=3, D=2
16.1	C	4	A=2, B=3, C=4, D=3
16.2	D	4	A=1, B=2, C=3, D=4
16.3	A	4	A=4, B=3, C=2, D=1
17.1	A	4	A=4, B=3, C=2, D=1
17.2	A	4	A=4, B=3, C=2, D=1
17.3	D	4	A=1, B=2, C=3, D=4
17.4	C	4	A=2, B=3, C=4, D=3
18.1	C	4	A=2, B=3, C=4, D=3
18.2	A	4	A=4, B=3, C=2, D=1
18.3	B	4	A=3, B=4, C=3, D=2
19.1	D	4	A=1, B=2, C=3, D=4
19.2	D	4	A=1, B=2, C=3, D=4
19.3	A	4	A=4, B=3, C=2, D=1
20.1	B	4	A = 0, B = 4
20.2	B	4	A = 0, B = 4
21.1	B	4	A=2, B=4, C=0
21.2	C	4	A=2, B=0, C=4
22.1	A	4	A=4, B=2, C=0
22.2	C	4	A=0, B=2, C=4
Total		276	/276

Your banding:
Score 221 – 276: Band A
Score 176 – 220: Band B
Score 131 – 175: Band C
Score 130 or under: Band D

ISC MEDICAL

MEDICAL SCHOOL INTERVIEW COURSE

Realise your potential ...

For full details about our Medical School Interview Courses and other resources available

visit our website: www.iscmedical.co.uk